10⁰⁰

THE SAVVY
WOMAN PATIENT

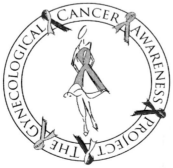

Also by the Society for Women's Health Research

*Women's Health Research: A Medical and
Policy Primer* (Health Press, 1997)

Other titles in Capital's Savvy series include the following:

*The Savvy Consumer: How to Avoid Scams and
Rip-offs that Cost You Time and Money*
BY ELISABETH LEAMY

*The Savvy Patient: The Ultimate Advocate
for Quality Healthcare*
BY MARK C. PETTUS, MD

Save 25 percent when you order any of these and other fine Capital
titles from our Web site: *www.capital-books.com.*

THE SAVVY WOMAN PATIENT

How and Why Sex Differences Affect Your Health

Society for Women's Health Research

Phyllis Greenberger, MSW, *and*
Jennifer Wider, MD, *Editors*

CAPITAL SAVVY SERIES

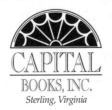

CAPITAL
BOOKS, INC.
Sterling, Virginia

Capital Books, Inc.
P.O. Box 605
Herndon, Virginia 20172-0605

Book design and composition by Susan Mark
Coghill Composition Company
Richmond, Virginia

ISBN 13: 978-1-933102-08-5
ISBN 10: 1-933102-08-X (alk.paper)

Library of Congress Cataloging-in-Publication Data

The savvy woman patient : how and why sex differences impact your health / Phyllis Greenberger and Jennifer Wider, editors.—1st ed.
    p. cm.—(Capital savvy series)
    Includes bibliographical references and index.
    ISBN 1-933102-08-X (pbk. : alk. paper)
    1. Women—Health and hygiene. 2. Women—Diseases. 3. Sex factors in disease. I. Greenberger, Phyllis. II. Wider, Jennifer. III. Title IV. Series.
    RA564.85.S399 2006
    613'.04244—dc22

                  2005019845

Printed in the United States of America on acid-free paper that meets the American National Standards Institute Z39-48 Standard.

First Edition

10 9 8 7 6 5 4 3 2

This book is dedicated to Florence Haseltine, PhD, MD, the inspirational visionary who founded the Society for Women's Health Research and whose understanding of the importance of sex differences in prevention, etiology, and treatment has led to new areas of scientific and clinical research and ultimately improved care for all women and men.

ACKNOWLEDGMENTS

The Society for Women's Health Research expresses appreciation to all the authors and organizations who contributed information for this book and the work they do in improving women's health.

CONTENTS

PART 3

WHERE TO GO FOR HELP

CONTRIBUTORS

Attila Barabas, MD, is chief resident at the University of Utah in the Division of Urology. He also graduated from the University of Utah medical school. Dr. Barabas is a member of the American Urological Association.

Rita Baron-Faust, editor of the *Weill-Cornell Women's Health Advisor,* is a best-selling author of numerous books, including *Mental Wellness for Women, Breast Cancer: What Every Woman Should Know, Being Female: What Every Woman Should Know About Gynecological Health, A Woman's Guide to Sleep* (co-author), and *The Autoimmune Connection* (co-author). She is a member of the Board of Directors of the American Autoimmune and Related Diseases Association.

Patricia A. Britz, MEd, MPM, is the former program director for the National Sleep Foundation (NSF) and is the director of information and education at the Brain Injury Association of America. She has twenty years of experience in program development and management in needs assessment, research, curriculum design, working collaboratively with health professionals, teaching, management, and evaluation. She spent ten years as educational administrator at St. Margaret Memorial Hospital in Pittsburgh, conducted staff training at the Hospice of Northern Virginia, and has worked at the National Academy of Sciences. During her tenure at NSF, Pat produced numerous public and professional educational materials and programs, including the *sleep for TEENS* toolkit, and she conducted the annual *Sleep in America* poll and the Pickwick Postdoctoral Fellowship program.

Melissa Brown, MD, MN, MBA, is an adjunct assistant professor of ophthalmology at the University of Pennsylvania School of Medicine and adjunct senior fellow at the Leonard Davis Institute of Health Economics at Penn. She is the director for the Center for Value-Based Medicine and co-chief editor of *Evidence-Based Eye Care.* Dr. Brown has served as president of the Montgomery County (PA) Medical Society and is on the Advisory Council for the National Institute for Aging. She has written more than 120 publications on medical issues.

Yvette Colón, MSW, ACSW, BCD, is director of Education & Internet Services at the American Pain Foundation (APF), a nonprofit education, support, and advocacy organization for people affected by pain.

She is responsible for the day-to-day operations of the Pain Information Center, as well as all electronic initiatives, including APF's website and PainAid, its online support community. She has published and lectured extensively on pain management, oncology, end-of-life social work practice, diversity and disadvantage in health care, and technology-based social work services. She is the co-chair of the Association of Oncology Social Work's Pain & Palliative Care Special Interest Group, a governing board member of the Intercultural Cancer Council, an appointed member of the Maryland Governor's Osteoporosis Prevention & Education Task Force, and editorial board member of the *Journal of Social Work in End-of-Life & Palliative Care.*

Terrie Cowley is a temporomandibular joint (TMJ) implant patient and co-founder and president of the TMJ Association, a nonprofit organization whose mission is education, research, and service. Through its newsletters and publications, Web site, e-mail, and other communication links, the Association has become a national and international resource for thousands of patients, providers, researchers, and other interested parties. Ms. Cowley has been indefatigable in alerting policymakers, the media, the National Institutes of Health (NIH) community, and Congress to the needs of TMJ patients, promoting research aimed at developing evidenced-based diagnostics, treatments, and, ultimately, prevention of TMJ problems.

Denise J. Fedele, DMD, MS, is a practicing dentist and serves as chief of professional development for dentistry at the VA Maryland Health Care System. Dr. Fedele also holds faculty appointments as clinical associate professor at the University of Maryland Dental School and the University of Medicine and Dentistry of New Jersey School of Osteopathic Medicine and is an assistant director for the Geriatric Fellowship at the UMDNJ-SOM. Dr. Fedele is a member of the American Dental Association (ADA) and is a recipient of the ADA Meritorious Award in Geriatric Oral Health.

Susan Finn, PhD, RD, FADA, chairs the American Council for Fitness and Nutrition. A registered and licensed dietitian, Dr. Finn is a fellow and former president of The American Dietetic Association (ADA). She initiated the ADA's Women's Nutrition & Health Campaign. Dr. Finn co-authored two books on nutrition, *The Real Life Nutrition Book: Making the Right Food Choices Without Changing Your Lifestyle* and *The American Dietetic Association's Guide to Women's Nutrition for Healthy Living.* She has made more than 500 appearances on radio and television shows such as ABC's *Good Morning America* and NBC's *Today Show*, delivering information about nutrition. Dr. Finn is a member of the American Society of Clinical Nutrition and the American Society for Parental and Enteral Nutrition.

Debra Gordon is an award-winning medical writer and editor who is widely published in magazines such as *Family Circle, Good Housekeeping, Prevention, Business Week, Managed Care Magazine,* and *Parents Today.* She is a contributor to numerous Web sites, including InteliHealth.com, DiscoveryHealth.com, Healthanswers.com, the Robert Wood Johnson Foundation, and the National Women's Health Resource Center. She is a contributor to the Reader's Digest book, *Medical Breakthroughs 2003,* editor of *The Woman Doctor's Guide to Health and Healing,* and author of *7 Days to a Good Night's Sleep.*

Linda Giudice, MD, PhD, is the chair of the department of obstetrics, gynecology and reproductive sciences at the University of California, San Francisco School of Medicine. She previously was the Stanley McCormick Memorial Professor of OB/GYN at Stanford University and director of the *Women's Health @ Stanford* Program and the Reproductive Endocrinology and Infertility Division at Stanford. Dr. Giudice chairs the Reproductive Health Drugs Advisory Committee of the U.S. Food and Drug Administration (FDA) and is immediate past president of the Society for Reproductive Endocrinology and Infertility. She is on the Executive Board of the Reproductive Scientist Development Program and is a member of the Frontiers in Reproduction Board of Scientific Counselors and the Board of Directors of the Society for Women's Health Research. She was recently elected presidential nominee (president in 2006) for the Society of Gynecologic Investigation, and she co-edited the textbook, *The Endometrium.*

Harriet Lin Hall, ARNP-BC, DNC, is a graduate of Capital University and University of Phoenix. She is a member of the Dermatology Nurses Association, American Academy of Nurse Practitioners, Florida Nurse Practitioner Network, and the Florida Nurses Association. Since 1998, Lin and Dr. Weinkle have been working side by side caring for skin cancer patients of Manatee and Sarasota counties.

Patricia Hurn, PhD, is professor and vice chairman of anesthesiology at Oregon Health & Science University in Portland and director of the OHSU Program for Gender-Based Biology in Medicine. She is a cerebrovascular physiologist with specific research interests in gender differences and the role of sex steroids in brain injury. Dr. Hurn's research team has explored the role of estrogen in protecting the brain-at-risk for stroke. She holds five active grants to study stroke, three of which center on gender differences in stroke and on estrogen as a protective agent in brain injury. Dr. Hurn is a member of the Medical Advisory Board of The Hazel K. Goddess Fund for Stroke Research in Women.

Michael E. Kalafer, MD, is an assistant clinical professor of medicine at the University of California, San Diego School of Medicine, and former medical director of the pulmonary and critical care medicine departments at Sharp Memorial Hospital in San Diego. He is also a principal investigator for the Early Lung Cancer Action Project. Dr. Kalafer has had a long-time interest in public health and has been a medical officer for the Centers for Disease Control and Prevention (CDC). He is board-certified in internal medicine, pulmonary medicine, and critical care medicine.

Lindsey Kerr, MD, is an associate professor of urology and co-director of the Pelvic Floor Center at the University of Utah. Formerly director of the Vermont Continence Center in Burlington, Vermont, she is on the Board of Directors of the National Association for Continence and has served as the organization's national spokesperson. Dr. Kerr is a member of the Society of Women in Urology (and has served as its president), the American Association of Clinical Urologists, and the American Urological Association. She has been awarded the Eagles Cancer Research Grant and has written numerous articles, chapters, and papers, appearing in such journals as *Urology*, *Journal of Urology*, and *Cancer Research*. Dr. Kerr is on the Board of Directors of the Society for Women's Health Research.

Ruth B. Lathi, MD, is a clinical assistant professor of obstetrics and gynecology at Stanford University Medical Center. She is fellowship trained in reproductive endocrinology and infertility. She conducts research on several topics including insulin signaling in the human endometrium and etiologies of recurrent miscarriage, infertility and polycystic ovarian syndrome. Dr. Lathi is a member of the American Society of Reproductive Medicine and the American College of Obstetrics and Gynecology.

Sherry A. Marts, PhD, is vice president of scientific affairs at the Society for Women's Health Research. Before joining the Society, Dr. Marts was a senior analyst at the consulting firm of Abt Associates, where she served as scientific research administrator for the HIV Network for Prevention Trials. She also was director of research grants at the American Health Assistance Foundation and worked in the office of the vice president for research and development at the American Red Cross biomedical research laboratories.

Peggy McCarthy, MBA, is owner and CEO of McCarthy Medical Marketing, Inc., a company that creates educational programs for health professionals and the public. She founded and served as volunteer executive director (from 1994 to 1999) of the Lung Cancer Alliance (formerly Alliance for Lung Cancer Advocacy, Support, and Education). The book, *LUNG CANCER: Myths, Facts, Choices, and Hope*, which she co-authored with Claudia Henschke, MD, and writer Sarah Wernick, has won two awards for providing excellent medical education for the public. She has developed and contributes to numerous Web sites and has appeared on television and radio to speak publicly about patient advocacy issues. She is a founding partner in C-Change (National Dialogue on Cancer).

Louise McCullough, MD, PhD, is assistant professor of neurology and neuroscience at the University of Connecticut. She is also director of stroke research and education for the University of Connecticut Health Center and the Hartford Hospital Stroke Center. Dr. McCullough is a board-certified vascular neurologist in addition to being an active basic science researcher. A former Goddess Fund Scholar, she studies the effects of estrogen on functional recovery after stroke. She also holds several active grants and is interested in examining the effects of sex on both clinical and experimental stroke.

Leah S. Millheiser, MD, is an instructor of obstetrics and gynecology at the Stanford University School of Medicine. She was recently awarded a Women's Reproductive Health Research (WRHR) Scholarship by the National Institutes of Health, which allows her to devote a significant amount of her time to research in female sexual health. She has also created the Female Sexual Health Program within the Division of Gynecology at Stanford University Medical Center. This clinical program focuses on the treatment of female sexual desire, arousal, orgasm, and sexual pain disorders and serves as an outlet for several clinical research trials.

Carol Nadelson, MD, is clinical professor of psychiatry at Harvard Medical School (HMS) and director of the Partners Office for Women's Careers at Brigham and Women's Hospital and HMS. In this position, she works with others to identify projects and advocate for women's careers and the advancement of professional women in the hospital. Dr. Nadelson recently stepped down from her position as editor-in-chief, president, and CEO of American Psychiatric Press, Inc. She was the first woman president of the American Psychiatric Association (APA) and a founding member of the first APA committee on women. Dr. Nadelson has presented nearly 1,000 lectures, written more than 200 papers and chapters, and co-edited 15 books.

Linda C. Niessen, DMD, MPH, is clinical professor in the department of restorative sciences and the Office of Communications and Development at Baylor College of Dentistry and serves as vice president, clinical education, for DENTSPLY International. She hosts *Dental Health Check*, a weekly television show on dental health. Along with television producer Sara Ivey, Dr. Niessen received the Chicago Dental Society's 2004 Cushing Award, an honor given to media for raising awareness of oral health issues. She is a past president of the American Association of Women Dentists and the American Association of Public Health Dentistry.

Barbara A. Phillips, MD, MSPH, is professor of pulmonary and critical care medicine in the departments of internal medicine and preventive medicine at the University of Kentucky College of Medicine. She directs the Sleep Clinic and Sleep Fellowship at the University of Kentucky College of Medicine and is medical director of the Sleep Disorders

Center at Samaritan Hospital in Lexington. Dr. Phillips is board-certified in internal medicine, pulmonary medicine, critical care medicine, and sleep medicine.

Diane Zipursky Quale is co-founder and president of the Bladder Cancer Advocacy Network (BCAN), the first national patient advocacy organization dedicated to bladder cancer. An attorney by training, Mrs. Quale has been an active participant in the cancer community since 2002, serving as the volunteer administrator of a retreat program for cancer patients and fundraiser for a small nonprofit cancer organization in Washington, D.C. She is a member of the National Cancer Institute's (NCI) Consumer Advocates in Research and Related Activities (CARRA) program and was recently invited to serve as an external reviewer on the Cancer Therapy Evaluation Program (CTEP) at NCI.

Vicki Ratner, MD, is an orthopedic surgeon at the Santa Teresa Community Hospital/Kaiser Permanente Medical Group. Founder of the Interstitial Cystitis Association, Dr. Ratner has served on the NIH Advisory Council, NIH Interstitial Cystitis Clinical Trials Group, the NIH Interstitial Cystitis Database Committee, and the Bladder Health Council of the American Foundation for Urologic Disease (AFUD). Dr. Ratner has written for and edited numerous urologic publications, including *Urology*, the *International Urogynecology Journal*, and the NIH's *Overcoming Bladder Disease: A Strategic Plan for Research*. She is a recipient of the F. Brantley Scott Award from the Bladder Health Council of the American Foundation for Urologic Disease.

Eileen Resnick, PhD, is scientific program manager at the Society for Women's Health Research. Before joining the Society, Dr. Resnick was a clinical trials specialist with PSI International, Inc., where she managed a portfolio of investigational drugs with clinicians in the Division of Cancer Treatment and Diagnosis at the National Cancer Institute. She also was program coordinator at the American Institute of Biological Sciences, where she managed peer review of scientific and medical grants for public institutions and private foundations.

Martin S. Rusinowitz, MD, is a neurologist in Bethesda, Maryland. He received his MD from Wayne State University. He has served as the chair, Medical Review Committee, and chair, Department of Medicine, at Shady Grove Adventist Hospital; and is assistant clinical professor of neurology at George Washington University School of Medicine.

Richard Schmitz, MA, is director of communications for the Society for Women's Health Research, where he manages the public education programs and oversees media outreach. Before joining the Society, he served as director of public relations for the National Association of Alcoholism and Drug Abuse Counselors. He has authored articles on brain health, with an emphasis on addiction, for publications such as *Family Therapy Magazine* and *Addiction Professional*.

Mark P. Schoenberg, MD, FACS, is a professor of urology and oncology and director of the Division of Urologic Oncology at Johns Hopkins Medical Institutions. He conducts basic and clinical research on the detection and management of patients with all forms of bladder cancer. His particular areas of clinical interest are surgical treatment of invasive tumors and lower urinary tract reconstruction in male and female patients. Dr. Schoenberg is a member of the American Association of Cancer Research and the American Urological Association and is a fellow of the American College of Surgeons. He also chairs the Scientific Advisory Board of the Bladder Cancer Advocacy Network (BCAN), the first national patient advocacy organization dedicated to bladder cancer.

Stephanie Shapiro is a junior at Dickinson College, majoring in art history. Ms. Shapiro has an extensive background in molecular biology and chemistry and has been a summer intern for Dr. Mark Schoenberg at the Bladder Cancer Research Center at the Johns Hopkins Medical Institutions since 2003.

Viviana Simon, PhD, is director of scientific programs at the Society for Women's Health Research. Dr. Simon has also worked at the Banting and Best Institute of Medical Research in Toronto, Canada, while completing a postdoctoral fellowship, and was a senior editor of human databases at Proteome Inc/Incyte Genomics, where she was in charge of product quality control.

Michael Spigler, CHES, is director of public education for the American Kidney Fund. The Fund provides direct financial assistance to kidney patients in need and education for those with or at risk for kidney disease. As the Fund's director of public education, he develops patient education materials, manages the toll-free national HelpLine, coordinates the Fund's organ and tissue donor awareness activities, and serves as co-editor of the Fund's *Professional Advocate* newsletter.

Suzanne Stone is vice president, finance & administration, for the Society for Women's Health Research and serves as a director of special policy projects. She has served as executive director of the Sjögren's Syndrome Foundation and the Society for Vascular Technology. She was vice president of education for both the Association for the Advancement of Medical Instrumentation and the Parenteral Drug Association. Ms. Stone has also worked in health policy analysis for the American Pharmaceutical Association, ECRI (formerly the Emergency Care Research Institute), and the American College of Physicians.

Nada Stotland, MD, is a professor of psychiatry at Rush Medical College and a professor of psychiatry and obstetrics/gynecology at the Illinois

Masonic Medical Center in Chicago. She has served as vice president of the American Psychiatric Association (APA) and as chair of APA's Joint Commission on Public Affairs. She is also past president of the Association of Women Psychiatrists. Dr. Stotland is the treasurer of the board of American Psychiatric Publishing, Inc.

Laura L. Tosi, MD, is an associate professor of orthopaedics and pediatrics at the George Washington University School of Medicine and Health Sciences and director of the Bone Health Program at Children's National Medical Center. Her clinical practice focuses on the orthopedic care of children and adults with musculoskeletal disabilities and issues related to bone health. Past president of the Ruth Jackson Orthopaedic Society, the professional association for women in orthopaedics, Dr. Tosi received its Presidential Special Merit Award in 2000 for her outreach on health topics in women's health. She is past chair of the Women's Health Issues Committee of the American Academy of Orthopaedic Surgeons and recently co-chaired a workshop for the Academy, entitled "The Influence of Sex and Gender on Musculoskeletal Health," to motivate change in the way musculoskeletal health research is conducted and, ultimately, to improve musculoskeletal care in men and women. She serves on the Interspecialty Medical Council of the National Osteoporosis Foundation.

Christin Veasley, BS, is the director of research and professional programs for the National Vulvodynia Association (NVA), a nonprofit organization that serves vulvar pain patients and medical professionals who care for women with vulvar pain disorders. Previously she worked as a research assistant in the department of neurology at the Johns Hopkins University School of Medicine investigating the neurophysiological mechanisms of pelvic inflammation and pain. As research director for the NVA, Ms. Veasley develops educational programs for the medical community, attends national health care conferences, meets with pharmaceutical industry representatives, and raises funds for the NVA's various programs and activities. She is also a contributing author for the *NVA News* and has volunteered extensively for faith- and medicine-based organizations.

Susan H. Weinkle, MD, is in solo private practice, specializing in Mohs micrographic surgery and cosmetic dermatology. She has held academic appointments at Stanford University Hospital, the University of California, Irvine Medical Center, and, most recently, at the University of South Florida. Board-certified in dermatology, Dr. Weinkle is a fellow of the American College of Mohs Micrographic Surgery and Cutaneous Oncology and a diplomat of the American Board of Dermatology. Dr. Weinkle also serves on the American Academy of Dermatology's Board of Directors.

Marisa Weiss, MD, is director of breast radiation oncology at Lanke-nau Hospital and has an active practice in the Philadelphia area. She also is founder and president of breastcancer.org, an Internet based nonprofit organization that provides medical information on breast cancer to women and their loved ones worldwide at no cost. Dr. Weiss was selected as Top Doctor of the Year 2005 by *Philadelphia Magazine* and has been an appointed member of the National Cancer Institute Director's Consumer Liaison Group since April 2000. She is the founder and past president of Living Beyond Breast Cancer® (LBBC), a national nonprofit education and support organization, and author of the acclaimed book, *Living Beyond Breast Cancer*. Her emphasis on improving the doctor-patient relationship has led to many appearances on national television and radio, including co-producing and/or guest appearances on the NBC *Today Show*'s Special Breast Cancer Series for seven consecutive years.

Nanette K. Wenger, MD, FACC, FAHA, MACP, is professor of medicine in the Division of Cardiology of Emory University School of Medicine and chief of cardiology at Grady Memorial Hospital. Dr. Wenger has held leadership positions in the American College of Cardiology, the American Heart Association, and the Society of Geriatric Cardiology. Among other honors, she has received the Gold Heart Award, the highest award given by the American Heart Association to volunteers; the American Heart Association's R. Bruce Logue Award for Excellence in Medicine; and the American Medical Women's Association's Elizabeth Blackwell Award, which recognizes a woman physician who has made the most outstanding contribution to the cause of women in the field of medicine. In addition, Women Heart: The National Coalition for Women with Heart Disease has established "The Wenger Awards" in honor of Dr. Wenger to recognize individuals and organizations that have demonstrated a commitment to and significant achievement in efforts to reduce heart disease in women. She is the senior editor of the medical text, *Women and Heart Disease,* and chairs the Board of the Society for Women's Health Research.

Beverly Whipple, PhD, RN, FAAN, is a professor emerita at Rutgers University. She is currently the secretary general of the World Association for Sexual Health. She has served as the vice president of the World Association for Sexology; president of the Society for the Scientific Study of Sexuality; president of the American Association of Sex Educators, Counselors and Therapists; and director of the International Society for the Study of Women's Sexual Health.

Jacqueline L. Wolf, MD, runs a clinical academic gastroenterology practice at Beth Israel Deaconess Medical Center. The focus of her clinical practice and research is women's health and gastrointestinal disorders in women and inflammatory bowel disease. Dr. Wolf is a member of the Inflammatory Bowel Disease Group at her medical center. She has participated in the women's health congress for many years, chairing or speaking at the gastroenterology portion. Dr. Wolf has developed a mentoring program for women in gastroenterology and medicine through the American Gastroenterological Association's Women's Committee. She is also secretary of the Society for Women's Health Research.

Mallory Zhang, MD, is a fellow in the gynecologic oncology program at Stanford University/UCSF. She is a graduate of Columbia University Medical School and completed her residency at Stanford University. Her research interests include ovarian cancer stem cell and immunotherapy for ovarian cancer. Dr. Zhang is a member of the American College of Obstetrics and Gynecology.

FOREWORD

The Society for Women's Health Research (SWHR) was founded and incorporated in the spring of 1990 to continue the efforts of a small group of people advocating for changes in research into women's health. A small group of us, including a public relations firm, began discussing possible avenues for our advocacy, including encouraging the National Institutes of Health (NIH) to increase its attention to conditions affecting women.

It was natural for us to think of the NIH. First, during the late 1980s, various patient groups were advocating that Congress pay more attention to diseases affecting their members. Some succeeded in having new institutes at NIH established (e.g., the National Institute of Nursing Research and the National Institute of Arthritis and Musculoskeletal and Skin Diseases). Most notable and vocal was the community dedicated to finding a cure for HIV/AIDS.

Additionally, my own interest in NIH's role in directing research came from several sources. I had been brought up in a research tradition; my father was a scientist who worked for the government. NIH had supported my graduate work and had provided me with research funding. And I had already begun advocating for change within NIH.

When I started working at NIH, the late Dr. Mort Lipsett told me that my role was to champion the field of obstetrics and gynecology. At that time, there were not a lot of people researching obstetrics and gynecologic problems. Later, former Congresswoman Pat Schroeder (D-CO) would remark, "There are three gynecologists and 39 veterinarians at NIH."

I first recognized this when a friend with whom I commuted developed ovarian cancer. Congresswoman Rosa DeLauro (D-CT) had been a staffer for Senator Christopher Dodd (D-CT), and we commuted from New Haven to Washington every week. Between 1985 and her election to Congress in 1990, I tried to find out what was available to her at NIH, but there was little to offer, in terms of in-house expertise and funding of academic scientists. Congresswoman DeLauro has been a friend of research at NIH and a great advocate in Congress. Fortunately for her and her constituents, Yale New Haven had a wonderful oncologist who took care of her. But it was so frustrating that there was very little to offer. Internists, not gynecologic oncologists, were conducting ovarian cancer research. My office at NIH received a huge number of calls from congressional staffers wanting to know what research was being done on gynecologic problems, and unfortunately, I always had to refer them elsewhere.

In the late 1980s, the National Heart, Lung, and Blood Institute was conducting early studies on postmenopausal hormone replacement (as it was then called). The initial study evaluated the effect of estrogen coupled with progesterone in a small sample of women. I was called in as a consultant while a larger trial was being designed, but it soon became apparent that I was more of a nuisance than a help. Since I was the only gynecologist involved, my input exhausted the others. I realized that more gynecologic muscle was needed at NIH. What to do? Well, if we were going to get more gynecologists at NIH, the bureaucracy needed to be convinced. For a variety of reasons, I chose to make our plight known to Congress.

I was impressed with the effectiveness of the HIV/AIDS community in getting change at NIH and having scientists hired to study AIDS. The same model could be used to put obstetrics and gynecology in the spotlight at NIH. I remember that a number of us met at the American College of Obstetricians and Gynecologists in the spring of 1989. We were all gathered around a large, dark wooden table shaped like a uterus. Everyone, and the advocacy groups they represented, was interested in the need for more gynecology research at NIH, but they thought the issue should be broadened to incorporate women's health generally. Reproductive health was minimized as a focus, because many national groups were already working in that area.

The Congressional Caucus played a critical role. Its executive director Leslie Primer took on this project and found a way for Congress to become active. She and her staff worked with Congressman Henry Waxman's (D-CA) committee to hold a hearing on why women were not included in many NIH clinical trials. (Of course, as a researcher in ob/gyn, I saw only women patients, so I did not notice that women were not included in clinical trials.)

The all-volunteer members of the Society's Board of Directors worked with the Congressional Caucus and Congressman Waxman to ask the Government Accountability Office (then called the Government Accounting Office, GAO) to examine the issue. The audit was released at an NIH reauthorization hearing in June 1990. To me, that hearing was a "tipping point." Those who worked on the issues could disappear, but this topic was not going to go away, and 15 years later, enormous changes have taken place. Along the way, we did expand research in obstetrics and gynecology, so my original concerns have been addressed.

With inclusion of women in clinical studies and the broadening of the ob/gyn program at NIH, it was time to move on. Actually, what happened involved a revisit of discussions held very early in the formation of the Society. During 1989, I had held many lunches and discussions with public opinion leaders around Washington. While at a Cosmos Club lunch, I had a discussion with Dr. Samuel Thier, then president of the Institute of Medicine, who emphasized that males and females were biologically different. He suggested that the Society look at sex differences as a long-range goal. That fit well with my prejudices, since I had always felt that the differences between males and females were the most interesting of all scientific questions.

Many of the Society's leaders began holding strategy working discussions, from which several action items emerged. One was that SWHR host a series of scientific research meetings highlighting sex differences, with morning and evening sessions exploring different topics in sex differences and genetic differences in individuals and afternoons devoted to informal networking. These meetings now occur annually and are extremely successful, bringing together geneticists with professionals from other disciplines.

Another Society goal was to promote networks of individuals looking at collaborative possibilities to examine sex differences over a wide range of related areas. Three of these networks have been established: on neuroscience, metabolism, and cancer biology.

A third goal was to obtain independent, unbiased validation of the importance of research on sex differences. Six years of work by the Society in this area resulted in the landmark 2001 Institute of Medicine (IOM) report, *Exploring the Biological Contributions to Human Health: Does Sex Matter?* This report not only validated the focus of the Society but also gave the scientists who wanted to do such work a solid underpinning and justification for their efforts. The importance of a study like this cannot be overestimated.

The chapters in this book illustrate the work of many scientists and clinicians who have found that sex differences are fascinating. One of the goals of the book is to offer a better understanding of diseases that affect men and women differently. Another is to show how much research is being done on all of the conditions that affect women and how all of our lives are being improved by that research and will continue to be improved by studies still to come.

I hope you enjoy the book, which is the result of a huge amount of work by the authors and the staff of the Society, including Suzanne Stone, who shepherded this project from conception to fulfillment.

—FLORENCE HASELTINE, PhD, MD,
FOUNDER, SOCIETY FOR WOMEN'S HEALTH RESEARCH

Do Sex Differences Matter?

This book brings the latest knowledge about how sex differences matter to you. Until the late 20th century, biomedical research and medical practice were characterized by general acceptance of the "male norm." Males were studied as representative of the species, and it was assumed that sex differences (outside of reproductive functions) could be explained by, for example, differences in body or organ size, body weight, or proportion of body fat. Anything that differed from the male norm was labeled "atypical" or even abnormal.

Courses in human physiology, anatomy, or pharmacology abounded with references to the "typical 70-kilogram man." He was, in many ways, a good research subject. Over the years, he remained white, middle-class, and middle-age. For the most part, he bore a remarkable resemblance to the researchers who were probing his biological mysteries. Until quite recently, he was the standard on which our knowledge of human biology is based. The "typical 60-kilogram woman" never seemed to make it to class.

As previously discussed, in the mid-1980s the medical research community began to recognize that the knowledge gap created by these policies had a negative effect on women's health. Women in the United States were routinely prescribed drugs that had not been tested for safety or effectiveness in women, and there was little understanding of the differences between men and women that might result in differences in safety or effectiveness of medical treatment. In 1985 the U.S. Public Health Service Task Force on Women's Health Issues concluded: "The historical lack of research focus on women's health concerns has compromised the quality of health information available to women as well as the health care they receive."

Due to the efforts of the Society for Women's Health Research, the regulations and guidelines were changed to include women in research studies. However, less progress was made in designing research studies to ensure the conduct of valid analysis by sex, which could reveal whether interventions affect women and men differently.

Does Sex Matter?

In April 2001, the U.S. Institute of Medicine (IOM) announced publication of a landmark report, *Exploring the Biological Contributions to Human Health: Does Sex Matter?* This event was the culmination of six years of work by the Society for Women's Health Research to obtain independent, unbiased validation of the importance of research on sex differences. In saying, "Yes, sex matters," the IOM clarified the definitions of "sex" and "gender:" sex indicates the biology of being male or female as determined by an individual's genes and hormones, while gender indicates the distinct social roles and behavior expected of men and women.

The IOM Committee on Understanding the Biology of Sex and Gender Differences was charged with reviewing and evaluating the current state of knowledge about, and scientific evidence for, sex and gender differences and their determinants; to identify gaps in research on sex and gender differences; and to make recommendations for filling those gaps. The IOM report validated the scientific study of sex differences as a means of improving health. It conveys three main messages:

- Sex matters. Sex is a crucial biological variable that "should be considered when designing and analyzing studies in all areas and at all levels of biomedical and health-related research."
- The study of sex differences must move from simply observing such differences to studying why and how they occur and whether or not they are important to health and disease prevention and treatment.
- The barriers to the advancement of knowledge about sex differences in health and illness must be eliminated.

The IOM Committee also reported that:

- "Sex begins in the womb." Sex differences appear early in the development of the embryo and continue to manifest throughout the life span, and there is a lack of data on sex differences across the life span.
- Sex affects behavior and perception. It is in this area that the interplay between genetic and biological factors and environmental factors is most evident.
- Sex affects health in all areas, including health promotion and disease prevention, diagnosis, and treatment. Men and women have different patterns of illness and statistically different life

spans. Again, this is an area where both biological and environmental factors come into play.

♦ Sex differences should be studied in the laboratory, in clinical research, and in the study of populations and public health.

The IOM Committee noted the potential for use of sex-based research in defending discrimination based on such differences and recommended that the scientific community be aware of this potential and work to reduce its impact. In addition, the scientific community should try to increase the public's awareness that human beings are not just their biology, and that the results of our genetic programming are often amenable to environmental influences and conscious efforts to change.

Progress in research on sex differences is fundamental to furthering our understanding of male and female biology as well as our ability to prevent, diagnose, and treat disease in men and women. Progress in sex-based biology will require work in many research disciplines and medical specialties and, among all research approaches, from molecular biology to the study of populations. The importance of sex-based biology to health care necessitates a "bench-to-bedside" translation that requires integration of research findings from studies at the cellular level, in animals, and in human subjects. Timely and accurate reporting of research results by sex, and support and funding for sex-based biology research and research resources, will be crucial. The Society for Women's Health Research will continue to seek ways to overcome these and other barriers to interdisciplinary research into sex differences.

Since the report was issued, interest in sex as a biological variable has increased among all participants in the biomedical research enterprise: funding agencies, basic and clinical researchers, publishers, health care providers, and health care consumers.

—SHERRY A. MARTS, PhD

INTRODUCTION

We are continually learning more about how sex differences can impact your health, so the Society of Women's Health Research decided to write this guide to help keep you (and the women you love) healthy throughout your lifespan and offer you the latest information about diseases that may affect your health differently than they affect men.

Although many people think that "sex" and "gender" are interchangeable synonyms, this is not the case for medical researchers and health care practitioners. Sex is a biological variable that determines whether you are female or male, while gender refers to culturally defined roles and behavior expected for females and males. Both sex and gender differences can affect one's health. For example, male and female brains process pain differently, which is a sex difference affecting the type and intensity of painful conditions women and men experience; and gender differences may play a part in the treatment each sex receives for their pain—health care providers who subscribe to the "strong, silent" view of men can overestimate the amount of pain a man is in when he complains and underestimate a woman's.

Part 1, Taking Care of Yourself, discusses women's special health considerations in staying healthy. Chapters in this section address wellness, nutrition, safe medicine use, and how to develop a family history.

Part 2, An A to Z Guide to Women's Health, includes chapters on the major diseases and conditions that affect women solely or differently from the way they affect men. Each chapter provides an overview of the condition, including risk factors, symptoms, and what is needed for a diagnosis, as well as critical sex differences in each of these areas. Special attention is given to how pregnancy, menopause, and other life-cycle episodes in women's lives matter.

And, finally, part 3 tells you where you can go for help.

We hope *The Savvy Woman Patient* will become an important health resource for you and your loved ones.

—PHYLLIS GREENBERGER, MSW, CEO AND PRESIDENT,
SOCIETY FOR WOMEN'S HEALTH RESEARCH

PART 1

TAKING CARE OF YOURSELF

CHAPTER 1

Women's Wellness through the Life Span

O ver the past 20 years, society has worked hard to eliminate gender differences in the workplace, at home, and in sports. Yet there's one area we *need* to keep separate, one area in which recognizing sex and gender differences is critical: health.

During most of modern times, the medical profession has used the white, male patient as a typical prototype, assuming that if we knew how a disease manifested itself in a man, how a drug worked in a man, why a procedure was successful in a man, we would know the same in terms of a woman.

But today, thanks to groundbreaking work by sex-based biological researchers, we know that sex *does* matter—and not just when it comes to reproductive health. Sex matters in nearly every avenue of mental, physical, and emotional health, from the different symptoms men and women exhibit during a heart attack to the ways in which they cope with pain. Sex differences are responsible for variations in bone composition, in drug metabolism, and in the rate at which the brain synthesizes neurotransmitters, chemicals important to mood and functioning.

Just consider these top 10 differences:

1. **Heart disease.** Heart disease kills 500,000 American women each year, over 50,000 more women than men; and strikes women, on average, 10 years later than it does men. Women are more likely than men to have a second heart attack within a year of the first one.
2. **Depression.** Women are two to three times more likely than are men to suffer from depression. In part, that is because women's brains make less of the neurotransmitter, serotonin.
3. **Osteoporosis.** At least 65 percent of those diagnosed with osteoporosis, or loss of bone mass, are women.

4. **Smoking.** Cigarette smoking is more harmful to women than it is to men. Women also have a harder time quitting smoking and have more severe nicotine withdrawal symptoms.

5. **Sexually transmitted diseases.** Women are twice as likely as men to contract a sexually transmitted disease and more likely to experience significant drops in body weight if they have AIDS, which can lead to wasting syndrome.

6. **Anesthesia.** Women tend to wake up from anesthesia more quickly than do men, an average of three to four minutes faster.

7. **Drug reactions.** Even common medications like antihistamines and antibiotics can cause different reactions and side effects in women and men.

8. **Autoimmune disease.** Three of four people suffering from autoimmune diseases such as multiple sclerosis, rheumatoid arthritis, and lupus are women.

9. **Alcohol.** Women produce less of the gastric enzyme that breaks down ethanol in the stomach. Therefore, after consuming the same amount of alcohol as men, women have higher blood alcohol levels, even allowing for size differences.

10. **Pain.** Morphine-like pain medications known as kappa-opiates are far more effective in relieving pain in women than they are in men. An example is meperidine, which is used to treat moderate-to-severe pain and for intravenous regional anesthesia and peripheral nerve blocks.

As Mary-Lou Pardue, PhD, chair of an Institute of Medicine (IOM) report on sex differences in health, said: "Sex does matter. It matters in ways that we did not expect. Undoubtedly, it also matters in ways we have not begun to imagine."

Unfortunately, our medical model is still a male-based one. Fifty years of clinical studies that focused mainly on men has left us with a lack of female-based data on everything from the best medication to treat hypertension in women to why women are more likely to develop an autoimmune disease. We are thankful that is beginning to change. Clinical trials for new medications must now include women. With more women scientists and doctors in the scientific workforce, new topics and new questions are being explored, even those that were often taken for granted.

The challenge, now, is to parlay this growing knowledge into actionable steps, to disseminate it to health care providers and consumers, and to ensure that the small momentum we have going does not buckle under the weight of politics and funding.

Sex Matters to Wellness

So what, you ask, does all this have to do with wellness through the life span? To answer that, consider an Institute of Medicine report published in 2001, *Exploring the Biological Contributions to Human Health: Does Sex Matter?* The report, initiated and supported by the Society for Women's Health Research, underscored the need to better understand the importance of sex differences and how to translate that knowledge into improved medical practice and therapies.

Among its key findings:

Every cell has a sex. Some of the reason for the sex of a cell is related to whether you have XX or XY chromosomes, some is related to the affects of hormones on cellular structure and growth, and some is related to whether you got your X chromosome from your mother or your father (recall that sperm carries X and Y chromosomes, while an egg only has X chromosomes). The result: "multiple, ubiquitous differences in the basic cellular biochemistries of males and females that can affect an individual's health."

Sex differences begin in the womb and continue through the life span. It seems obvious, but these differences go far beyond the egg and sperm meeting. Some research indicates that differences in the intrauterine environment triggered by a fetus's sex may lay the groundwork for later health. These differences continue throughout life and lay the groundwork for biological differences in health and disease.

Sex affects behavior and perception. Basic biological differences in the male and female brain help explain some of the different play behavior we see in boys and girls; boys tend to focus on objects and choose gross motor activities, and girls tend to focus on people and relationships and choose activities that use discreet, finer motor skills. While early play behavior can be strongly influenced by society as well, some of the distinctions are based on the genetic makeup of each individual. And these differences in both perception and the behavior it influences manifest throughout the life span, such as in how women handle stress.

Sex affects health. In fact, sex should be considered a "biological variable" in all biomedical and health-related research, the IOM report notes, much as ethnicity, preexisting conditions, and current health status are.

Raising a Healthy Daughter

Congratulations! It's a girl! As visions of frilly dresses, mother-daughter teas, and sports bras dance through your head, take a deep breath and think about this: How you raise your daughter over the next 10 years will have a strong impact on her lifelong emotional, and physical health.

The notion that much of our lifelong health is determined in the first decade of life (indeed, even before we leave the womb) is just emerging. But there is enough existing evidence to encourage you to give your daughter the healthiest start possible. In many instances, what you do yourself will have the greatest impact on her future health. Specifically:

- **Relax about dirt.** Throughout childhood, boys are more likely to develop asthma than are girls, but the trend reverses after puberty, until at 18, more girls than boys have asthma. One contributing factor to the country's growing endemic of asthma and allergies may be our national obsession with cleanliness. Studies find, for instance, that children who attend daycare or grow up on farms are less likely to develop these chronic conditions. The message: Do not obsess over the dirt!

- **Watch the sun.** Skin and sun damage in our early years come back to haunt us when we hit our thirties and see those first wrinkles appear. Those of us who grew up during the baby-oil-and-bake years did not know any better; now we do. Most frightening: the most lethal form of skin cancer, melanoma, is the most frequent cancer in women between the ages of 25 and 29, and the second most frequent cancer, after breast cancer, in women between the ages of 30 and 34. The message: Stick a bottle of sunscreen with an SPF of at least 15 in the car, the diaper bag, the kitchen. Slather it on her first thing every morning—even if you're just going to the store. The sun is just as damaging through glass or clouds as it is on the beach in July. Some experts recommend avoiding sunscreen for babies under six months, so check with your doctor first.

- **Quit smoking.** Secondhand smoke contributes to numerous health conditions in children and, later, adults, including asthma, bronchitis, colds, and respiratory syncytial virus (RSV) (the most common cause of lower respiratory tract infections in children). The message: If you smoke, quit—if not for your own health, then for your daughter's.

♦ **Eat healthy and move!** Overweight children are more likely to become overweight adults and are more likely to have cardio-vascular problems and diabetes than are normal-weight children. Sadly, today's children are all too often too fat. In fact, children's health experts point to an epidemic of overweight children as one of the greatest health threats facing our kids today. One reason: too much food and too little physical activity. The message: You need to lead by example. If your daughter sees you loading your plate with vegetables, she will, too. If you invite her on a walk after dinner instead of plopping down in front of the TV, she will come to associate exercise with pleasant memories.

♦ **Pour the milk.** Want to ensure your daughter has a set of healthy bones? Pour the (skim) milk now. The message: Teach your daughter early on that nonfat dairy is an excellent way to build bone and get valuable nutrients—without packing on the pounds.

So, there you have some important steps to build a strong foundation of physical health for your daughter. Now, what about her emotional health? Studies find that around age 12, otherwise strong, independent girls begin to fade, becoming less assured and more vulnerable to peer pressure and self-doubt. A University of Illinois study that followed 900 boys and girls from fourth through seventh grade found that while girls had better grades than boys in language arts, social studies, math, and science, girls said they felt much more stress and anxiety and less confidence in their abilities than did boys. They were also more likely to underestimate their ability, all of which eventually leads them to take fewer risks and shy away from subjects like math and science. As the study's lead author, Ewa Pomerantz, PhD, told a newspaper reporter: "Even the highest-achieving girls are depressed more, worrying more, and have a lower self-esteem."

This kind of thinking can follow a girl into adulthood, preventing her from reaching her full potential in school, the workplace, even relationships. You can help your daughter maintain independent thought and self-assurance. For instance, expose her to unique situations at home and in the community. If your daughter questions her ability in math or science, set up an informational interview with a female engineer or math professor. Encourage her to explore so-called "unfeminine" avenues, such as learning to change the spark plugs and tires on her car or taking karate.

Teach her that it is okay to make mistakes, but do not continually rescue her when things go wrong. Help her understand why negative events

Raising Emotionally and Physically Healthy Children

There is obviously no one right way to raise a child. But years of research have teased out some common threads when it comes to bringing up emotionally and physically healthy children. The National Mental Health Information Center recommends that parents:

- Do their best to provide a safe home and community for their child, as well as nutritious meals, regular health checkups, immunizations, and exercise.
- Understand child development stages so you do not expect too much or too little from your child.
- Encourage your child to express her feelings and respect those feelings. Let her know that everyone experiences pain, fear, anger, and anxiety.
- Help your child express anger positively, without resorting to violence.
- Promote mutual respect and trust. Keep your voice level down— even when you do not agree. Keep communication channels open.
- Listen to your child. Use words and examples your child can understand. Encourage questions.
- Provide comfort and assurance. Be honest. Focus on the positives. Express your willingness to talk about any subject.
- Look at your own problem-solving and coping skills. Do you turn to alcohol or drugs? Are you setting a good example? Seek help if you are overwhelmed by your child's feelings or behaviors or if you are unable to control your own frustration or anger.
- Encourage your child's talents and accept limitations.
- Set goals based on the child's abilities and interests—not someone else's expectations.
- Celebrate accomplishments. Do not compare your child's abilities to those of other children; appreciate the uniqueness of your child.
- Spend time regularly with your child.
- Foster your child's independence and self-worth.
- Help your child deal with life's ups and downs. Show confidence in your child's ability to handle problems and tackle new experiences.
- Discipline constructively, fairly, and consistently. Learn what works best for your child and express approval of positive behaviors.
- Love unconditionally. Teach the value of apologies, cooperation, patience, forgiveness, and consideration for others.
- Do not expect to be perfect; parenting is a difficult job.

occur and how to resolve and learn from them. And, above all, keep the lines of communication open—by simply being there when she wants to talk, scheduling special mother/daughter events (a weekly breakfast, perhaps?), and learning to listen—before you react.

Navigating Adolescence

Sex-based biology definitely comes into play during adolescence. Teenage girls are twice as likely as boys to be depressed and nearly twice as likely to commit suicide. They are more likely to have body image problems and develop eating disorders. And they are more likely to battle with self-esteem issues than are boys, a particularly dangerous sex difference, since self-esteem is directly linked with such risk-taking behaviors as premarital sex, smoking, and substance abuse.

Those sex differences also manifest themselves when it comes to girls' vulnerability to risky behavior. Consider these statistics from the Center for Alcohol and Substance Abuse (CASA):

- Girls may develop symptoms of nicotine addiction faster than boys and become addicted to nicotine even before they become regular smokers.
- Girls progress from regular alcohol use to alcohol abuse at a faster rate than males and are more susceptible to health disorders such as liver disease, cardiac problems, and brain damage from drinking, which occur more quickly and with lower levels of alcohol consumption than they do in males.
- Teenage girls are more likely than boys to become addicted to cocaine and to be hospitalized due to nonmedical use of medications, such as acetaminophen or antidepressants.

Girls are also catching up to boys in rates of smoking, drinking, and substance abuse and are starting these behaviors at ever-younger ages. Girls often use drugs for different reasons from boys, get their drugs from different sources, have an easier time gaining access to substances, and are targeted by the media in different ways.

So what is a mother to do? Talk to your daughter. Study after study finds that, despite popular perceptions, parents have more influence on their kids' lives in terms of their risky behavior than any best friend. In fact, CASA's studies on adolescent girls find that the worse a girl's relationship with her parents, the more likely she is to use drugs. Even more: 61.6 percent of girls said having conversations with their parents about smoking, drinking, or drug use made them less likely to try any of those substances.

The same approach works when it comes to enhancing your daughter's self-esteem: Be involved in her life, talk to her, and support her. Encourage her to follow her dream and pay attention to her, whether she has done something wonderful—or something terrible.

Healthy Living

Now let us turn the focus to you. Regardless of your age, you need to follow certain basic underpinnings to manage your health today—and tomorrow.

Let us start with your weight. Just as our children are getting fatter, so, too, are women. Today, almost 62 percent of women are overweight; of these, 33 percent are obese. Body mass index, or BMI, is a measurement that takes into account your weight and height. For women age 20 and older, a BMI below 18.5 means you are underweight; 18.5 to 24.9 means you have a normal weight; and 25 to 29.9 is overweight. Anything 30 and above is considered obese.

You can easily find your own BMI by using the BMI calculator online at the Centers for Disease Control and Prevention (CDC) at www.cdc.gov, or by using this formula:

$$\text{BMI} = \left(\frac{\text{Weight in Pounds}}{(\text{Height in inches}) \times (\text{Height in inches})} \right) \times 703$$

Source: CDC

While BMI does not *measure* body fat, it does *correlate* with body fat. Thus, the higher your BMI, the higher the percentage of body fat you are likely to have. Next to cigarette smoking, nothing affects your health more negatively than being overweight. Women who are overweight have a greater risk of:

- ◆ **Breast cancer.** Approximately one-third of postmenopausal breast cancers are associated with weight gain after menopause. One possible reason is that fat cells serve as a storehouse for androgens, hormones that convert to estrogen, which, in turn, stimulate the growth of breast cells.
- ◆ **Endometrial cancer.** The more overweight you are, the greater your risk for endometrial cancer, the most common gynecolog-

ical cancer. Blame those androgen-storing fat cells again because estrogen stimulates the lining of the uterus.

◆ **Birth defects.** If you are overweight or obese when you get pregnant, you have a greater risk of giving birth to a baby with a variety of birth defects, including spina bifida, a neural tube defect in which the spinal column does not close completely.

◆ **Obstetric and gynecologic complications.** Being overweight or obese increases your risk of menstrual abnormalities, infertility, and miscarriage. It can also increase your risk of hypertension, toxemia, gestational diabetes, urinary infection during pregnancy, having a Cesarean section, and delivering an overly large baby.

◆ **Cardiovascular disease.** If you are overweight you are much more likely to have high levels of triglycerides and low-density lipoprotein (LDL) cholesterol ("bad" cholesterol) and low levels of high-density lipoprotein (HDL) cholesterol ("good" cholesterol), significantly increasing your risk of heart attack, stroke, and other cardiovascular diseases.

◆ **Type 2 diabetes.** You are more likely to develop type 2 diabetes and its precursor, metabolic syndrome, if you are obese, and you are more likely to have problems managing the condition once you are diagnosed, thereby increasing the risk of complications.

◆ **Urinary stress incontinence.** If you are overweight or obese, you are more likely to experience urinary stress incontinence. This condition can seriously affect your quality of life and is a leading cause of nursing home admissions in the elderly.

Bottom line: being overweight hurts you in so many more ways than just your waistline.

However, losing excess weight and maintaining a health weight is not easy—regardless of what popular diet gurus tell you. One of the few long-term studies examining what makes for successful weight loss and weight control—the National Weight Control Registry (NWCR)—tracks more than 4,500 men and women who have successfully maintained a 30-pound weight loss for at least a year. The average registrant has lost approximately 60 pounds and has maintained that loss for roughly five years. So far, the study finds:

◆ Successful weight losers say they make substantial changes in eating and exercise habits to lose weight and maintain the loss.

◆ Two-thirds of these successful weight losers were overweight as children, and 60 percent report a family history of obesity.

- Approximately half of the participants lost weight on their own without any type of formal program or help.
- Walking is the most frequently cited physical activity registry members performed.

Members said that their weight loss significantly improved their self-confidence, mood, and physical health. And—here is some more good news—42 percent said maintaining their weight loss was less difficult than initially losing the weight.

There is no secret when it comes to losing weight. The successful members of the weight loss registry reduced their caloric intake and increased their caloric, or energy, expenditure, generally by moving more. That means exercise, which we discuss next.

10 Painless Ways to Cut Calories

1. Switch from sodas to water.
2. Keep a container of cut-up vegetables with some low-fat dressing in the fridge for hunger attacks.
3. Eat several small meals throughout the day so you are never starving.
4. Order a side salad in lieu of French fries when you are eating out.
5. Eat a big salad before your main course; you will fill up on the salad and eat less of the other foods.
6. Opt for nonfat or low-fat dairy—ice cream, milk, yogurt, and cheese.
7. Bake, do not fry.
8. Carry a snack pack with you containing dried fruit, trail mix, a piece of fruit, and a bottle of water to avoid impulsive vending machine raids.
9. Eat a handful of nuts a day. Studies find you will eat fewer calories overall.
10. Substitute plain coffee with skim milk for fancy coffee drinks. You will save hundreds of calories a day.

Moving through Your Life

It is not easy to be physically active in today's society. In fact, it is almost as if the world we live in is designed to keep our bottoms pinned to our chairs. Just think about it: we have labor-saving devices for *everything*, from changing TV channels to turning on lights to raising the blinds! We do not have to get out of our car to buy our dinner, deposit our paycheck, pick up our dry cleaning, or drop off a prescription. Nor do we have to walk down the hall to talk to our co-workers any longer; we can just e-mail!

Small wonder government statistics show that more than 60 percent of women do not get the recommended amount of physical activity, and that one in four women is not physically active at all. That number jumps in women over 55—nearly 40 percent of whom say they do no leisure-time physical activity.

There are many benefits to exercising. Regular exercise lowers blood pressure, reduces levels of "bad" cholesterol while raising levels of "good" cholesterol, and slows your resting heart rate so that organ works more efficiently. It does not take much; in one study, women who walked briskly for three or more hours a week slashed their risk of heart disease 35 percent more than women who walked less frequently.

Physical activity also reduces your risk of colon cancer, kidney stones, gallstone surgery, and diverticular disease (your colon has small pouches that bulge outward through weak spots, and diverticulosis exists when the pouches become infected or inflamed). And weight-bearing exercise, like walking, riding a bike, or lifting weights, not only strengthens muscle, but bone as well, increasing bone density and preventing or slowing osteoporosis.

Exercise can also lower the risk of the disease most women fear most: breast cancer. A study of 26,000 women found that those who exercised at least four hours a week had 37 percent fewer breast cancers than sedentary women. Researchers think moderate to high activity levels lower a woman's lifetime exposure to estrogen, a primary risk factor for breast cancer.

Exercise has numerous emotional benefits, too. It helps you fall asleep faster and sleep longer and deeper, and it can relieve depression. One small study found that just 30 minutes of daily walking on a treadmill at various intensities worked faster than drugs to lift depression. Then there are exercise's well-studied stress-reducing benefits. In study after study, aerobic exercise (for example, walking) reduces anxiety, improves depression, helps you cope with stress better, and contributes to positive mood, self-esteem, and mental functioning. Not bad for a brisk march around the block.

We do not expect you to begin training for a triathlon. But just a few changes in your daily routine can help you get the recommended 30 minutes a day of physical activity so critical to your overall health (you will need at least 60 for weight loss). For instance:

♦ Walk around the block while your child is at piano practice or around the soccer field while she is at practice.

- Use a 15-minute break at work to walk briskly up and down the stairs.
- Turn off the TV and use that half-hour to weed the garden or rake leaves.
- Give up automatic devices for manual ones. That means cutting the grass with a manual mower, not a riding one, raking leaves and shoveling snow, not blowing them away.
- Park your car at the outer edge of the parking lot and walk to the store or office.
- Always get out of your car when running errands or picking up food; make drive-throughs off limits.

One thing that may help: Surround yourself with people who are also physically active. A national study conducted by Stanford University researchers found that if women did not see other people exercising in the neighborhood, they did not feel like exercising themselves.

Tackling the S Word: Stress

The word, "stress," is so overused in our vocabulary that it has basically lost its meaning. Overall, the U.S. Department of Labor reported a 20.3 percent increase in days missed at work because of anxiety, stress, and neurotic disorders between 2000 and 2001, with the American Institute of Stress estimating that a million U.S. workers miss work every day because of stress-related complaints.

Yet stress, and how you handle it, plays an important role in your health throughout your life. Give into it and drown in it, and you are more likely to develop conditions such as hypertension, angina, gastric reflux, constipation, irritable bowel syndrome, depression, anxiety, and fatigue.

Women's bodies respond to stress differently from men's. We produce more stress hormones and have less ability to turn off this production. And that is not all! Japanese researchers who studied 8,656 women found highly stressed women were more than twice as likely to suffer strokes than were women reporting low stress and had a coronary disease risk more than two times higher than normal, while their overall chance of dying from heart disease was more than 1.5 times greater than average.

You are also more likely to get fat, since the stress hormone, cortisol, not only triggers appetite, but can encourage deposition of fat in the abdomen, creating life-threatening visceral fat and increasing your risk of heart disease and diabetes. Research now correlates chronically elevated levels of cortisol with blood sugar problems, fat accumulation, compromised immune function, exhaustion, bone loss, and even heart disease.

Memory loss has also been associated with high cortisol levels. Continued stress can indeed have a negative impact on your health.

Work is one of the greatest stressors for women. In one government survey, 60 percent of employed women cited stress as their number one problem at work. And in a four-year study of more than 21,000 nurses published in the *British Medical Journal*, Harvard researchers concluded that job stress can sap a woman's health just as surely as smoking or a sedentary lifestyle can. Jobs that are repetitive and boring and that provide little control, leaving women feeling powerless, seem to cause the most stress. A five-year study of more than 10,000 British government employees found such jobs can nearly double one's risk of heart disease.

Work stress is not the only stress in our lives, of course. Add aging parents, children (whether small or grown), relationship issues, financial woes, even today's "macro" stress over terrorism and safety, and you can understand why we often feel like we are running with our emotional meters on empty.

There is no way you will ever rid your life of stress entirely, nor would you want to. After all, think how boring a stress-free life would be. Plus, a lot of stress is related to positive events: a marriage, a new baby, a new house, a promotion.

The key is learning how to manage the stress in your life, along with trying to reduce the amount of negative stress encroaching on your well-being. Start by identifying your primary stressors. Sit down in a quiet place with a pad of paper and a pen. Divide the page vertically into two sections and label the left side, "Stressors," and the right side, "Solutions." Now list everything in your life—from credit card debt to your mother's cancer to your daughter's weekly activities—that adds to your stress. Look carefully at each one. In the right-hand column, write three ways in which you could either eliminate this stressor or manage it better.

For instance, take credit card debt. Financial woes are a form of chronic stress, which is the grinding, everyday stress that is the prime contributor to health problems. Make a plan to pay down your debt, put it in writing, then post it on the refrigerator so you will see it first thing every morning. It could include things like:

♦ Only eat out once a month.
♦ Brown-bag my lunch.
♦ Fire the housekeeper.
♦ Cut up the credit cards.
♦ Pay cash for all purchases.

You get the picture.

Get These Tests

You know the saying: "An ounce of prevention is worth a pound of cure." The federal government has recommended certain medical tests at certain times (see the chart below). Medical specialty societies and voluntary health agencies may have different recommendations.

---

*The American College of Obstetrics and Gynecology also recommends that women age 30 and older can be screened for cervical cancer with the Pap test alone or with the Pap test plus a test for high-risk types of human papillomavirus (HPV). This test for HPV is also used in women with slightly abnormal Pap test results to determine if more testing or treatment might be needed.

Screening Test	Ages 18–39	Ages 40–49	Ages 50–64	Ages 65+
Full checkup, including weight and height	Discuss with your doctor or nurse	Discuss with your doctor or nurse	Discuss with your doctor or nurse	Discuss with your doctor or nurse
Thyroid test (TSH)	Start at age 35, then every 5 years	Every 5 years	Every 5 years	Every 5 years
Blood pressure test	Start at age 21, then once every 1–2 years if normal	Every 1–2 years	Every 1–2 years	Every 1–2 years
Cholesterol test	Discuss with your doctor or nurse	Start at age 45, then every 5 years	Every 5 years	Every 5 years
Bone mineral density test		Discuss with your doctor or nurse	Discuss with your doctor or nurse	Get a bone density test at least once; talk to your doctor or nurse about repeat testing
Blood sugar test	Discuss with your doctor or nurse	Start at age 45, then every 3 years	Every 3 years	Every 3 years
Dental exam	1–2 times every year	1–2 times every year	1–2 times every year	1–2 times every year
Pap test and pelvic exam*	Every 1–3 years if you have been sexually active or are older than 21	Every 1–3 years	Every 1–3 years	Discuss with your doctor or nurse

Screening Test	Ages 18–39	Ages 40–49	Ages 50–64	Ages 65+
Chlamydia test	If sexually active, yearly until age 25	If you are at high risk for chlamydia or other sexually transmitted diseases, you may need this test	If you are at high risk for chlamydia or other sexually transmitted diseases, you may need this test	If you are at high risk for chlamydia or other sexually transmitted diseases, you may need this test
Other sexually transmitted disease tests (STDs)	Talk to your doctor or nurse if you or your partner have had sexual contact with more than one person or if either of you has ever had an STD	Talk to your doctor or nurse if you or your partner have had sexual contact with more than one person or if either of you has ever had an STD	Talk to your doctor or nurse if you or your partner have had sexual contact with more than one person or if either of you has ever had an STD	Talk to your doctor or nurse if you or your partner have had sexual contact with more than one person or if either of you has ever had an STD
Mammogram		Every 1–2 years	Every 1–2 years	Every 1–2 years
Fecal occult blood test			Yearly	Yearly
Flexible sigmoidoscopy (with fecal occult blood test)			Every 5 years	Every 5 years
Double contrast barium enema (DCBE)			Every 5–10 years (if you are not having a colonoscopy or sigmoidoscopy)	Every 5–10 years (if you are not having a colonoscopy or sigmoidoscopy)
Colonscopy			Every 10 years	Every 10 years
Rectal exam	Discuss with your doctor or nurse	Discuss with your doctor or nurse	Every 5–10 years with each screening (sigmoidoscopy, colonoscopy, or DCBE)	Every 5–10 years with each screening (sigmoidoscopy, colonoscopy, or DCBE)
Vision exam	Once between ages 20 and 39	Every 2–4 years	Every 2–4 years	Every 1–2 years

(continued)

Screening Test	Ages 18–39	Ages 40–49	Ages 50–64	Ages 65+
Hearing test	Starting at age 18, then every 10 years	Every 10 years	Discuss with your doctor or nurse	Discuss with your doctor or nurse
Mole exam	Monthly mole self-exam; by a doctor every 3 years, starting at age 20	Monthly mole self-exam; by a doctor every year	Monthly mole self-exam; by a doctor every year	Monthly mole self-exam; by a doctor every year
Influenza vaccine	Discuss with your doctor or nurse	Discuss with your doctor or nurse	Yearly	Yearly
Tetanus-diphtheria booster vaccine	Every 10 years	Every 10 years	Every 10 years	Every 10 years

Source: National Women's Health Information Center, www.4woman.gov.

Now let us talk about reframing the way you view stressful events. A growing body of research finds that if you shift your attitude, you can reduce the levels of stress hormones your body releases in response to stressful events. For instance, suppose you are stuck in traffic. You could get steamed up about it, curse and bang on the steering wheel, cranking up production of stress hormones. Or you could switch on a classical radio station or the news, slip in a book on tape, or simply let your mind wander to resolve a problem at work and relish this as time alone for you.

One of the best things women can do to manage stress is call a friend. Research finds that when women are stressed, they are more likely to "tend and befriend" by getting together with friends, talking about their feelings, and connecting with others. So pick up the phone, attend this month's book club meeting, or just call a neighbor for a walk around the block—and talk it out.

Menopause and Perimenopause

This is a time of life that used to be kept in the proverbial closet. But, thanks to the impact of the largest generation of women ever to reach menopause at one time—the baby boomers—menopause has become one of the hottest topics around. There is even an off-Broadway play about it!

This transitional time of life, when a woman bids goodbye to her reproductive years, is not an ending but a new beginning. For many women, it is a time when they are firmly established in their careers and do not have young children to care for, a time when they can truly focus on themselves.

In a survey on menopause conducted by the North American Menopause Society (NAMS), the majority of women said many areas of their lives had improved since menopause, including their family or home life, sense of personal fulfillment, and relationships with their partner and friendships.

Women report that they see this as a time to take control of their lives and their health, with three-quarters of the surveyed women reporting that they made lifestyle changes at middle age or menopause, including changes in diet or nutritional habits, exercise, and stress level.

The women said they also saw themselves as role models for the next generation, with 69 percent saying they had discussed menopause with their daughter or a younger woman.

Here are the top 10 highlights about the menopausal transition:

1. **Menopause is not a disease.** In fact, the actual "menopause" is only one day in a woman's life—the day on which she has gone 12 months without menstruating. The transition period we so often call "menopause" is actually perimenopause. After a woman reaches menopause, she is considered menopausal. Natural menopause generally occurs between ages 40 and 58, with a U.S. average age of about 51.

2. **There is no "menopause test."** Researchers are studying whether looking at a woman's ovaries with ultrasound may help predict when menopause will occur. But for now, you need to learn the signs of perimenopause. Generally, the first sign is that your periods become erratic, often for five or six years before you actually reach menopause. They may get shorter or longer in duration, come more or less frequently, and are often much heavier. Other signs include nighttime sweating, hot flashes, headaches (especially around your period), mood swings, vaginal dryness, reduced sex drive, and fuzzy thinking. Although there is no one test to tell if you are in perimenopause, your doctor may perform some tests to rule out other reasons for your symptoms, such as thyroid problems and diabetes.

3. **Perimenopause does not mean feeling bad.** About 10 to 20 percent of women sail through menopause without breaking a sweat. Another 65 to 70 percent experience changes in their bodies that range from mildly troublesome to seriously disruptive. At the other end of the spectrum are women who find the

transition to menopause overwhelming and hard to handle. Some research shows that women who experience hot flashes are at greater risk for developing depression than others.

4. **Hormone therapy still has a place in treating menopausal symptoms.** Although hormone therapy (HT) is not a panacea and is not for every woman, it still is the most effective medical therapy available to relieve hot flashes and vaginal dryness. Today, there are numerous forms of hormone therapy, ranging from pills to creams to patches that come in different doses and combinations of estrogen and progestin. Only you and your doctor can determine which, if any, is best for you. Overall, most medical organizations recommend that women use hormone therapy to treat specific symptoms and for the shortest time possible. Most of all, treatment should be customized to a woman's individualized needs and medical profile. Hormone therapy should not be used to treat chronic conditions such as heart disease in older women who have not been on HT. Some recent studies have questioned whether there is a protective role for younger women; more research is needed.

5. **Menopause is not the reason your brain is fuzzy.** Stress and lack of sleep are. So do not blame your forgetfulness on your hormones; instead, go to bed an hour earlier and try some of our recommendations for stress reduction.

6. **Your health needs change after menopause.** Estrogen has been proven to protect your bones and cardiovascular system. That may be why a woman's risk of heart disease increases after menopause. So it is more important than ever that you maintain the healthy lifestyle you have been following throughout your life, following the nutritional guidelines outlined in chapter 3 and getting at least 30 minutes of physical activity a day.

7. **You can still have an enjoyable and active sex life after menopause.** The NAMS survey found that 51 percent of women said their sex lives remained the same after menopause, while 16 percent said it improved, and 17 percent said it was worse. If you are having problems with vaginal dryness, definitely talk to your doctor; vaginally applied hormone therapy may help relieve symptoms. And if you are having relationship problems, consider a therapist. You have a lot of living yet to do, and it is nice to have someone to share the years with.

8. **Lifestyle changes can help with menopause symptoms.** Studies find that regular exercise, quitting smoking, and losing weight can all help reduce the severity and frequency of hot

flashes. Other changes that can help include stress management, wearing fewer layers of clothing, avoiding caffeine and alcohol, and keeping the temperature set as cool as possible.

9. **You can still get pregnant.** In fact, 51 percent of pregnancies in women age 40 and older are unintended, with 65 percent ending in abortion. Until your period stops for good, your ovaries are releasing eggs, so you can still get pregnant. Talk to your health care professional about birth control options.

10. **You cannot blame your weight gain on menopause.** Instead, you can blame it on a slowing metabolism, a normal result of aging. That is why it is so important to maintain a healthy diet and, if possible, increase the amount of physical activity you do every day.

Medicare and You

Once you hit that golden age 65, you get some help maintaining your health. The government health insurance program for the elderly and disabled, Medicare, offers numerous preventive health screenings and tests. Specifically:

- **Diabetes screening.** You are covered if you have high blood pressure, high cholesterol, obesity, or a history of high blood sugar, all of which put you at high risk for diabetes. Based on your findings, you may be eligible for up to two diabetes screenings a year.
- **Cardiovascular screening.** Medicare covers screening for blood tests that measure cholesterol and triglyceride and other lipid levels once every five years.
- **A one-time "Welcome to Medicare" physical exam.** When you begin Medicare coverage, you are invited to receive this physical exam within the first six months of the advent of your part B coverage (medical insurance; Part A is hospital insurance). It includes a thorough review of your health and education and counseling about preventive services you need, like certain screenings and shots, and referrals for other care if necessary. Your doctor checks your weight and height, gives you a vision test, and conducts an electrocardiogram (EKG) to assess your heart rhythm. You will also get a written plan letting you know what other screenings and tests you need. You pay 20 percent of the Medicare-approved amount after you have met the Part B deductible.

- **Annual mammograms.** Medicare covers annual mammograms for women over age 40. You pay 20 percent of the Medicare-approved amount after you have met the Part B deductible.
- **Pap tests.** Medicare covers Pap tests and pelvic exams once every 24 months. There is no charge for the Pap lab test; you pay 20 percent of the Medicare-approved amount after you have met the Part B deductible for the collection of the Pap and pelvic and breast exams.
- **Colorectal cancer screening.** Medicare covers the full range of colorectal cancer screening tests, including fecal occult blood test, flexible sigmoidoscopy, screening colonoscopy, and barium enema. You pay 20 percent of the Medicare-approved amount after you have met the Part B deductible for everything except the fecal occult blood test.

Medicare also covers annual flu shots, a pneumonia shot, and hepatitis B shots as well as bone mass screening (once every two years) and annual glaucoma tests.

Communicating with Your Health Professional

Whether your primary health professional is an internist, family practitioner, a gynecologist, nurse practitioner, or naturopath, how the two of you interact and communicate makes a big difference in your overall health.

Despite our growing reliance on tests and procedures, medicine is still very much an art. And the communication between you and your health care professional is one of the primary elements in creating the final "design."

Take your medical history, for instance. If you hide anything—the fact that you were once hospitalized for depression, that you smoke, or that you really do not exercise much—you are asking your doctor to do her job with one hand tied behind her back. Conversely, if your doctor just hands you a scribbled prescription and does not explain carefully how to take the medication, what side effects you might expect, etc., you might be left in the dark, without a full understanding of your own health needs.

Unfortunately, studies find too little of this two-way communication going on between health care professionals and patients. One reason is that doctors tend to talk in their own language (they call a heart attack a "myocardial ischemic event" and heartburn after eating a "postprandial esophageal reflux"). If you do not understand what your doctor says, you are not alone; a 1999 American Medical Association (AMA) study found that less than half the U.S. adult population understands many commonly used medical words. Another study of nearly 1,000 women with breast cancer found that nearly half said the information they received on several medical aspects of their condition was "incomprehensible or incomplete," significantly affecting their quality of life.

It is not that we are stupid. It is just that most Americans, indeed most nonmedical people, have relatively low levels of health literacy. Health literacy has nothing to do with reading and everything to do with understanding complex medical information. An Institute of Medicine report defines health literacy as "the ability to obtain, process, and understand basic health information and services needed to make appropriate health decisions," and it estimates that nearly 90 million Americans have problems with it.

Studies find that people with low health literacy are hospitalized more, have more difficulties using metered dose inhalers (for asthma and other lung conditions), and have worse HbA1c levels, an indication of how they're managing their diabetes, than do those with higher literacy levels. Research also suggests that people with low health literacy are less likely to comply with recommended treatments. It is a major reason, experts suspect, that only about half of all patients take prescribed medications as directed.

While you cannot change your doctor (although you *can* change doctors), there are things you can do to maximize your communication and to get the information you need. Start by following the "Ask Me 3" program, designed to help patients better understand the health information they get from their health care professionals and created by the Partnership for Clear Health Communication. It works like this: When you see your health care provider (and do not forget to include your pharmacist and dentist in that group), ask these three questions:

1. What is my main problem?
2. What do I need to do?
3. Why is it important for me to do this?

If it helps, write down these questions and take them with you to every doctor appointment. If you still do not understand your condition or the suggested treatment after you have gotten answers to these questions, stop, take a deep breath, and then say, "I appreciate all you have told me.

But I am still not clear on . . . . Is there another way you could explain it to me?"

There are other things you can do, too. For instance, bring a friend or family member to your doctor visit. Make a list of questions and concerns to ask your doctor or nurse *before* your visit. Put all medications you are taking, including vitamins, herbs, and supplements, in a bag and bring them to your next appointment. Turn to your pharmacist for help when you have questions about your medications.

You can also ask your doctor to draw a picture of the part of your body with the problem, to write down your instructions, and to be specific. For instance, if your doctor says you should get more exercise, ask how much? What kind? For how long?

Most important: Be honest and open with each other. Remember that everything you tell your health care professional remains confidential. And every little detail—no matter how unimportant it might seem—provides important clues for the diagnosis and treatment of your health condition.

Evaluating Risk

Much of what your health care provider tells you and many news reports about medical research tend to focus on *risk*. Drinking more milk can reduce your *risk* of osteoporosis. Eating more fruits and vegetables can reduce your *risk* of breast cancer. Taking hormone therapy may increase your *risk* of breast cancer. So it is important to understand just what researchers mean when they talk about *risk*.

There are two forms of risk when it comes to your health: relative risk and absolute risk. Most articles discuss relative risk. *Relative* risk is the amount of the increase or decrease in whatever the study was designed to evaluate—breast cancer, heart disease, etc.—over an entire population. So, for instance, if a news report says that a certain medication doubles the risk of a heart attack, it simply means that twice as many people taking the drug will have a heart attack as those *not* taking the drug.

Absolute risk, however, is the average person's risk of experiencing that side effect. So, for instance, if *you*, personally, have a 5 percent risk of having a heart attack during your lifetime, then taking the drug increases your individual risk by another 5 percent, resulting in a relative risk of 10 percent. In other words, 10 percent is 5 percent doubled.

Recently one report indicated that use of oral contraceptives may double a woman's risk of developing a heart attack or stroke. If you are a healthy young woman taking oral contraceptives, your risk for these cardiovascular events is probably extremely low. If you double *your* low risk, you will still have a low risk.

Bottom line: Always try to learn the *absolute* risk of a procedure or therapy, along with any side effects, before making any treatment decisions.

In the End

The key to wellness throughout your life is the same as for every other major challenge that comes your way: taking it one day a time. Every day, make five healthy choices. By the end of the year, you'll have made 1,825 healthy choices, which will undoubtedly enhance your overall health and well-being.

—DEBRA GORDON

CHAPTER 2

Using Medicine Safely

Most people assume that the effects of prescription drugs are the same for everyone. But an ever-increasing number of studies show that the safety and effectiveness of many widely used drugs vary depending on the sex of the user. In fact, eight of 10 drugs removed from the market by the U.S. Food and Drug Administration (FDA) between 1997 and 2000 posed greater health risks to women than they did to men, according to a report by the General Accountability Office, Congress's nonpartisan audit agency. While sex and medicine issues are still a fairly new concept, it is becoming increasingly clear that physicians and patients should consider a patient's sex when choosing a drug therapy and deciding on dosages.

Safety Differences in Drugs Based on Sex

To take just one example of sex-based differences in drug therapy, common medications, including antibiotics, antihistamines, antidepressants, antipsychotics, and some heart medications, alone or in combination, cause more women than men to develop potentially fatal irregular heartbeat or arrhythmias.

These drugs may act by prolonging the QT interval, the part of the electrocardiogram (EKG) that represents the time it takes for the heart to relax after each beat. Physicians can measure the length of the QT interval in fractions of a second. If it takes longer than normal, it is called a prolonged QT interval. In rare cases, QT prolongation can cause a life-threatening heart rhythm disturbance, called torsade de pointes, and sudden death. In other cases the prolongation does not have serious consequences. The findings suggest that women, doctors, and pharmacists should be alert to cardiovascular side effects brought on by drugs or combinations of drugs.

Pregnancy poses special concerns for women taking medicine. For example, we are learning more about the potential risks of anticonvulsant drugs, which are used by more than a million American women with epilepsy and millions more to treat chronic medical problems affecting the central nervous system, including migraine, severe pain caused by damaged nerves (neuropathic pain), and bipolar and associated mood disorders.

While the majority of women who become pregnant while taking these medications deliver healthy babies, new research shows that some anticonvulsants increase the risk of major malformations (including heart, spinal cord, and cleft lip/cleft palate abnormalities) in fetuses exposed to them during the mother's pregnancy. The Epilepsy Foundation urges women to increase their chances of a successful pregnancy and long-term health by discussing medicine options and possible therapeutic changes with their health care providers before pregnancy. This advice should be followed for women taking other medicines as well.

Other Sex Differences

In addition to potential sex differences in the safety profile of medications, sex differences in the effectiveness of certain drugs have been demonstrated. For example, researchers at the University of California at San Francisco, led by Jon Levine, MD, found that morphine-like painkillers, called kappa opioids, provide more powerful and longer-lasting relief to women than they do to men. In fact, at some doses kappa opioids can actually make the pain worse for men and afford phenomenal pain relief to women.

General anesthesia, drugs that render a person unconscious during surgery, can also behave differently in men and women. At least two studies suggest that women may be less responsive to anesthesia than men. The research shows that women wake up three to four minutes faster than men after taking the same dose of medication per pound of body weight. Women also tend to suffer more side effects, such as headaches, nausea, and vomiting.

Why the Response to Drugs Differs

Exactly why drugs affect men and women differently remains unclear. And, in fact, the answer may turn out to be different for every class of medication. Nonetheless, research points to a number of possible mechanisms for these sex-based differences.

The varying rates at which men and women metabolize drugs may be involved. Studies show that some liver enzymes involved in processing the drugs are more active in women than they are in men, which may affect the levels of drug in the body, drug effectiveness, or the severity of its side effects. In addition, evidence suggests that a drug's ability to enter some cells in the body may vary between the sexes, which could lead to differences in overall activity of the drug.

Anatomy also affects the way drugs are processed. On average, women have lower body weight, smaller organ size, reduced blood flow, and a higher proportion of fat than men. Overall differences in hormonal activity between the sexes affect the way drugs are processed, absorbed, and cleared by the body as well.

In addition, organs seem to function differently depending on whether they are inside a male or female body. Evidence suggests that "female" kidneys are slower to act than "male" kidneys, a difference that may affect how fast the body gets rid of certain drugs. In addition, liver functioning, which can influence the incidence of adverse events, may vary among men and women. What's more, the rate at which drugs pass through the gastrointestinal system, which affects how much of the drug is absorbed into the bloodstream, seems to differ between the sexes.

Building Awareness

Despite mounting evidence that men and women respond differently to the same drug, most physicians and patients are still not aware that sex matters when medications are prescribed. Why the lack of awareness? One of the reasons is that the FDA and the pharmaceutical industry only recently began to analyze the effects of sex on safety data. In fact, reporting of sex-based data analyses in medical journals, while increasing, is still not routine. This shortcoming of the system keeps sex-specific risks as well as benefits buried beneath heaps of other data.

Women are at higher risk of adverse drug reactions (ADRs) than men, in part because they are more likely to use more than one medication or dietary supplement at any one point in time. A recent review of 48 studies in the United Kingdom revealed that ADRs to newly marketed drugs are 60 percent more common in women than they are in men. This sex difference was observed in all women older than age 19. Other studies have found less pronounced, yet significantly higher risks of ADRs among women.

Women need not look further than their own medicine cabinet for potentially problematic combinations. For instance, oral contraceptives, when taken in combination with the antibiotics rifampin, tetracycline, or penicillin, can fail and result in pregnancy. Considering that women suffer from urinary tract infections (UTIs) more than men do, women should be aware that some antacids can inactivate drugs often prescribed for UTIs, called fluoroquinolones, allowing infections to progress unchecked.

Similarly, because depression affects more women than it does men, there is a greater potential for women to suffer serious consequences when combining selective serotonin reuptake inhibitors (SSRIs) with other types of antidepressants, pain medications, or illegal drugs such as ecstasy and cocaine.

Herbal and Dietary Supplements

Dietary supplements, used more often by women than men, can also interact with other drugs to cause serious problems. And because there are no regulatory requirements for testing most of these compounds in humans, doctors and pharmacists know very little about their risks. Although no FDA-reviewed data exist regarding the risks associated with combining dietary supplements and drugs, numerous reports have indicated that administering some of these compounds together may be harmful. For example, a number of herbs have been shown to interact with heart medications and blood thinners like warfarin. The FDA has specifically warned women who take birth control pills against the concurrent use of Saint John's wort because it decreases the effectiveness of oral contraceptives. Combining Saint John's wort with antidepressants; some cough syrups; a protease inhibitor used to treat HIV/AIDS; the commonly used chemotherapy drug, irinotecan; and the heart medication, digoxin, can also cause serious ADRs.

How to Get Information

Pharmacists can help women avoid undesirable effects of medications by providing them with information about the drugs they are taking. The Public Citizen Health Research Group in Washington, D.C., suggests that women ask their pharmacists for FDA-approved drug information, which contains data on drug interactions. The FDA-approved drug information may supplement the information provided in computer-generated leaflets. All over-the-counter (OTC) medications should also contain an FDA-approved insert. Pharmacists should emphasize to women that, although the FDA-approved inserts provide additional information about the drug, the information is geared to a scientific audience.

The FDA suggests that women also use the following guidelines to help prevent undesirable side effects and interactions:

♦ Tell your doctor about everything you take, including prescription and nonprescription drugs and dietary supplements.

- Stop taking all herbs at least two weeks before surgery, because many interfere with anesthesia and affect blood clotting.
- Drugs may interact with certain foods and beverages, so ask your doctor or pharmacist if you should make any dietary modifications.
- Let your doctor know about any side effects you may experience. Keep track of them when you take your medications.

—VIVIANA SIMON, PhD, AND EILEEN RESNICK, PhD

Reprinted with permission from the American Pharmacists Association.

CHAPTER 3

The Role of Nutrition in a Woman's Life

Whether she is a middle-aged woman experiencing the effects of menopause; an older woman concerned about hypertension, cholesterol levels, and bone density; an adolescent building strong bones and developing a healthy body image; or a pregnant woman concerned about the future health of her baby—nutrition is a key component of a woman's health. As Bernadine Healy, MD, former head of the National Institutes of Health (NIH) and chief architect of the groundbreaking Women's Health Initiative, observes, nutrition is undoubtedly the single biggest factor influencing the health and well-being of women at any stage of life.

Research is revealing new information about conditions women are most vulnerable to, including cardiovascular disease, breast cancer, osteoporosis, diabetes, and overweight/obesity. Although these are distinct ailments, they share at least one common thread—the impact nutrition can have on their prevention and treatment. Studies show that nutrition plays an important role in health promotion *throughout* a woman's life span. Lifestyle choices such as diet and physical activity influence the health and well-being of the *whole* woman.

Cardiovascular Health

As we are learning with so many diseases, the earlier prevention begins the better, and cardiovascular disease (CVD) is no exception. Prevention must begin in childhood, perhaps even in utero. The "fetal origins" theory suggests that fetal undernutrition is independently associated with a susceptibility to heart disease in later life. In other words, if a mother's nutritional status is poor, she may actually put her baby at risk for heart disease later in life. Although this theory is still under debate, some studies have detected early heart disease in young children and teens.

For example, autopsy studies from the Bogalusa Heart Study have demonstrated a strong association between risk factors such as obesity, high cholesterol, and hypertension and vascular lesions in children. And a study reported in late 2004 in the *Journal of the American Medical Association* showed that for young women, a low cardiovascular risk profile is associated with lower long-term CVD. The risk profile included blood pressure, cholesterol level, body mass index (BMI), diabetes, and smoking. The authors concluded that prevention and control of all major CVD risk factors by lifestyle approaches—from conception, weaning, childhood, and youth—are necessary to increase the proportion of the population at low risk for CVD. Thus, a woman may actually lower her risk of heart disease later in life by making wise dietary and fitness choices as a young person.

Unfortunately, however, as children get older, the quality of their diet declines. In 1998, only 24 percent of girls and 23 percent of boys (ages six to 11) consumed the number of servings of fruit recommended in the food guide pyramid. Only 18 percent of adolescent girls and 14 percent of adolescent boys had diets that met pyramid guidelines for fruit intake. Clearly, if this trend persists, there is good reason to be concerned about the health of the next generation of women.

Breast Health

Dietary fat intake and obesity have been examined extensively in breast cancer research. If fat intake does, in fact, have any effect on the risk of breast cancer, it is probably in childhood and adolescence, when the breast is developing. The rationale is that breast cancer occurs in more than 85 percent of cases in the milk ducts, which are formed before a woman begins her period. This is the time breast tissue experiences the most intense growth.

Dietary fat is also thought to affect breast density. Dense breast tissue makes mammograms more difficult to read, and National Cancer Institute research indicates that cancer rates are higher in women with dense breast tissue. A study of menopausal women with extensive areas of dense breast tissue shows that after two years on a low-fat, high-carbohydrate diet, breast density is reduced significantly.

Obesity can contribute to a woman's risk of breast cancer at various stages of life. For example, a 2002 study of Finish women suggests that gaining and retaining a significant amount of weight from pregnancy may cause changes in breast tissue that place women at higher risk for developing breast cancer later in life. Other research demonstrates that preventing weight gain or losing weight and maintaining the loss, between age 18 and menopause, reduces the risk of postmenopausal breast cancer.

In women who already have breast cancer, studies show that obesity can have a negative influence on early-stage breast cancer—a time when the disease is believed to be most treatable. In addition, breast cancer patients who gain weight after diagnosis have decreased quality of life, an increased risk of recurrence, and poorer survival rates.

What can women do to help lower their risk of breast cancer? Mayo Clinic researchers observed 30,000 women from the Iowa Women's Health Study for 13 years and found that women who closely followed diet and exercise guidelines developed by the American Institute for Cancer Research—including five or more servings of fruits and vegetables a day—had a 31 percent lower risk of developing cancer (and also reduced their risk of heart disease by 22 percent).

Bone Health

Thirty years ago, doctors thought weak bones and osteoporosis were a natural part of aging, but as Surgeon General Richard Carmona observed when introducing his 2004 report on bone health: "Osteoporosis isn't your grandmother's disease. You are never too old or too young to improve your bone health."

The only time in a woman's life to build solid bone mass is during her youth. Too often, though, lack of exercise and fear of gaining weight from calcium-rich dairy products sabotage this priority. After age 30, prevention strategies switch to preserving the bone that is already there. Calcium and weight-bearing exercise are required for optimal bone health.

Nutrition experts agree that "food first" should be the primary approach to protecting bone health throughout life. Women not only need calcium to build bones during childhood and adolescence, they also need it to ensure that therapies for preventing and treating osteoporosis are effective. But calcium is not the only nutrient that affects bone health. Protein; vitamins D, K, C, and A; the B vitamins; and minerals like magnesium, potassium, phosphorus, and zinc are critical, too. The synergistic effect of these nutrients demonstrates just how important balance and variety are in the diet.

Exercise is also important for bone health in both younger and older women. Regular exercise helps girls build bone during the critical teen years. And studies show that even moderate physical activity is associated with higher bone mineral density in postmenopausal women.

Diabetes

Today, there is increasing interest in the theory that obesity, diabetes, and heart disease are part of one common mechanism. The process may begin early in life and persist through childhood into adulthood. This theory underscores the value of prevention. Findings from the Diabetes Prevention Program (DPP), which ended in 2001, showed that people at high risk for type 2 diabetes can sharply lower their chances of getting the disease with diet and exercise.

In 1997, the National Institute of Diabetes and Digestive and Kidney Diseases, along with the Office of Research on Women's Health and other sponsoring agencies, launched the Look AHEAD (Action for HEAlth in Diabetes) Study. This long-term, randomized clinical trial is examining how lifestyle changes such as decreased caloric intake and exercise play a role in achieving and maintaining weight loss over time. Look AHEAD is focused on type 2 diabetes, the disease most affected by overweight and obesity, and on the outcome that causes the greatest morbidity and mortality: cardiovascular disease.

Healthy Weight

Women tend to gain weight at certain times during their lives—puberty, postpregnancy, and after menopause—when hormones fluctuate. Some women (and their doctors) accept weight gain as inevitable, but it is important to recognize that extra weight can create serious health risks. We often talk about successful weight loss with words like "how much" and "how fast." In fact, successful weight loss should be measured by the ability to lose even a small amount of weight, maintain the loss, and reap the health benefits associated with it.

Unfortunately, people enrolled in weight loss programs typically regain most of what they lose in three to five years. According to the National Weight Control Registry, people who keep the weight off report making substantial changes in eating and exercise habits to lose weight and to maintain their loss. On average, registrants report consuming about 1,400 calories each day (24 percent of calories from fat) and using about 400 calories each day in physical exercise. Walking is the most frequently cited physical activity.

Although some people cannot stick with a structured exercise plan, many are willing to adopt a more physically-oriented lifestyle. Research from Johns Hopkins University and the University of Pennsylvania suggests that taking a lifestyle approach to exercise can make a positive difference in fitness and disease risk. In addition, work being done at the Cooper Clinic demonstrates that even when exercise does not lead to weight loss, it has a positive effect on such chronic conditions as high blood pressure, diabetes, cardiovascular disease, and cancer.

Researchers and health care providers have accomplished a great deal over the past 10 years in improving the health of women, but we are only just beginning to uncover the important role nutrition plays in preventing and treating disease. With every new discovery, we are confirming two important principles of women's health: first, that nutrition and physical activity influence health at every stage of a woman's life and, second, that to promote and protect women's health effectively, we must look at how lifestyle choices affect the *whole* woman.

—SUSAN FINN, PHD, RD, FADA

CHAPTER 4

How to Develop a
Sex-Based Family History

Take a look in the mirror. What do you see? your mother's eyes, your grandfather's nose? Are your features a mix of your family's traits?

The resemblance does not end there. If you look deeper, you may also see your grandmother's heart condition or your father's diabetes. Just as your traits were passed from generation to generation, diseases can be passed down, too.

Parents pass on different things to their offspring through their genes. Our genes are made up of a substance called deoxyribonucleic acid (DNA) and are located on chromosomes. Everyone has 46 chromosomes, which contain all sorts of information from hair and eye color to the likelihood of developing a specific disease.

You might not realize it, but knowing the medical history of your family is extremely important for your health and the health of your loved ones. Have you ever stopped to think why your mother's side of the family lived long lives and your father's side died at younger ages? Do you know what they died from? You need to! Some of what influences the state of your health has been inherited from your ancestors.

In the Dark

The majority of Americans are in the dark when it comes to their family's medical history. Only three in 10 people actually compile and record the health histories of their relatives, according to a 2004 survey conducted by the Centers for Disease Control and Prevention (CDC) in Atlanta, Georgia.

As a result, the Surgeon General launched the "Family Health Initiative" and is encouraging people to download free computer software to keep track of their family's medical history. The program generates a family tree that patients can take with them to doctor appointments, and, together, the patient and doctor can tailor personalized preventive measures based on this information.

The Challenges Facing Women

If you are a woman, you will undoubtedly face extra challenges when creating a family medical history. Awareness of certain diseases in the past was more limited than it is now. So while you may have thought that your grandmother died of old age, she might have suffered from symptoms that were never recognized properly by the medical community.

Take heart disease, for example. Most people do not realize it, but heart disease is the number one killer of women, and if the risk factors are ignored, it can cut your life short. But the symptoms of a heart attack can present differently in women from how they do in men. While the classic symptoms include squeezing chest pain; tightness in the chest; shortness of breath; and pain spreading to the shoulders, neck and arm, women are more likely to experience indigestion, dizziness, nausea, or vomiting.

The trial of sorting through a woman's family history is compounded by the fact that sex differences in diseases were not really defined in the past. Certain disorders that were once thought of as predominantly male were often overlooked in women.

So, getting back to Grandma—the doctors may have missed these symptoms long ago, and her cause of death might not have been recorded properly. If you sit down to create a family history, you might not have all the information!

If you are wondering how all of this affects your life, it is really very simple. As a woman, you may need to do some extra work when compiling your family's health history. Things may not be exactly what they seem. Dig a little deeper: get the medical records, talk with family members, and contact doctors if necessary.

If you do not know the exact cause of death, find out if a relative had risk factors for a certain disease. If you are not sure why your aunt died at an early age, try to figure out which conditions she suffered from during her lifetime. Was she overweight or diabetic? Did she have high cholesterol or high blood pressure? Does cancer run on her side of the family? All of this information is important; it will help you identify and possibly prevent health risks you may face in the future.

Putting Together Your
Sex-Based Family History

Putting together a family medical tree is an important step in safeguarding your own health and the health of your loved ones. This information can help uncover patterns of diseases that run in your family or isolate a specific disease of which you might not have been aware.

Creating your family tree can be daunting and will likely involve interviews with family members. Start with your own generation and move backward. Speak with grandparents, great aunts and uncles, and other family members who may know the history of previous generations. You will want to record as much information as possible, and pay particularly close attention to the following items:

♦ date of birth and death;
♦ cause of death;
♦ patterns of major diseases (including heart disease, cancer, diabetes, stroke, autoimmune disease, and neurological and mental illness, etc.);
♦ race and ethnicity (certain diseases are seen more frequently among specific races or ethnicities);
♦ history of chronic illness (asthma, hypertension, etc.);
♦ history of childhood diseases (cystic fibrosis, type 1 diabetes, hemophilia, etc.);
♦ history of allergies (environmental and drug); and
♦ history of mental illness or behavioral problems (addictions, depression, anxiety disorders, etc.).

Remember, it may not be easy to uncover all of the necessary information. Paternalism, or the practice of protecting patients from their own medical conditions, may have played a role, especially for older female patients. Women of earlier generations might have been told that they suffered from a "female problem," and the truth of their medical condition might not have been fully divulged. If the female problem turned out to be gynecological cancer, which often has a hereditary component, the information becomes vital to the health of other people in the family.

If your relatives are unsure about the cause of death, look at medical records, death certificates, old family letters, or official papers. Speak with your family's doctor for more tips on gathering information; she or he may have records in the office you can look at.

It is also important to pay attention to life-cycle issues in female relatives. At certain times in a woman's life, her hormone levels fluctuate. During adolescence, pregnancy, and menopause, a woman's hormones undergo changes. Studies have revealed a connection between hormone levels and common female conditions, including migraine headaches, thyroid problems, premenstrual syndrome (PMS), chronic fatigue syndrome, fibromyalgia, and allergies. Some of these conditions may run in your family, and it is important to determine at what stage of life a female relative was diagnosed with a particular disease.

Be sure to include your health during pregnancies for future generations. We are learning more about the way a mother's diet, environment, or health status during pregnancy can influence her children's health. Scientists are studying how environmental factors, such as diet, stress, and maternal nutrition, can change gene function in the fetus, which may play a role in vulnerability for cancer, stroke, diabetes, mental illness, and other diseases. For example, researchers have found that a diet rich in omega-3 fatty acids during pregnancy and while nursing—coupled with ensuring that the baby's diet after weaning is also rich in these fatty acids—may reduce daughters' risk of developing breast cancer later in life. Although we do not know what factors may turn out to be important, adding a brief diary that includes notes on your diet, environmental impacts such as allergies or workplace exposure to chemicals, and any changes in your health that occur during your pregnancy will make your family history more complete.

Identifying Your Risk and Taking Precautions

Many diseases run in the family and knowing what you are at risk for can actually protect you. Conditions including diabetes, obesity, heart disease, and certain cancers can all be inherited. The more you know about your family's health, the better off you will be. Identifying the diseases that affect your relatives can aid in calculating your own risk.

Take breast cancer, for example. The American Cancer Society recommends a baseline mammogram for all women starting at age 40. A woman who has a family history of breast cancer may need to take certain precautions. She may begin to have mammograms at an earlier age, and she may opt for other screening methods including ultrasound or magnetic resonance imaging (MRI) as well. Women who are at high risk may decide to take hormone-blocking medications, an option that needs to be discussed thoroughly with a physician.

Screening methods are not the only precautions a person with a family history of breast cancer can take. Dietary choices and fitness levels can contribute both negatively and positively to a person's risk for cancer and other conditions. Studies have shown that increasing intake of foods rich in antioxidants (certain fruits and vegetables) and decreasing intake of foods high in saturated fat (such as red meat) can help ward off disease. Lifestyle choices such as avoiding tobacco products, exercising regularly, and limiting alcohol can all help lower a person's risk of disease too.

Tracking the pattern of disease is so important in this case. Because breast cancer is fairly common, having more than one relative with cancer diagnosed after menopause would not necessarily place a woman in the high-risk category. Cancers with a genetic component typically affect first-degree relatives at early ages, before menopause. Certain diseases are linked to each other and may signal a genetic root as well. For example, women with a common gene mutation for breast cancer may see relatives on their tree with ovarian, prostate, or stomach cancers. It is important to look at both the maternal and paternal side.

Genetic Counseling

Genetic counseling is available for people whose families have a strong history of disease. The counselors provide information and support to families at risk for a variety of inherited conditions. By examining a family's medical tree, they can help detect a family with a strong history of disease. The counselors are trained to analyze inheritance patterns and make recommendations based on the information.

Genetic counselors can serve as patient advocates and can refer the patient and family to local support services. Some counselors are involved in research studies in genetics. To find a counselor in your area, the National Society of Genetic Counselors can be of assistance.

—Jennifer Wider, MD

PART 2

AN A TO Z GUIDE TO WOMEN'S HEALTH

In this section of the book, top medical experts discuss major diseases that affect women solely or differently from the way they affect men. Special attention is given to how pregnancy, menopause, and other life-cycle episodes in women's lives matter. Scattered throughout are the stories of real people who have suffered from, survived, or are managing the various diseases.

Each chapter provides an overview of the condition, including risk factors, symptoms, and treatments, as well as critical sex differences in each of these areas. When relevant, gender differences are highlighted as well. Sex differences refer to those differences that occur because of biological differences, such as different hormones, while gender differences refer to those behaviors that our society defines as more typical of women or of men. For example, gender differences incorporate the facts that men tend to visit doctors less often than women do, and women are more likely than men to develop skin cancer on the upper thighs because of differences in bathing suits.

This section is meant to be used as a resource for you and your friends and families; and you may find that you will use this material to educate your health professional as well. Although the biology of sex differences is a rapidly growing field, many providers are not yet aware of the many ways sex differences can affect one's health.

—JENNIFER WIDER, MD

CHAPTER 5

Autoimmunity

What Is the Immune System?

The immune system is your body's front line of defense against bacteria, viruses, and other foreign invaders. The first barrier is actually your skin; invaders can enter when you get a cut or other injury. (You can also get infections from airborne pathogens, which enter the body through mucosal surfaces such as the respiratory tract.) Once inside the body, bacteria and other intruders encounter cellular patrols, the neutrophils and macrophages, which are dispatched by the bone marrow. There are billions of these cells circulating in your bloodstream and patrolling your tissues at any given time. Macrophages (which literally means "big eaters") suck in the intruder, chew it up, and destroy it with enzymes within the cell. They can also send a chemical alarm that calls into action white blood cells, known as lymphocytes, to search out the rest of the invaders of foreign cells (antigens).

There are several types of lymphocytes. Helper T cells identify and eliminate antigens and signal other lymphocytes, the B cells, to produce proteins, called antibodies, that attach to each specific antigen to mark it for destruction. The effect is almost like a game of paintball or laser tag. Some antibodies stick to the surface of an antigen like a glowing target; other antibodies may actually attack. There are also cytotoxic (cell-killing) T cells that produce molecules that destroy cells marked as antigens and suppressor T cells that dial down the intensity of other immune responses. T cells are supposed to tolerate the body's own (self) antigens. Self-reactive T cells also exist and are usually eliminated in your thymus gland. But sometimes by accident these rogue T cells are not eliminated. When this happens, B cells get a signal to produce autoantibodies, antibodies that attach to and can provoke an attack on the body's own tissues. In susceptible women, this can result in autoimmune disease.

During their assault on foreigners, macrophages and white blood cells also produce chemicals that not only destroy the invaders (or the cell marked by a self-antigen), but cause inflammation as well. Inflammation normally helps to heal injuries in the body, but in some autoimmune diseases, such as rheumatoid arthritis (RA), inflammation continues for too long and can become destructive. Many of the medications used to treat autoimmune disease, such as corticosteroids, are designed to dampen inflammation and adjust the immune system reactions that provoke it. In addition, the body produces a number of chemicals, or cytokines, that promote inflammation, notably tumor necrosis factor alpha (TNFα) and interleukin-1 (IL-1). Drugs specifically designed to inhibit these cytokines, such as TNFα blockers etanercept and infliximab, are used to treat multiple autoimmune diseases, including RA and Crohn's disease. Other antibodies, proteins, and chemicals are involved in autoimmune diseases, and scientists are working on treatments to inhibit them as well.

What Is Autoimmune Disease?

Autoimmune disease results when the immune system accidentally launches an attack on the body's own organs and/or tissues. Autoimmune diseases can affect almost any area of the body. Some antibodies or T cells attack tissue in an organ or gland. In RA, excessive inflammation causes the lining of the joints to become swollen, inflamed, and painful, eventually destroying the joint itself. In systemic lupus erythematosus, the skin, kidneys, brain, and lungs all can be targets of inflammatory and destructive molecules. Even your blood can be affected; autoantibodies can cause dangerous blood clots in antiphospholipid syndrome or speed up the normal turnover of platelets in the spleen in immune thrombocytopenia, causing bleeding and heavy periods. Other autoimmune diseases affect the pancreas (type 1 diabetes), adrenal glands (Addison's disease), connective tissues (scleroderma), skin (psoriasis), and muscles (myasthenia gravis).

Because these diseases affect multiple body systems (often at the same time), and women may have more than one disease (as many as four to five diseases), there may be a wide range of early symptoms. Illnesses often overlap and mimic each other. For example, fatigue and joint pain can be symptoms of RA, lupus, and autoimmune thyroid disease. Symptoms can also come and go, creating a time lag between the symptoms experienced and the clinical signs of disease needed to make a diagnosis.

If you have early RA, for instance, your joints may be red and painfully swollen for weeks, but on the day you see your doctor, your joints may look perfectly normal. The gap between when a disease develops and when a formal diagnosis is made can be considerable. The signs of autoimmune disease can be vague, or they may be misdiagnosed and treated as another condition. Many women have been told that their symptoms are "all in their head." A survey by the American Autoimmune Related

Diseases Association (AARDA) found that more than 45 percent of patients were labeled hypochondriacs in the earliest stages of their illness. Women may spend years bouncing from specialist to specialist, spending thousands of dollars before they get a correct diagnosis. By that time, there may be major damage to joints or organs. Ongoing research is looking for blood markers and other techniques to diagnose these diseases earlier, before major damage occurs.

Risk Factors

GENETICS

There are more than 80 autoimmune diseases, and genetics links many of them. Some share common genes; for example, scientists in Britain recently discovered a single gene that may increase susceptibility to type 1 diabetes, Hashimoto's thyroiditis, and Graves' disease. Researchers in Japan found a genetic defect shared by RA, psoriasis, and lupus. Because of the shared genes phenomenon and the fact that these diseases run in families, scientists have now come to think of autoimmunity as a single category of disease.

Many scientists do not believe that a single specific gene leads to autoimmune disease, but rather that several genes can increase a woman's susceptibility. The Multiple Autoimmune Disease Genetics Consortium (MADGC) was established to study the genes of family members of people with RA, lupus, MS, autoimmune thyroid disease, type 1 diabetes, psoriasis, inflammatory bowel disease, and Sjögren's syndrome.

ENVIRONMENT

A number of environmental factors, including drugs, viruses (such as Epstein-Barr virus), bacteria, and even food, also appear to trigger autoimmune diseases in susceptible people. For example, gluten, a protein in wheat and other grains, triggers an autoimmune reaction in the small intestine leading to celiac disease (celiac sprue). Recent research suggests that exposure to toxins such as asbestos may provoke autoimmunity as well.

WHY YOUR SEX MATTERS

Another factor linking autoimmune diseases is their strong prevalence in women; 75 percent of those affected by these diseases are women. In some cases, that proportion tops 90 percent.

Female-Male Ratios in Selected Autoimmune Diseases

Hashimoto's thyroiditis	10:1
Graves' disease	9:1
Sjögren's syndrome	9:1
Systemic lupus erythematosus (SLE)	9:1
Rheumatoid arthritis	2.5:1
Scleroderma	3:1
Multiple sclerosis (MS)	2:1

Source: Baron-Faust, Rita, and Jill P. Buyon. *The Autoimmune Connection*. New York: McGraw-Hill, 2003.

Why are women affected more often than men? For one thing, women have stronger immune responses than men and tend to produce more antibodies and autoantibodies. Female hormones, particularly estrogen, may play a role. Estrogen can stimulate certain immune responses; it may act partly as an on-off switch in some autoimmune diseases, and it may affect other hormones that influence autoimmunity. For example, some autoimmune diseases such as Hashimoto's thyroiditis or myasthenia gravis may arise (or worsen) during pregnancy, while RA and multiple sclerosis get better. Some disease symptoms flare when estrogen is elevated during the first part of the menstrual cycle; in MS and myasthenia gravis, symptoms can worsen premenstrually when progesterone spikes. Other diseases, such as Sjögren's syndrome, often occur after menopause, when estrogen levels are low.

An example of a hormone that can be influenced by estrogen is corticotropin-releasing hormone (CRH), which releases stress hormones when you are under stress or pregnant. These stress hormones affect immune activity. Research indicates that when these stress hormones are high, susceptible women may be more likely to develop some autoimmune diseases, including lupus, and when these hormones are low, susceptible women may be more likely to develop other autoimmune diseases, including RA and multiple MS.

On the other hand, women produce androgens (male hormones), such as testosterone, that may have a protective effect. In recent years, scientists have found that women with lupus and Sjögren's have low levels of testosterone. The androgen dehydroepiandrosterone (DHEA) is even used as a treatment for lupus, and androgen eye drops are being tested for alleviating dry eyes in women with Sjögren's.

Autoimmunity may also have roots in women's ability to carry a fetus in the womb. A fetus is technically half a "foreign" body, because it contains genes and proteins from the mother and the father. During pregnancy, a woman's immune system does not attack the non-self-antigens.

After delivery, studies show that fetal cells can remain in the mother's circulation for more than 20 years. Since these cells no longer enjoy privileged status; they may confuse the immune system and provoke an immune reaction akin to the rejection of a transplanted organ. Evidence of these persistent fetal cells (referred to as microchimerism) has been found in women with scleroderma, Sjögren's, and autoimmune thyroid and liver diseases. Women may also develop autoimmune diseases in greater numbers because they are exposed to possible triggers more often.

This chapter explores seven of the most common autoimmune diseases, all of which are more common in women than in men and discusses two associated disorders. Two other autoimmune diseases—autoimmune hepatitis and primary biliary cirrhosis—are discussed in chapter nine.

Rheumatoid Arthritis

WHAT IS RHEUMATOID ARTHRITIS?

More than two million Americans—about 75 percent of them women—are affected by rheumatoid arthritis (RA), a chronic inflammation of the lining of the joints (synovium). Although it can occur at any age, women typically first notice symptoms between the ages of 30 and 50. RA is the most common rheumatic autoimmune disease and can lead to permanent joint damage and can cause chronic pain, loss of function, and disability. RA can also be a systemic disease, affecting other parts of the body.

RISK FACTORS

RA appears to be caused by a combination of genetic vulnerability, environmental triggers, and hormonal influences. People with the genetic marker, a portion of DNA that is used to identify an individual disease or trait, known as HLA-DR4, appear to have an increased risk of developing RA and of having more severe disease. Some of the suspected environmental triggers include Epstein-Barr virus and bacteria, including streptococci (which causes strep throat and rheumatic fever), salmonella (which causes food poisoning), *Escherichia coli* (*E. coli*, which causes urinary tract infections), *Helicobacter pylori* (which causes stomach ulcers), and *Borrelia burgdorferi* (which causes Lyme disease). Cigarette smoking is also linked to RA.

WHY YOUR SEX MATTERS

While women are two to three times more likely to get RA than men, men tend to be affected more severely. Studies show that women who have never had a child are twice as likely to develop RA as women who have. The disease often improves during pregnancy (when estrogen levels are high) but worsens after delivery (when estrogen levels drop). The peak age for RA appears to be after age 40, when estrogen levels are fluctuating or declining. Recent research suggests that if RA is diagnosed after menopause, it may progress at a faster rate. This has spurred research into the role that estrogen may play in RA; some scientists are studying whether oral contraceptives might be protective.

Women with RA may have reduced fertility, which can predate their diagnosis. Some drug treatments used for RA can also affect fertility. Menopausal symptoms in women with RA can be treated with low-dose estrogen, but hormone therapy needs to be individualized (as it does for any menopausal woman).

The risk of premature atherosclerosis (thickening of artery walls by cholesterol-laden plaques) and coronary artery disease is greater among women with RA. Some research indicates that women under age 50 with RA have three times the risk of death from heart attack and congestive heart failure as healthy women of the same age. Corticosteroids such as prednisone, one of the mainstays of RA therapy, can also increase cholesterol and the risk of diabetes, infections, and osteoporosis. Women taking corticosteroids may need bone-building drugs or cholesterol-lowering medications. In addition, RA has been linked to low bone density independent of corticosteroid therapy.

SYMPTOMS

The first symptoms of RA may include swelling, stiffness (often worse in the morning), and general aching of the joints. RA affects joints on both sides of the body, in contrast to osteoarthritis, a disease of wear and tear that may strike joints in one area. The joints affected by RA also may be warm or red. Other common symptoms are fatigue, weakness, muscle pain, and depression.

In 50 percent of women, symptoms come on gradually and can wax and wane. As the disease progresses, inflamed cells in the joint release enzymes that can digest bone and cartilage, often causing the joint to lose its shape and alignment and increasing pain and loss of movement. Early diagnosis and treatment are important in minimizing joint destruction, so it is essential to see a doctor if telltale symptoms persist for a number of weeks.

Around 20 percent of women with RA may develop raised, firm lumps just under the skin, known as rheumatoid nodules. These nodules often occur in areas where there is repeated pressure on the skin, such as the elbows. Because RA can be systemic, these nodules may arise in the eyes, heart, or lungs.

Up to half of women with RA may develop inflammation in the lining of the lungs (pleurisy), making it painful to take a deep breath. Inflammation may also develop around the sac enclosing the heart (pericarditis); symptoms include chest pain, dry cough, and fever. Even blood vessels may become inflamed in RA; a sign of this vasculitis can be tiny broken blood vessels in the nail bed.

DIAGNOSIS

Doctors may need to perform several tests to diagnose RA properly. The work-up will most likely include a complete medical history, physical exam, and lab tests and x-rays. During the physical exam, your doctor will look for evidence of joint swelling, tenderness, redness, misalignment, or loss of motion. Expect to describe your pain, including the times of day it is most and least severe. Blood tests include a test for an antibody called rheumatoid factor (RF); approximately 70 to 80 percent of people with RA have positive tests for rheumatoid factor (but it may not be detected early on in RA). It is important to note that RF can be present in other conditions (including lupus and even infections), so testing positive is only one factor in making a diagnosis. Other blood tests look for evidence of inflammation, including an erythrocyte sedimentation rate (ESR or SED rate), which measures the speed at which red blood cells fall to the bottom of a test tube, and C-reactive protein (CRP), which is elevated with systemic inflammation. A complete blood count may reveal anemia, a low red blood cell count, which often occurs in RA. X-rays are used to determine the degree of joint erosion, cartilage loss, and joint distortion.

TREATMENT

Your doctor will prescribe treatments to attack RA on several fronts: to relieve pain and reduce inflammation and to stop or slow joint damage. The choice of medications takes into account how severe your symptoms are and how far the disease has progressed. Nonsteroidal anti-inflammatory drugs (NSAIDs) are commonly used to combat pain. These include aspirin and its chemical cousins, ibuprofen and naproxen, diclofenac, and indomethacin, and newer NSAIDs, called COX-2 inhibitors. However, COX-2 drugs carry an increased risk of heart attack and stroke and should not be used if you have or are at increased risk for cardiovascular disease. Recent studies show that all NSAIDs also carry slight cardiovascular risks and should not be used at high doses for prolonged periods.

Corticosteroids such as prednisone are used to combat inflammation and modulate immune overreactivity. Disease-modifying antirheumatic drugs (DMARDs), including methotrexate and leflunomide, may be used to slow joint destruction. The newest DMARDs are "biologic" agents that inhibit the cytokines that promote inflammation and joint destruction. These include the TNFα blockers.

Joint replacement surgery is often needed for RA patients with severely damaged joints. Just about any joint in the body can now be replaced, and the surgery dramatically improves function and pain. Exercise and stress reduction are important for RA patients. Patients and their health care providers are turning increasingly to alternative and complementary therapies such as massage and acupuncture.

FUTURE APPROACHES TO RA TREATMENT

Researchers are looking at agents that block the processes by which arthritis begins. One strategy being tested is the use of cancer drugs, such as rituximab, to selectively destroy B cells that contribute to the disease process of RA. Another biological drug being tested for RA, alefacept, targets specific T cells.

Stem cell transplantation is another novel therapy under study. Stem cells are primitive cells in the bone marrow that can multiply into specific blood cells. In this experimental treatment, a patient's immune system is destroyed with high doses of chemotherapy drugs and then reconstituted with stem cells from the person's own red blood cells (autologous stem cells).

Studies are also being done on new markers that could be used to diagnose RA earlier, before joint destruction has begun (or perhaps in women at high risk before the disease process is fully underway). One such experimental test looks for autoantibodies, called cyclic citrullinated peptides (CCPs); one study found that 93 percent of those who tested positive for CCPs went on to develop RA after three years, but only 25 percent of those who tested negative developed the condition.

Autoimmune Thyroid Disease

The thyroid is a small, butterfly-shaped gland in your neck that plays a major role in your body. Thyroid hormones influence almost every organ and regulate metabolism, the rate at which your body turns food into energy. Endocrinologists often liken thyroid disease to living in a house with a broken thermostat. Having excess thyroid hormones turns up metabolism and body heat and causes weight loss, heat intolerance, and anxiety. Low levels of thyroid hormone turn down metabolism and make you feel cold, tired, and depressed.

WHAT ARE THYROID DISEASES?

Autoimmune thyroid diseases are actually the most common of all autoimmune diseases, affecting 10 million Americans. Hashimoto's thyroiditis results from an underactive thyroid gland and affects women 10 times more often than it does men. Graves' disease, which results from an overactive thyroid, is five times more common in women.

RISK FACTORS

In Hashimoto's thyroiditis, T cells attack cells in your thyroid gland, causing inflammation that interferes with thyroid hormone production. In Graves' disease, antibodies attack the receptors for thyroid-stimulating hormone (TSH), triggering overproduction of thyroid hormones. Researchers do not yet know what triggers these processes. Some theories include excess iodine in the diet, fetal cells that persist in a woman's blood circulation after pregnancy, and even severe stress.

Family history is a major risk factor; if you have close relatives with autoimmune thyroid disease, you are five to 10 times more likely to develop it than the average person. Autoimmune thyroid diseases also occur frequently with other autoimmune conditions such as RA and lupus. In some cases, other endocrine disorders such as adrenal insufficiency and type 1 diabetes may be risk factors for autoimmune thyroid disease.

WHY YOUR SEX MATTERS

Estrogen and progesterone can both exacerbate thyroid inflammation. Women with Hashimoto's disease often have heavier menstrual periods that last for longer than a week. Hashimoto's can disrupt the normal hormonal communication between the ovaries and endocrine glands, causing the ovaries to fail to ovulate, even though the uterine lining continues to be stimulated. As a result bleeding can occur between periods. Women with Graves' disease may have a decreased menstrual flow and a shorter cycle.

Both Hashimoto's disease and Graves' disease can lead to infertility and miscarriage. However, women who have trouble conceiving because of thyroid disease often regain fertility after being treated. Untreated hyperthyroidism can also lead to bone loss, since excess thyroid hormones activate bone-eating cells.

Autoimmune thyroid disease improves during pregnancy and worsens in the year after giving birth. If a woman has mild thyroid inflammation, pregnancy may tip the balance; there's also an increased risk of Graves' disease during the postpartum period. Thyroid function should be checked before, during, and after pregnancy. Your obstetrician will use TSH tests to tell whether your thyroid hormone dose needs to be increased as your pregnancy progresses.

The fetus relies in part on maternal thyroid hormones, especially before the 10th week of pregnancy, when the fetal thyroid begins to develop. In Graves' disease, autoantibodies can cross the placenta and cause temporary neonatal hyperthyroidism. Women with untreated thyroid deficiency during pregnancy may be up to four times more likely to have children with lower IQ scores as well as deficits in motor skills and attention, language, and reading abilities. Fortunately, all newborns in the United States are tested for thyroid hormone levels.

Postmenopausal hormone therapy can affect thyroid hormones; women taking estrogen or estrogen and progestins need to have their TSH levels monitored and the dose of replacement thyroid hormone (levothyroxine) adjusted if needed. Women over age 65 can be at increased risk of subclinical hypothyroidism, so TSH testing and possible replacement thyroid hormones may be necessary for this age group.

Burnout or What?

By Peggy McCarthy, owner and CEO of a company that creates educational programs for health professionals and the public

I was 57 years old and owned my own business. I had been traveling because of my job about 70 percent of the time. In the past year I had had three weekends free, and at home, because much of the work involved weekend meetings. I often made two cross-county trips a week. I had been living this lifestyle for about 15 years.

It was the holiday time at the end of the year, time when I usually tried to retreat to my home for a few days of rest and relaxation. But this year, I suddenly realized after a few days of rest that I was not bouncing back in my usual way. Normally I am a high-energy, very positive person. This particular year I realized I was depressed. I knew that I had been working far too hard and had far too much on my plate, too many responsibilities. Maybe I had finally burned out and was ready for a change.

After a week at home, I made the decision that I would meet with a counselor to discuss my future plans. I thought I might sell my business or simply close it down. I had never really been depressed in my life, and the feeling was not comfortable. I knew I was not able to make good decisions feeling this way, so I gave myself a year in which I would think, discuss, and make plans. Whatever I ended up doing, I wanted it to be done "gracefully." I did not want to inconvenience my staff or my clients in any way.

It took me about a month to interview potential therapists. I wanted someone I felt I could work well with. In fact, before I hire any medical person to work with me as my physician or therapist, I always interview him or her. I find this works the best with any professional consultant, be it medical, legal, financial, or other.

By February I had engaged a really lovely woman as my therapist, and I went for my first hourly session with her. She asked me to describe what was going on in my life. I spent the hour talking about my work and the projects we were developing. At the end of the session she said, "I don't think you are burned out. Yes, you are working too many hours but you obviously love what you do and get tremendous pleasure out of doing it. I think you may have a medical problem that is causing this depression. Have you ever had your thyroid checked?"

Lights flashed for me!!! Three years earlier I had to have a physical for an insurance policy. The insurance doc who did the physical had briefly mentioned that my thyroid was a bit enlarged on one side. I was too busy and didn't give it another thought until this particular February afternoon with my therapist.

A week later I had been diagnosed with Hashimoto's disease and began therapy with thyroid hormone. Within a few weeks all signs of the depression that I was feeling had gone away. However, I continued seeing the therapist for some time. I realized I could not continue to live the lifestyle I was living without having other, potentially more serious physical consequences from the abuse my body was taking.

Since that time I have cut my travel to a maximum of three trips per month. I started doing yoga when I was in my 20s and had been diagnosed with Raynaud's disease, another autoimmune disease, just like Hashimoto's. I began doing yoga again, daily. I had always had a healthy diet but had put on extra pounds, so I lost some weight. I made it a priority to walk as much as possible, something that was harder to find time to do on the west coast than in New York where I had lived previously. And I continue to plan for my next phase of life, knowing that I still want to move into it as gracefully as possible.

(Reprinted with permission by Peggy McCarthy)

SYMPTOMS OF HASHIMOTO'S THYROIDITIS

An underactive thyroid slows metabolism and decreases production of body heat; the most common symptoms are weight gain and intolerance to cold. Other common symptoms include fatigue, constipation, dry skin, hair loss, heavy and irregular menstrual periods, and difficulty concentrating. Some of these symptoms may appear suddenly and others, especially hair loss (on any area of the body), may be very gradual. Depression is a key symptom of Hashimoto's that is often overlooked, and persistent depressive symptoms may warrant TSH tests. Major depression is a separate illness and does not occur with thyroid disease.

However, thyroid hormones can interact with the mood stabilizer lithium used as a long-term treatment for bipolar disorder, making it less effective. It's not clear why, but lithium itself may cause the thyroid to become underactive as a side effect, so thyroid hormone levels need to be monitored in women taking this drug.

SYMPTOMS OF GRAVES' DISEASE

An overactive thyroid increases metabolism, causing weight loss. Also, because your body needs more blood for increased energy use, your heart pumps faster causing a rapid pulse, palpitations, and sometimes an irregular heartbeat. Your gastrointestinal system may also speed up, resulting in more frequent bowel movements. Increased metabolism causes your body to produce more heat, which may cause you to feel warm and flushed and have increased sweating. People with Graves' disease may find it hard to fall or stay asleep, and sleep loss can lead to fatigue. They may also have muscle weakness, especially in the hips, thighs, and shoulders. Hyperthyroidism can also cause a person to feel more energetic, even hyperactive or jumpy, to be irritable, or to experience mood swings. Menstrual flow can become lighter, and some women can lose their period altogether.

Roughly half of the women with Graves' disease develop eye inflammation and protruding eyes (Grave's orbitopathy). Eye muscles can become weakened from increased pressure behind the eye and hamper eye movement, leading to impaired or double vision. Graves' orbitopathy can also damage the optic nerve. In some cases, the eyelids may not close completely during sleep, causing the cornea to become dry and prone to ulceration. Fortunately, less than 1 percent of people with Graves' disease have serious or permanent eye problems.

DIAGNOSIS

Both a physical exam and blood tests are needed to diagnose thyroid disease. The thyroid may enlarge (goiter) in both Hashimoto's and Graves' diseases. Your doctor will physically examine the thyroid, often while you are swallowing water, to get a sense of the gland's size and texture.

Blood tests to measure TSH are the best indicators of thyroid function. Low TSH indicates hyperthyroidism; elevated TSH signals hypothyroidism. Other blood tests can determine the existence of thyroid antibodies; up to 80 percent of women with Hashimoto's have antithyroid antibodies. If you have a goiter, a test to measure radioactive iodine uptake may be done to look for abnormal thyroid function. If nodules are present, ultrasound can be used to image the gland, and a thyroid scan can determine if overactive thyroid nodules are causing Graves' disease.

TREATMENT

Hashimoto's is easily treated with synthetic replacement thyroid hormones. However, it may take some time to find just the right dose, and yearly blood tests are needed to ensure thyroid hormones remain at the right level. While 10 percent of women with Hashimoto's thyroiditis have a spontaneous remission, others may have progressive thyroid failure and will need increased doses of medication. Even with careful monitoring, women with Hashimoto's run a slight risk of having excess thyroid hormones and should be checked (especially after menopause) for bone loss and heart rhythm problems.

Treatment for Graves' disease involves calming down the overactive thyroid or destroying the gland so that it does not pump out excess thyroid hormones. This can be achieved with antithyroid drugs or radioactive iodine or by surgically removing the gland. After the gland is destroyed, replacement thyroid hormones are given. Until these replacement hormones become fully effective and are adjusted properly, beta blockers, such as propanolol, may be needed. Such drugs block the effects of thyroid hormones, slow elevated heart rate, and lessen anxiety. In many cases, eye inflammation and protrusion in Graves' disease are mild and do not require therapy. If orbitopathy is more severe, corticosteroids may be prescribed to reduce inflammation and lessen swelling. Swollen eye tissue can be removed with surgery, and swollen muscles around the eye can be repaired; surgery to enlarge the bony opening around the eyes is done only if other treatments are unsuccessful.

What Is Sjögren's Syndrome?

As many as four million Americans—about 90 percent of them women—may have Sjögren's syndrome, in which the immune system attacks the body's moisture-producing glands and tissues. These include the lacrimal glands that produce tears and the salivary glands as well as mucus membranes in the nose and vagina. In some cases, Sjögren's can also affect the kidneys, gastrointestinal (GI) tract, lungs, liver, and blood vessels. In 50 percent of cases, Sjögren's syndrome occurs alone (primary Sjögren's), and 50 percent of the time it occurs in the presence of another autoimmune disease such as RA, lupus, scleroderma, or thyroid disease.

Sjögren's develops when moisture-producing glands are damaged by activated immune cells, making them less able to respond to signals from the brain to produce tears or saliva. In addition, inflammatory cytokines may damage the nerves and neurotransmitters (chemical substances in the brain) that stimulate the tear ducts or salivary glands. The dry eyes that characterize Sjögren's are also caused by damage to tiny glands behind the eyelashes (called meibomian glands) that secrete an oil that prevents tears from evaporating too quickly.

RISK FACTORS

Like RA and other autoimmune disorders, Sjögren's can also run in families. Although it can develop at any age, it is most prevalent after age 40. Like other autoimmune diseases, Sjögren's syndrome appears to be influenced by genetic vulnerability, environmental triggers (such as the Epstein-Barr virus), and hormones.

WHY YOUR SEX MATTERS

The underlying cause of evaporative dry eye may be low levels of male hormones. Androgens decline after menopause, although not to the extent that estrogen production drops. Researchers are studying androgen therapy as a treatment for primary Sjögren's and androgen eye drops for dry eye symptoms. Studies have shown that estrogen therapy appears to worsen dry eye.

Women with Sjögren's syndrome often experience vaginal dryness, which can lead to painful intercourse. Vaginal lubrication does not come from moisture-producing glands but from fluid that is passed from the bloodstream through the vaginal walls. Vaginal dryness in Sjögren's patients is often mistaken for menopause-related vaginal atrophy or degeneration. Symptoms related to dryness can be helped by moisturizers. Lubricants can make sex more comfortable. Local estrogen therapy in the form of creams, a ring, or suppository tablet also helps dryness by reversing the atrophy of vaginal tissues that occurs after menopause.

SYMPTOMS

The hallmarks of Sjögren's syndrome are dry eyes, dry mouth, and fatigue. Classic dry eye symptoms include a dry, gritty, or burning sensation; itching; light sensitivity; eyelids that stick together; and mucus accumulation in the corners of the eyes on awakening. Women with dry mouth may have difficulty chewing or swallowing, burning mouth or tongue, and increased dental decay (due to low saliva production). Sjögren's can also cause swollen parotid glands (the largest of the salivary glands, in front of the ears), joint pain, dry nose, and fatigue and can lead to peripheral nerve problems, lung inflammation, and kidney dysfunction. Women with Sjögren's may also have a slightly increased risk of lymphoma, a malignancy of the lymph glands, so swollen lymph nodes should be investigated.

DIAGNOSIS

Because symptoms of Sjögren's syndrome, such as joint pain and fatigue, may overlap with those of RA and other autoimmune diseases, it is often misdiagnosed or missed altogether. Physicians may treat dry eye and overlook other symptoms, such as dry mouth or dry vagina, which may signal Sjögren's. Dentists may see women with dry mouth and numerous cavities and never ask if they suffer dry eyes as well. A woman may visit her doctor for menopausal symptoms in her late 40s and not be diagnosed with Sjögren's syndrome until much later. In fact, the average time from the onset of symptoms to a diagnosis can sometimes exceed six years.

During a work-up, blood tests are performed to check for specific autoantibodies, including RF and antinuclear antibodies (ANAs), present in 70 percent of patient with Sjögren's, as well as variety of autoimmune diseases including lupus (see page 58). Your sedimentation (SED) rate will be measured, and you will be given tests to look for elevation in normal blood proteins known as immunoglobulins, common in people with Sjögren's syndrome.

For women with dry eyes, special tests are performed to measure tear production and the volume of tears produced. The most common of these is the Schirmer's test, in which small pieces of filter paper are placed between your eyeball and lower lid to measure the amount of moisture produced within five minutes. A slit-lamp examination uses a special lamp and a magnifying device to reveal the normal layer of tears along the lower eyelid, which may appear thickened. Another test, called rose bengal staining (involving a harmless vegetable dye), helps to determine the quality of the oily layer of tear film and its distribution over the surface of the eye. Other tests may be done to assess the condition of the cornea.

A dentist or oral pathologist can measure saliva production in dry mouth. This is done by putting an acidic or sour substance in the mouth to stimulate saliva production. In some cases, a biopsy of the tiny salivary glands in the lower lip may be needed to detect immune cell infiltration.

The symptoms of Sjögren's syndrome are treated individually. Over-the-counter (OTC) and prescription medications are available to relieve the dry eye and dry mouth symptoms. OTC products include preservative-free artificial tears, artificial saliva, saline nasal sprays, and vaginal lubricants. An ophthalmologist may recommend eyedrops containing cyclosporine for dry eye. In some cases, tiny silicone plugs (punctal plugs) are inserted in the tear ducts to prevent tears from draining away. Non-drug strategies include the use of a humidifier and protective goggles to prevent tear evaporation.

Two oral prescription drugs are used to treat dry mouth, pilocarpine hydrochloride and cevimeline, which are taken after meals to improve salivary flow. Studies suggest they may also improve dry eye and dryness in other areas of the body. Artificial saliva can provide topical relief for dry mouth.

Other manifestations of Sjögren's, such as kidney or lung problems, are treated separately with medication.

FUTURE APPROACHES TO SJÖGREN'S SYNDROME

One promising avenue of therapy for dry eye is eyedrops containing androgens. The National Institutes of Health is also exploring the use of androgens, in the form of dehydroepiandrosterone (DHEA), to treat primary Sjögren's syndrome. Some medications used to treat RA may also be useful in Sjögren's.

What Is Systemic Lupus Erythematosus?

As many as 1.5 million people, 90 percent of them women, may have systemic lupus erythematosus (SLE), a chronic inflammatory disease that can affect almost any organ or organ system of the body, including the skin, joints, lungs, blood, and kidneys. It is the leading cause of kidney disease in young women. Around 10 percent of patients initially develop a form of lupus that involves only the skin, discoid lupus, but then go on to develop systemic lupus. In some cases, lupus is mild and can be managed with medications. In others, lupus can cause serious and potentially life-threatening problems. It can affect just about any area of the body; antibodies may attack not only the cells in various organs but also parts of cells, including the DNA and cell nuclei.

Recent animal research reveals that antibodies to DNA (and other autoantibodies) bind to specific receptors on the surface of cells, called

Fc receptors. A specific Fc receptor appears to be defective in lupus, allowing accumulation of damaging antibodies, which may help set the stage for lupus. In addition to antibodies, structures, called immune complexes, play a major role in lupus. Immune complexes are lattice-like structures formed when antibodies bind to their targets. They can build up in blood vessels and cause inflammation and blockages. Immune complexes are normally cleared partly by proteins, called complement, but women with lupus may produce too little complement to keep up with immune complex formation, or the complement they produce is used up too quickly. The resulting accumulation of immune complexes can cause damage to blood vessels and organs such as the kidneys. Low levels of androgens may also factor into lupus.

RISK FACTORS

Risk factors for SLE appear to be a combination of genetic vulnerability and environmental triggers, including infections, certain drugs and antibiotics (especially those in the sulfa and penicillin groups, which may worsen lupus), and ultraviolet light.

While some studies suggest a role for microchimerism, other research suggests that maternal cells that get into a fetus's blood circulation and persist into adult life may increase the risk of developing lupus. Biopsies of heart muscle have found maternal cells in babies with neonatal lupus; however, this research is highly speculative.

So far, researchers have identified about a dozen genes that are associated with lupus, and some of these genetic defects appear to run in families. About 10 percent of lupus patients have a close relative with the disease, and about 5 percent of the children born to women with lupus will develop it. Lupus most often occurs in women between the ages of 15 and 40, but it can occur in both sexes and at any age. African Americans, American Indian, and Asian American women develop SLE more frequently than Caucasians.

WHY YOUR SEX MATTERS

Since there is some increased risk of lupus becoming more active during or immediately after pregnancy, pregnant women or those trying to become pregnant should be monitored closely. Women with lupus run a higher risk of getting pre-eclampsia, a dangerous form of high blood pressure during pregnancy. Antiphospholipid syndrome (APS), an autoimmune disease that promotes clotting, can coexist with lupus and complicate pregnancy. Additionally, women with central nervous system, kidney, or heart and lung involvement may be at greater risk during a pregnancy and require close medical supervision. The good news is that most women who are in remission for six months before becoming pregnant do well during their pregnancy.

Antibodies in the mother's blood travel across the placenta during pregnancy to protect the growing fetus from infection. But bad antibodies travel along with the good ones, so women with lupus who have certain antibodies (anti-SSA/Ro and SSB/La) may give birth to children with neonatal lupus, which is usually temporary. Neonatal lupus is a misnomer; it is not a systemic disease like SLE. Most often, neonatal lupus only causes a skin rash that resolves without treatment within eight months after birth.

In two percent of women with anti-SSA/Ro antibodies, neonatal lupus can cause a permanent condition, called congenital heart block, in which there is a blockage in the electrical signal that travels from one part of the heart to another. In congenital heart block, an area in the middle of the heart, called the AV node, which is critical to transmitting electrical impulses that regulate heartbeat, is damaged by maternal autoantibodies (or other yet unknown factors). This causes an abnormally slow heartbeat in the newborn, requiring a pacemaker. In less than 20 percent of these cases, the condition can be fatal. Some babies may have both heart block and the skin rash. The proportion of women with anti-SSA/RO antibodies whose babies will develop a neonatal lupus rash in unknown. However, as mentioned earlier, the rash is transient and usually disappears by eight months, when the mother's antibodies are cleared from the baby's circulation.

Lupus and the Heart

Lupus poses an increased risk for cardiovascular disease in women, especially before age 45. But the factors that cause this increased risk of premature atherosclerosis are unclear. Some studies indicate that the natural estrogen found in women's bodies, which is usually protective against cardiovascular disease, may promote blood clotting in younger women with lupus who have antiphospholipid antibodies.

Symptoms

The most common symptoms of SLE include achy or swollen joints, prolonged fatigue, fever, anemia, and skin rashes, including the telltale butterfly-shaped rash across the cheeks and nose. Additional symptoms may include chest pain on deep breathing, sensitivity to sunlight, hair loss, and Raynaud's phenomenon (a condition where fingers turn white or blue in the cold due to spasms in tiny blood vessels that restrict blood flow).

DIAGNOSIS

Lupus is often perceived as difficult to diagnose, because its signs and symptoms can accumulate over time. Many physicians refer to the criteria established by the American College of Rheumatology (ACR). While the ACR criteria are mostly used for clinical trials, they can aid in a diagnosis. To meet the criteria, a woman must have four or more of the following symptoms (not necessarily at the same time):

♦ a rash over the nose and cheeks that looks like a butterfly (malar rash);
♦ red raised patches (discoid rash) on the skin (often on the scalp or earlobes);
♦ skin sensitivity to sunlight;
♦ ulcers (usually painless) in the nose or mouth;
♦ arthritis (tenderness, pain, and swelling) in two or more joints;
♦ inflammation of the lining of the lung or heart;
♦ excessive protein in the urine;
♦ blood cell disorders, including hemolytic anemia, a low white blood count, or thrombocytopenia (a low number of platelets—cells needed for clotting);
♦ positive test for antinuclear antibodies (ANAs); and
♦ evidence of other autoantibodies, including anti-double-stranded DNA antibodies (anti-dsDNA), anti-SSA/Ro, anti-SSB/La, and antiphospholipid antibodies (APLs);

Blood tests to detect antinuclear antibodies (ANAs) are positive in more than 95 percent of women with SLE. Recent studies suggest that these antibodies may actually be present for years before symptoms develop. However, women with other autoimmune diseases can also have ANAs, so a combination of other tests, a physical examination, and a detailed medical history are necessary to make a diagnosis. For example, since the kidneys can be involved in SLE, a urine dipstick test is important. This test measures the amount of protein in the urine, which can indicate if the kidneys are losing too much protein. A new screening test for lupus looks for molecules called SR proteins and may pick up the 20 percent of cases that might not be detected through standard screening tests. Whether it will prove to be helpful in diagnosing SLE awaits more study.

TREATMENT

Therapy for lupus centers on reducing symptoms and lowering the number and severity of disease flare-ups, halting the progression of the disease, and minimizing organ damage.

Nonsteroidal anti-inflammatory pain medications (NSAIDs) commonly are used to ease joint pain. They must be used with caution in lupus patients, since they can worsen kidney disease. Another mainstay of treatment includes corticosteroids and other drugs that suppress inflammation. (As in other autoimmune diseases, corticosteroids increase the risk of infections, diabetes, osteoporosis, osteonecrosis, and hypertension.) Many lupus patients are helped by antimalarial drugs, most commonly hydroxychloroquine, which help dampen inflammation. This drug is most useful for relieving discoid lesions, hair loss, joint pain, and perhaps even fatigue. Some studies suggest it may also have positive effects on bone mass and perhaps protect against blood clots and high cholesterol. Immunomodulating drugs, including azathioprine and cyclophosphamide, are used when there is more serious kidney or organ involvement. These drugs may help suppress the immune system by reducing the number of immune cells more active in lupus.

Women who have clotting problems (such as clots in leg veins) or antiphospholipid antibodies and who have suffered a blood clot are given anticoagulant medications.

Women may also be treated with DHEA, a natural steroid hormone. Research has found that many women with lupus have low levels of androgens, which may have anti-inflammatory properties. DHEA may be helpful for women with mild lupus, particularly those with skin rashes, hair loss, and joint pain. While DHEA is sold as a dietary supplement, a pharmaceutical-grade preparation has not shown clear-cut effectiveness in clinical trials, so it has yet to win U.S. Food and Drug Administration (FDA) approval for treating lupus.

Women with lupus are also cautioned to use sunscreens and avoid excessive sun exposure.

Regular monitoring of the disease is essential to detect increases in symptoms as well as development of new ones that could require a change in treatment.

FUTURE APPROACHES TO LUPUS

Researchers are investigating new drugs and biologicals that target specific cells of the immune system, with the hope of being able to obstruct or suppress the production of specific antibodies and harmful cytokines. Early research is also underway into correcting the defect in Fc receptors that allows accumulation of autoantibodies. Lab experiments in mice suggest that increasing the activity of these receptors could potentially reverse or halt part of the autoimmune process in lupus, paving the way for a future gene therapy.

Right now, results of a major study indicate that oral estrogens are safe for carefully selected women with lupus. It was believed that hormones caused disease flares, and for years women with lupus were told to avoid estrogen. But the recently concluded Safety of Estrogens in Lupus Erythematosus, National Assessment (SELENA) trials found that hormone therapy did not significantly increase the rate of severe lupus flares and was associated with only a higher risk of mild and moderate flares. The SELENA trial also found that oral contraceptives did not increase severe, moderate, or even mild flares. With the exception of women with unstable SLE, or those at increased risk of clots, experts say birth control pills can be prescribed safely for women with lupus.

What Is Scleroderma?

The term scleroderma is taken from two Greek words, "sclero," meaning hard and "derma," meaning skin. Scleroderma affects up to 300,000 people in the United States, 80 percent of whom are women. In scleroderma, autoimmunity leads to excessive production of collagen in the skin and other connective tissues, causing hardening and scarring (fibrosis). Smaller blood vessels are also damaged by the disease, causing many of the complications, including high blood pressure. About two-thirds of women with scleroderma have localized scleroderma, which affects only the skin. The rest have a systemic form of the disease, affecting not only the skin, but also internal organs such as the lungs, kidneys, and esophagus. Systemic scleroderma can be widespread (diffuse) or limited, affecting just a few areas.

Scleroderma affects the tiny blood vessels in the fingers and other areas of the body, causing them to narrow and restrict blood flow. This frequently happens in the small blood vessels of the hands, making them extremely sensitive to cold, a problem called Raynaud's phenomenon. In Raynaud's, narrowed blood vessels go into painful spasms when exposed to the cold, causing a brief stoppage of blood flow that turns the fingers white, then blue, and then red as blood flow resumes. Raynaud's occurs in most people with scleroderma, but it can also occur in RA and lupus as well as in otherwise healthy people. When blood vessels in the kidneys are narrowed, it leads to high blood pressure. Up to 40 percent of people with scleroderma develop pulmonary hypertension, or high blood pressure in the lungs.

In scleroderma, the immune system attacks cells that produce collagen, a substance that normally makes your skin elastic and supports the joints, ligaments, and tissues that surround internal organs. Collagen is usually made in small amounts, but the immune attack causes it to be overproduced, replacing normal tissue in the skin or other organs. Small blood vessels in the skin and organs are also damaged early on in this process. It is not known what triggers the immune system attack.

With localized and systemic scleroderma, damage to small blood vessels within the skin can lead to skin ulcerations. Complications of scleroderma can range from very mild to life-threatening, depending on the areas affected. Chronic heartburn and gastroesophageal reflux disease (GERD) are frequent complications of scleroderma, due to fibrosis (or formation of scar tissue) of the esophagus. This damage leads to weakening of the valve that keeps acid in the stomach, causing the acid to back up into the esophagus. Systemic fibrosis can also affect the lungs and heart. Early diagnosis and proper treatment can minimize symptoms and lessen the risk of more serious complications.

RISK FACTORS

Scleroderma can develop at any age (even in childhood), but it most commonly arises between the ages of 25 and 55. A family history of scleroderma increases the risk; relatives of people with scleroderma have a two times greater risk of developing the disease. A family history of rheumatic diseases also appears to be a slight risk factor. Other risk factors include occupational exposure to silica dust, organic solvents such as polyvinyl chloride, and some drugs.

WHY YOUR SEX MATTERS

Female hormones are believed to play only a slight role, if any, in scleroderma. As in some other autoimmune diseases, fetal cells that persist in a woman's circulation after pregnancy may be a factor. One theory is that these fetal cells may provoke an immune reaction akin to the rejection of a transplanted organ, which leads to scleroderma. Researchers have found that women with scleroderma have 20 times the number of circulating fetal cells as women with children without scleroderma. However, since some patients have not been pregnant, microchimerism cannot explain all cases of scleroderma. It is, however, an interesting avenue for further research, since there are no other strong candidates (genetic or environmental) for potential triggers for the disease.

SYMPTOMS

Early symptoms of scleroderma can include puffy hands, joint pain, and Raynaud's phenomenon. As many as 95 percent of people with scleroderma experience Raynaud's. Other common symptoms include skin thickening on the hands and forearms (which eventually may cause the hands to be frozen in a claw-like position); tight, mask-like tightening of facial skin; and ulcerations on fingertips or toes due to lack of blood supply. Because scleroderma can stiffen the esophagus, heartburn and difficulty swallowing are frequent symptoms. Shortness of breath may signal lung involvement. Scleroderma can also produce hair loss, abnormally dark or light patches of skin, widening of small blood vessels in the skin (telangiectasias), tiny calcium deposits in the skin (calcinosis), and fatigue. Symptoms of limited scleroderma have often been referred to as CREST—for calcinosis, Raynaud's, esophageal dysfunction, and telangiectasias. However, as understanding of the disease has progressed, this term has become less widely used.

DIAGNOSIS

A variety of tests, along with a complete physical examination, is needed to diagnose scleroderma. If there is tightness, thickening, or hardening of the skin, your physician may order a skin biopsy. Blood tests for antinuclear antibodies (ANAs) are positive in 85 percent of people with scleroderma; other antibody tests are less specific for the condition. Protein may appear in your urine if there is kidney involvement. Chest x-rays can reveal lung fibrosis, while pulmonary function tests can assess the severity of lung damage. If you have symptoms of GERD, gastrointestinal studies such as a barium swallow (which involves drinking a small amount of liquid containing barium, which appears white on x-rays) and endoscopy (using a fiberoptic scope) may be done to check for damage to the esophagus.

TREATMENT

There is no cure for scleroderma, but complications of the disease can be treated. Joint pain can be eased with nonsteroidal anti-inflammatory drugs. Thickened skin is treated with a variety of agents, including D-penicillamine, and moisturizers and lubricants can keep skin from tearing. If cracks or ulcers in the skin become infected, topical or systemic antibiotics are used. Physical or occupational therapy, including range-of-motion exercises, can help maintain hand flexibility. The arthritis that can occur in scleroderma is treated with some of the same drugs used to treat RA.

Raynaud's phenomenon can be treated with drugs to help dilate blood vessels, including calcium channel blockers and medications that improve blood flow, such as pentoxifylline, or clopidogrel to prevent blood clots.

Drugs that reduce stomach acid production, including proton pump inhibitors, are used to treat reflux and may also help heal the structures and precancerous lesions in the esophagus that can result from GERD. People with GERD are also helped by lifestyle changes, including eating slowly, chewing food thoroughly, drinking plenty of water, not eating within two hours of going to bed, and sleeping with the head of the bed elevated.

High blood pressure and kidney problems in scleroderma are often treated with drugs, called angiotensin-converting enzyme (ACE) inhibitors, such as captopril or enalapril. Three new drugs have been approved to treat pulmonary hypertension in scleroderma: bosentan, which aids blood vessel function and two derivatives of prostaglandin (a substance that occurs naturally in the body), epoprostenol, and treprostinil. Immunosuppressants, drugs that inhibit immune cells, and certain anti-cancer agents (including cyclophosphamide) have been useful for pulmonary fibrosis and are being tested further.

FUTURE APPROACHES TO SCLERODERMA

Researchers are exploring the use of immunosuppressive agents that selectively target overproduction of collagen. Antibodies that inhibit growth factors to reduce collagen production are also being studied. Stem cell transplantation is another therapy under active investigation.

Studies show that many women with scleroderma remain sexually active, and sildenafil and other longer-acting drugs are being tested to improve problems with decreased sensation and vaginal lubrication caused by restricted blood flow.

What Is Multiple Sclerosis ?

Multiple sclerosis (MS), a chronic disease of the central nervous system, affects more than 400,000 people, two-thirds of whom are women. In MS, autoantibodies, immune cells, and inflammation eat away myelin, the protective tissue wrapped around nerve cell fibers in the brain and spinal cord; sometimes the nerve fiber itself is damaged or broken during the attack. The damage to myelin interferes with communication between nerve cells, causing symptoms ranging from dizziness and blurred vision to paralysis. As myelin is stripped away, it is replaced by scar (sclerotic) tissue at multiple sites around the nervous system (hence the name multiple sclerosis).

This is a gradual process, and myelin may regenerate itself in the beginning and inflammation can come in spurts; this may underlie relapsing-remitting MS, in which the disease worsens and then gets better. The majority of people with MS have the relapsing-remitting form. Around 10 percent of people have the primary-progressive form of MS, which is characterized by a continual worsening of the disease. Half of those with relapsing-remitting disease eventually develop the progressive form (secondary-progressive MS). In rare cases (less than 5 percent), people have a progressive-relapsing form of MS.

RISK FACTORS

As with other autoimmune diseases, a combination of genetic vulnerability and environmental triggers (such as Epstein-Barr virus) may play a role in MS. There appears to be a genetic link with MS; several studies show that the risk of developing MS increases almost 20 times if a close family member has the disease. MS also seems to be more prevalent in people of northern European descent and uncommon in those of Asian descent. However, it is not clear whether this is due to genetic or environmental factors. And there are likely multiple genes involved.

A recent multinational study found that a variation in a gene that controls an inflammatory cytokine, called interferon (IFN) gamma, may play a role in MS. Unlike the beta interferons used to treat MS symptoms (see page 69), IFN gamma plays a role in the immune attacks that produce MS symptoms. One gene variant that causes high levels of IFN gamma to be produced (causing more attacks on myelin) was found to be more common in women, which may help to explain why more women have MS than men. In any case, genes are only part of the picture; the identical twin of a person with MS has only a one in three chance of developing the disease, and more than 80 percent of people with MS do not have a close relative with the disease.

Respiratory infections are known to trigger MS relapses, and there are dozens of potential viral suspects in MS, in addition to the Epstein-Barr virus (EBV) (which causes infectious mononucleosis). However, some of the strongest evidence is for EBV. Antibodies to EBV and other viruses (evidence we have had an infection) are elevated in people with MS, and EBV antibodies are increased during MS exacerbations. So far, however, there is no solid, scientific evidence that a virus actually causes MS.

WHY YOUR SEX MATTERS

Female hormones, especially estrogen, could play a role in MS. During pregnancy there are fewer MS relapses when estrogen is elevated. It is thought that estriol, a weak form of estrogen that is produced during pregnancy, may even help protect against MS. Early studies in animals show that testosterone may be protective, and researchers think this could explain why men develop MS less often and typically later in life than women. (However, when men get MS, it is usually more severe and progressive.) A recent study from Italy indicates that the hormone testosterone is reduced in women suffering from MS, and that estrogen may help control nerve damage in MS. Studies are underway to study the effects of estriol on MS, and preliminary data have been positive.

MS does not appear to have any effect on a women's ability to get pregnant or to have a healthy pregnancy. And women with MS do not have any higher rate of birth defects. At this time it is not known whether the wide shifts in hormones during perimenopause or the decline in estrogen after menopause affect the severity or course of MS.

SYMPTOMS

MS can produce a wide variety of symptoms: the most common are actually fatigue and depression (as well as wide mood swings), which are not often associated with MS. (In fact, depression may be due to undiagnosed brain lesions.) Early symptoms that raise a red flag for MS include blurred or double vision or a sudden blindness in one eye. Many MS patients experience muscle weakness in their extremities and difficulty with coordination and balance, sometimes severe enough to impede standing or walking. People with MS can also experience abnormal nerve sensations such as numbness, prickling, or a "pins and needles" feeling. There can also be tremors, dizziness, and spasticity (involuntary movement of muscles or stiffness). Approximately half of all people with MS experience cognitive problems such as difficulties with concentration, attention, memory, and poor judgment, but such symptoms are usually mild and are frequently overlooked. Less commonly, people experience headaches, seizures, or speech and swallowing difficulties. Heat often makes symptoms worse. As the disease progresses, one may experience loss of bowel and bladder control, and in severe MS, paralysis may result.

DIAGNOSIS

Making a diagnosis of MS is not easy, and the symptoms often mimic those of other conditions. Specific diagnostic tests are required to rule out other diseases and establish a definitive diagnosis of MS. You can expect to have your reflexes, balance, coordination, and vision checked, and diagnostic tests performed. Magnetic resonance imaging (MRI) of the brain is the most frequently used test and can clearly show the white "plaques" (patches of scar tissue and inflammation) characteristic of MS. (An MRI may be done using the contrast agent gadolinium to spotlight areas of demyelination.) Several new MRI techniques may help quantify and characterize MS lesions that are too subtle to be detected using conventional MRI scans.

Other diagnostic tests include evoked potential tests, which measure how quickly and accurately your nervous system responds to certain stimulation, and a spinal tap, which checks your cerebrospinal fluid for antibodies and proteins that result from the breakdown of myelin.

The severity of MS is scored using the Extended Disability Status Score (EDSS), which measures vision, sensation, coordination, strength, and walking ability. A score of 0 indicates a normal neurological exam. A score of 1.0–1.5 indicates an abnormal neurological exam, but no disability; 2.0–2.5 shows mild disability; 3.0–3.5 shows mild to moderate disability; and someone with a score of 6.0 generally needs assistance from a cane to walk.

The National Multiple Sclerosis Society established criteria that require evidence (either on MRI or clinical signs) of two separate neurological disturbances occurring at least 30 days apart for a diagnosis of MS. However, a woman who experiences a single MS attack can be started on disease-modifying medications that can slow disease progression and potentially prevent permanent disability.

TREATMENT

There are now six disease-modifying drugs approved for relapsing-remitting MS. Three of these drugs are based on natural beta interferons, which have been shown to dampen immune reactions and improve MS exacerbations: interferon beta 1-a and interferon beta 1-b, all given by self-injection. Glatiramer acetate is a synthetic protein to which the immune system responds as it would myelin, so it acts as a "decoy" for attacks on myelin. Mitoxantrone is actually chemotherapy drug that suppresses the activity of T cells, B cells, and macrophages and seems to lessen attacks on myelin. It can also affect the heart, so patients must have normal cardiac function and regular cardiac tests to receive the drug, which is given intravenously. Some interferon products have begun to be used in some cases of secondary-progressive MS, and one of them and the glatiramer acetate are being tested against primary-progressive MS.

Since MS relapses, or "flares," are due to inflammation in the central nervous system, the most common treatments for exacerbations are intravenous, high-dose corticosteroids, most commonly methylprednisolone. It is important to note that corticosteroids can increase the risk of atherosclerosis, diabetes, and osteoporosis.

Other treatments target MS symptoms, such as depression, pain, tremor, bladder or bowel dysfunction, and fatigue. Stimulants such as modafinil can help combat fatigue, as can the antiviral medication amantadine and antidepressants. Antiseizure medications and tricyclic antidepressants are effective for nerve pain, and antispasmodic drugs and muscle relaxants are used to relieve spasticity. Physical therapy and exercise can help preserve function. One study of early MS patients found that six months of regular exercise (either practicing yoga or riding a stationary bicycle) improved energy levels.

Many people find aids such as foot braces, canes, and walkers help them remain independent and mobile. However, studies show that two of three people with MS are able to walk on their own 20 years after their diagnosis, and those numbers should improve as more and more people are treated earlier.

FUTURE APPROACHES TO MS

Investigators are continuing their search for early diagnostic tests for MS. A recent study revealed a distinct pattern of proteins and protein building blocks (peptides) in the blood of a small group of newly diagnosed MS patients, raising the hope that a simple blood test may be used one day to diagnose MS before any nerve damage is evident on MRI. In addition, a potential blood test for antimyelin antibodies is in clinical trials.

Preliminary research suggests that the cholesterol-lowering drugs called statins, which have anti-inflammatory properties, can modulate immune responses in MS patients. A recent review found that all statin drugs have side effects, including potentially serious muscle wasting, so they should not be taken in hopes of treating MS symptoms until more research is done to confirm their effects and determine the proper dose.

In addition, drugs used to treat Alzheimer's disease, such as donepezil, are being tested to see if they can improve the cognitive decline that can occur in MS. Scientists are also investigating ways to reverse the damage to myelin (and myelin-producing cells) or trigger myelin to regenerate.

Associated Disorders

Some women with autoimmune disease may also suffer from disorders such as fibromyalgia or chronic fatigue syndrome (which are not generally thought to be autoimmune). Since the symptoms are often similar, notably joint pain and fatigue, women with autoimmune diseases may be mistakenly diagnosed with these "fellow travelers" or the symptoms may be diagnosed as a disease flare.

WHAT IS FIBROMYALGIA SYNDROME?

Fibromyalgia syndrome (FMS), a disorder characterized by pain or hypersensitivity in the muscles, ligaments, and tendons of the body, affects

2–4 percent of women in the general population. Up to 25 percent of women with RA, lupus, and Crohn's disease meet the American College of Rheumatology diagnostic criteria for FMS, which usually strikes women between the ages of 20 and 40.

RISK FACTORS

It is not known what causes fibromyalgia, but recent research suggests that pain sensitivity may be greater in women with FMS. Studies show that areas involved in processing pain and certain brain chemicals may be different in people with FMS. In vulnerable women, a stressor or trauma—such as a physical injury, an autoimmune disease, extreme emotional stress, or hormonal alterations (such as being hypothyroid)—may provoke a disturbance in the central nervous system. Studies also reveal higher levels of certain inflammatory cytokines in women with FMS. Fibromyalgia can run in families, and several genes may contribute to a predisposition to pain amplification. In some cases, FMS can arise after an infection, especially infectious mononucleosis and Lyme disease.

WHY YOUR SEX MATTERS

Around 2–4 percent of women in the general population may be affected by this disorder, and up to 25 percent of women with autoimmune diseases may also have FMS. Fibromyalgia symptoms also overlap with other disorders that can occur in women with autoimmune diseases, including chronic fatigue syndrome (CFS), irritable bowel syndrome, and interstitial cystitis. Women are more than twice as likely as men to experience depression during their lifetime, and the incidence of depression and anxiety in women with FMS may run as high as 40–70 percent.

SYMPTOMS

Women with FMS often complain of widespread, chronic pain and pain sensitivity around the body. Women with FMS may also suffer from fatigue, sleep disturbances, depression, anxiety, difficulty concentrating, and memory problems. Other symptoms can include migraine headaches, abdominal pain, bloating or alternating constipation and diarrhea, and temporomandibular jaw pain.

DIAGNOSIS

To meet the criteria for fibromyalgia set by the American College of Rheumatology, there must be a history of chronic widespread pain involving all four quadrants of the body, as well as areas overlying the bones of the skull, backbone, ribs, and chest, and pain produced by applying pressure at 11 of 18 specific "tender points" located at the neck, shoulders, lower back, hips, and knees.

A fibromyalgia work-up includes blood tests for liver, kidney, and thyroid function; a complete blood count; and a sedimentation rate or level of C-reactive protein to detect inflammation. Unless pain has come on suddenly or there is evidence to suggest an autoimmune disease, testing for autoimmune markers is not usually done. If there is pain and stiffness in weight-bearing joints, x-rays or other imaging may be done to look for evidence of arthritis, either RA or osteoarthritis.

TREATMENT

FMS can be treated with low doses of antidepressants, which reduce pain signals from nerves. These drugs include tricyclic antidepressants, selective serotonin reuptake inhibitors (SSRIs), and antidepressants that also affect norepinephrine. However, numerous studies show that exercise may be the most effective prescription for treating FMS. Exercise not only helps to combat deconditioning and relieve pain, it may also act as an antidepressant. Physical therapy and other treatments for pain, including injections of cortisone or local anesthetic at tender points where pain radiates to other areas (trigger points), can reduce discomfort. Women with FMS are also helped by cognitive-behavioral therapy and learning relaxation techniques and other stress-reducing measures.

What Is Chronic Fatigue Syndrome?

While fatigue is a common symptom of many autoimmune diseases, chronic fatigue syndrome (CFS) is a separate disorder. CFS is characterized by prolonged, debilitating fatigue and multiple complaints, including headaches, muscle and joint pain, and difficulties with memory and concentration. It may affect as many as two million Americans, 75 percent of whom are women. The hallmark symptom, profound fatigue, can come on suddenly or gradually. While CFS can feel like the flu, its symptoms linger for at least six months and may even persist for years. While some patients recover fully, most recover partially or recover and relapse.

RISK FACTORS

CFS can occur with autoimmune diseases, but it is not believed to be autoimmune itself. The syndrome may involve as yet unknown interactions between the immune and central nervous systems. Although researchers once thought that elevated antibodies to Epstein-Barr virus indicated a greater likelihood of developing CFS, further research has not shown this to be the case.

WHY YOUR SEX MATTERS

CFS affects women three times more often than men and occurs most often between the ages of 40 and 49, although it can occur at any age. There do not appear to be any risk factors associated with race or socioeconomic class. Some studies have shown, however, that allergies are significantly more common in people with CFS.

SYMPTOMS

CFS symptoms can include fatigue and weakness, muscle and joint aches, headaches, inability to concentrate, allergy-like symptoms, and tender lymph nodes. These symptoms plateau early and may linger or come and go frequently for more than six months. In about a third of cases, CFS develops after a bacterial or viral infection with flu-like symptoms. Other common symptoms include gastrointestinal complaints, skin rashes, dizziness, numbness and tingling in extremities, dry eyes, chills, or night sweats. Some CFS patients also report mild to moderate symptoms of anxiety or depression.

DIAGNOSIS

The criteria set by the CDC for a diagnosis include unexplained fatigue lasting at least six months, associated with a marked reduction in activity and not alleviated by rest. In addition, a person must have four of seven possible symptoms, including memory impairment, tender lymph nodes, muscle pain, pain in multiple joints, new-onset headaches, unrefreshing sleep, and malaise (feeling unwell) lasting more than 24 hours after exertion. If an autoimmune disorder is suspected, lab tests may be done.

TREATMENT

Since the underlying cause (or causes) is unknown, there is no specific treatment for CFS. Exercise (including tai chi, yoga, and stretching), cognitive behavioral therapy, nonsteroidal anti-inflammatory drugs, low-dose tricyclic antidepressants, and medications to combat fatigue have all been shown to be helpful. According to the CDC, other therapies such as massage, acupuncture, chiropractic, and light therapy may also be beneficial. While many claims are made for herbal remedies and dietary supplements, they have not been evaluated in controlled trials.

—RITA BARON-FAUST

A Witness

By Kellie Martin, actor, producer, director, and spokesperson for the American Autoimmune Related Diseases Association

I'm a sister, a daughter, a stepdaughter, a wife, a potential mother, an actress, a woman and a friend. But most of all, I'm a witness to the havoc autoimmune diseases wreak on those they strike, the devastation they level on families and loved ones, and the terrible price we pay for one of the biggest problems associated with autoimmune diseases . . . getting a correct diagnosis in a reasonable amount of time before major damage is done.

I'm a witness to my sister, Heather. Heather and I were always best friends. For 19 years, I watched my little sister grow into a beautiful woman. I was there when she was born, and I was there when she died.

A few days after finishing her sophomore year at college, Heather couldn't get out of bed. The doctor said it was the flu. This doctor was new to my family. He'd never had to handle anything more than a sore throat for us.

When Heather's abdominal pain, fever, nausea, and insomnia got worse, the doctor prescribed an anti-nausea medication. She had a violent allergic reaction to it. She started to convulse. She lost control of her neck muscles, and her eyes rolled back in her head.

That was Heather's first visit to the emergency room, but she was treated only for the convulsions. They didn't deal with anything else . . . her stiff joints, intense muscle pain, fatigue, her inability to eat. She was so weak, she couldn't hold a spoon. Later, she couldn't eat because she had sores in her mouth, and it hurt her too much.

The following night, Heather had to go back to the emergency room for abdominal pain and horrible cramping in her legs. They gave her a painkiller and sent her home. The next day, my mom had to take her back again. They went to the emergency room three times in three days. Then they finally put Heather in the hospital. My mother had to beg the doctor to admit her.

At the hospital, the nurses took blood from Heather three times a day, and each day, a new specialist was called in to see her . . . an internist, an infectious-disease specialist, a hematologist. As a last resort, they gave Heather a test for lupus. But they still thought Heather had an unusual virus, so the doctors discharged her.

My mom and I carried Heather into the house and put her in bed. We knew she'd feel better in her own room with her dog, Sparky. She was relieved to be home, but she got weaker every day. It seemed like she was sent home, not to get better, but because no one knew how to help an incapacitated 19-year old who had been completely healthy two weeks earlier.

The doctor told us he believed that Heather had a virus that was attacking her joints and muscles. My mom asked if the results had come back from the lupus panel. The doctor said that he'd gotten a verbal response that the test was negative. He told us to go home and put a cool cloth on Heather's forehead for her fever. He smiled, patted her on the head and left.

That night, for the first time in her life, Heather crawled into bed with our mother. That was highly unusual; Heather wasn't afraid of anything. She was much more like a big sister, even though I'm three years older. Heather was the rock of our family.

We took Heather to another doctor's office, where her condition was diagnosed two minutes after her examination. The doctor looked really disturbed when he saw Heather's hospital charts and medical history. He ordered a second lupus panel because the first one never appeared in her file. The next day, Heather was admitted to the hospital because of dehydration and kidney failure—both caused by lupus.

We were given a list of treatments that Heather would be getting: steroids, vitamins, fluids. During her first week at the hospital, the blood vessels in Heather's lungs began to burst. Her breathing became more labored. The doctors also found that the lupus had affected Heather's liver and bone marrow. The list of treatments increased to antibiotics and chemotherapy.

Heather liked to be in control, and while her body was so out of control, she wanted to make decisions . . . even though she knew she had no choice. When they said she had to go into the intensive-care unit, it was her choice to go in. But, after that, nothing was her decision, because she was sedated from then on and her body started its descent.

The night before Heather went into ICU, though, she had an amazing burst of energy. It was exactly like the old Heather. She didn't want to rest, she wanted to talk . . . about school, basketball, friends, boyfriends, everything. She sang songs, talked on the phone. That night was such a gift.

I'm still trying to make sense of what happened to Heather. Because of her experience, I've gotten sort of a crash course in lupus and autoimmune disease. I've learned that my stepmother also has lupus, and that one of my best friends from college has just been diagnosed with scleroderma. Those are very close relations in my life.

You may think autoimmune disease hasn't touched your family. I'll bet that all you have to do is scratch the surface, and you'll find it has.

Until we can find a cure for autoimmune diseases, I'm told our best hope is early, prompt diagnosis. Something my sister was not fortunate enough to receive. But, something that is well within our reach.

(Reprinted with permission by Kellie Martin; originally published in *Jane*)

CHAPTER 6

Bone and Muscle Health

As our country's population ages, maintaining the best possible quality of life is essential. Everyone, men and women alike, seeks the goal of the ancient Greeks: "To die young—at the oldest possible age." Bone and muscle health are critical to maintaining an active and rewarding lifestyle for people of all ages. The fitness of bones and joints determines, to a greater extent than any other factor, how well people do as they age.

Bone and muscle disease, and the resulting pain and disability, affect our capacity to perform functions of daily life and maintain independence. The extent of such disability has recently been documented in a major long-term study, the Women's Health and Aging study, which involved some 1,000 women over age 65, all of whom were living in one community at the time the study began in 1992. The study revealed that 32 percent of American women age 70 and older have difficulty performing, or are unable to perform, basic self-care activities. Musculoskeletal pain was the most common self-reported cause of disability among these women; the second and third causes, weakness and balance difficulties, were directly related to musculoskeletal health. Among women who were unable to provide basic self-care, 37–58 percent attributed their difficulties to musculoskeletal pain. Pain stemming from musculoskeletal disorders likewise restricts women's ability to walk, leading to further physical deterioration and loss of independence.

This chapter discusses the most common bone problems in women, including sports injuries, osteoarthritis, and osteoporosis, as well as a section on musculoskeletal health during pregnancy.

Bone Basics

The musculoskeletal system includes bones and the muscles and the connective tissues that bind them together. When this system works properly, there is full-range, painless motion. The human body has 206 bones, whose primary function is to support the body. The ends of the bones are covered with cartilage, which serves as a cushion between the bones. The bones come together at joints, which allow the skeleton to be flexible. The bones are connected at the joints by fibrous tissue called ligaments, and they are lined with a thin membrane, called the synovium. The synovial membrane produces fluid that provides nutrition for the cartilage and lubricates the joint, reducing friction and wear and tear. Muscles, which are responsible for movement, are attached to bones by tendons.

In addition to supporting the body, bones encase and protect certain organs. For example, the rib cage shields the lungs and heart. Bones also serve as a storehouse for fat and for such minerals as calcium and phosphorus. These stored minerals are released into the bloodstream and are carried to all parts of the body as needed. Inside the bones is a cavity filled with soft tissue, called marrow, which produces the red blood cells.

Bone growth is ongoing during the first 25 years of life. During adolescence, a growth spurt changes the skeletal structure. Legs become relatively longer, hips and chest become wider, and the torso lengthens. Men and women both gain 50 percent of their bone mass between the ages of 10 and 20. Most young women have completed their growth by age 14. Between age 20 and 30, bone mass increases only slightly.

Bone, like all other tissue, is made up of cells and mineralized matrix that are constantly dying and being renewed. The process by which old bone breaks down and is replaced by new bone is called remodeling.

Heredity has the strongest role in determining bone mass and the rate of bone formation and loss. However, bone growth and loss are also affected by lifestyle factors, the most important of which are diet and exercise. Taking measures to ensure bone health needs to start in childhood; individuals who have calcium deficiency during their adolescence may not achieve their optimal bone mass. Unfortunately, as many as 85 percent of adolescent girls, compared with just 43 percent of adolescent boys, consume less than the recommended daily allowance of calcium. Estimates of daily calcium consumption by adult women are even lower.

Exercise is also essential. Recent research suggests that exercise may be even more important than dietary calcium in helping children reach the highest possible peak bone mass. For example, researchers in Canada reported that girls who engaged in jumping, a high-impact exercise, for 10 minutes a day, three times a week, over a 20-month period, had approximately 3–4 percent more bone mass than did girls who did not do the exercise. Although these differences seem minor, small differences in bone density can make a significant difference in reducing fracture risk. Girls in both study groups were similar in terms of body composition, size, overall physical activity, and calcium intake.

The bones in the adult female skeleton are the same shape as the bones in the male skeleton; the sole difference is that women's bones are generally smaller. One exception is the pelvis. A woman's pelvis is usually broader than a man's and has a larger space in the middle. This shape allows for the head of a baby to pass from the uterus through the pelvis during childbirth.

Despite these similarities, the factors that affect bone health are different for men than for women. Women are nearly twice as likely to develop osteoarthritis and osteoporosis as are men. Despite ongoing bone remodeling, once an individual reaches peak bone mass, no additional bone growth occurs. As a person ages, more bone is broken down than is replaced. The resulting loss in bone mass is a normal occurrence for both men and women. The rates of loss, however, differ. Women, for example, have a sharp drop in bone mass as a result of the hormonal changes associated with menopause; however, after age 60, women's rate of bone loss is identical to that of men. By age 80, both men and women have experienced a significant decrease in total bone mass. Attaining maximum peak bone mass is extremely important, because this mass is the "capital" in an individual's bone bank.

What Is Osteoporosis?

Osteoporosis is characterized by progressive bone loss and an increased risk of fracture. It literally means "porous bone." Because the changes in bone are at the microscopic level, and the disease initially produces no pain or other outward symptoms, osteoporosis often goes unnoticed for years. As a person ages, it causes loss of height and, in some cases, a dowager's hump, or rounded back. Osteoporosis affects some 28 million Americans. The term, bone mineral density, or BMD, is used to describe bone strength. The lower the BMD, the more porous and weaker the bone.

CAUSES AND RISK FACTORS

Although the exact cause of osteoporosis is not known, a number of factors do increase the risk. There is clear evidence of a genetic predisposition to osteoporosis. For women, excessive loss of bone occurs when certain hormones essential for bone formation and maintenance decrease substantially following menopause. If the body does not receive enough dietary calcium to meet its needs, it takes calcium from the bones to make up the difference. In premenopausal women, the sex hormone, estrogen, protects bones from being robbed of calcium by other demands of the body and helps produce and maintain collagen, an important component of bone. Once estrogen levels are depleted, it can no longer play this protective role. Another hormone, calcitonin, may facilitate the uptake of calcium from the blood into the bone and, at the same time, inhibit the loss of calcium from the bone. Other known risk factors include being underweight, tobacco use, excessive alcohol use, and certain medications.

On the basis of criteria set forth by a World Health Organization (WHO) expert panel, 54 percent of postmenopausal white women in northern parts of the United States have osteopenia, or low bone mass, and an additional 30 percent have osteoporosis in at least one skeletal site. Osteoporosis occurs in all racial groups. For example, 13–16 percent of Hispanic women have osteoporosis; as many as 49 percent of Mexican American women age 50 and older have low bone density; about 10 percent of African American women over age 50 have osteoporosis; and an additional 30 percent have low bone density. Between 80 and 95 percent of all fractures experienced by African American women over age 64 are related to osteoporosis.

Diagnosis

Osteoporosis is diagnosed on the basis of a medical history and physical examination, skeletal x-rays, bone densitometry, and laboratory tests. Bone densitometry is an x-ray technique that compares a patient's BMD to the BMD that someone of the patient's sex and ethnicity should have reached at about age 20–25, when bone density is at its highest. Doctors use several types of bone densitometry to detect bone loss in different areas of the body. Dual beam x-ray absorptiometry (DEXA) is one of the most accurate methods, but other techniques can also identify osteoporosis. These include single photon absorptiometry, quantitative computed tomography (CT), and ultrasound.

WHO has defined osteoporosis as bone mineral density measuring two and one-half standard deviations or more below the young adult mean. The test is often performed in women at the time of menopause. Bone densitometry is used not only to diagnose osteoporosis but also to monitor the effects of treatment.

Prevention

Once bone mass is lost, it is difficult or impossible to replace. For this reason, preventing osteoporosis is vital. It is important to do everything you can to build peak bone mass by age 25 and then to ensure that the inevitable loss of bone occurs as slowly as possible. Prevention entails a variety of measures, including the following:

♦ Monitoring calcium and vitamin D intake. Calcium requirements depend primarily on age. The Institute of Medicine offers the following guidelines for daily calcium intake:

- children from 4 to 8: 800 milligrams (mg)
- children from 9 to 18: 1,300 mg
- men and women age 19–50 (including pregnant and nursing women): 1,000 mg
- pregnant and nursing women under age 18: 1,300 mg
- men and women over age 50: 1,200 mg

Dairy products, especially those low in fat such as skim milk and low-fat yogurt, are an excellent source of calcium. An eight-ounce glass of skim milk provides 300 mg of calcium and only 90 calories.

Women who are lactose intolerant and vegans, as well as anyone who wants a varied, calcium-rich diet, can turn to dark-green leafy vegetables such as kale, broccoli, and mustard greens; soy milk and other soy products such as tofu; salmon (with edible bones); and calcium-fortified fruit juices and breakfast cereals.

Vitamin D is essential for calcium absorption and for muscle strength. There is, moreover, increasing evidence that a vitamin D deficiency may increase fracture risk. The skin manufactures vitamin D when exposed to the sun; however, widespread use of sunscreens has reduced the role of natural light in preventing vitamin D deficiency. In addition, older people who are rarely out of doors need a supplemental source of this essential vitamin.

♦ Overall nutrition. A high protein intake has been shown to be associated with a lower risk of hip fracture in men and women between age 50 and 69, although not in older individuals. Contrary to earlier reports, there is no conclusive evidence that the carbonation in beverages has an adverse effect on bone health. It is possible, however, that the caffeine in some carbonated beverages increases calcium excretion. Drinking large quantities of carbonated beverages rather than milk also deprives the body of a major calcium source. Finally, recent research has indicated that vitamin B12 may be an important link in preventing osteoporosis. Good sources of this vitamin include low-fat dairy products, fish and lean meat, and eggs. The ability to absorb B12 from food decreases with age, so a vitamin supplement may be advisable for older women.

♦ Exercising. Women of all ages should engage in regular weight-bearing exercise. Walking is one of the best methods ways to maintain bone strength. Other weight-bearing exercises include jogging, hiking, tennis, bicycling, dancing, aquatic exercises (but not swimming), and weight training. Choose an exercise that combines movement with impact on the limbs. Start exercising slowly, especially if you have been inactive. Because falls are the most common cause of fractures, do some balance activities to reduce your risk. The benefits of tai chi in particular have been documented. Consult your doctor before beginning any exercise program.

♦ Cutting out smoking and reducing alcohol intake. Eliminate smoking and excessive alcohol use; these cause bone loss and increase your risk of a fracture.

TREATMENT

Controlled trials involving thousands of women have shown that a number of medications are effective in reducing bone fracture risk in women with osteoporosis. Treatment is often a team effort involving a family physician or internist, an orthopaedic surgeon, a gynecologist, and an endocrinologist.

Hormone therapy (HT) is often recommended to prevent bone loss and reduce fracture risk in postmenopausal women. This therapy may consist of estrogen alone (ERT) or estrogen plus progestin. Such therapy can be effective; for example, a study done as part of the Women's Health Initiative (WHI) showed a 34 percent reduction in hip fracture risk among women taking estrogen plus progestin, compared with women of a similar age who were not taking this drug. Because there also was an increased incidence of breast cancer and various types of circulatory problems found in women in the WHI study, hormone therapy is no longer the agent of choice for prevention of osteoporotic fractures in women over age 50. If you had been taking HT and stopped or are at menopause and do not intend to start HT, you need to talk with your doctor about alternatives to prevent bone loss.

New antiestrogens known as specific estrogen receptor modulators (SERMs) have been introduced. A three-year trial of the SERM, raloxefine, showed that it was associated with a 2–4 percent increase in spine and hip bone mineral density, a 30 percent reduction in the incidence of new vertebral fractures in women with existing vertebral fractures, and a 50 percent decrease in new vertebral fractures in women without pre-existing fractures.

Bisphosphonates are currently the drugs of choice to prevent bone loss after fracture. These products, called antiresorptive drugs, slow the rate of bone loss and increase bone density. They include alendronate, risedronate, and etidronate. Etidronate was among the first bisphosphonates to be developed. Although it increases bone mineral density slightly and reduces vertebral fracture risk somewhat, it may actually impair bone mineralization over the long term. For this reason, it is not a first-line agent for treatment of fragility fractures. Alendronate and risedronate have both shown convincing evidence of effectiveness. Women in clinical trials with these two medications have shown BMD increases of 3–10 percent and a reduced risk of vertebral fracture of up to 50 percent. In addition, these are the only two therapies that have been shown to reduce hip fracture risk. The older bisphosphonates are taken once a week. The U.S. Food and Drug Administration (FDA) has recently approved another bisphosphonate, ibandronate, which can be taken in a single, monthly dose. Ibandronate has been shown to reduce spinal fracture risk by up to 50 percent and to increase bone density at all sites, but no hip fracture data are yet available.

The only FDA-approved product that builds new bone, as opposed to slowing the rate of bone loss by limiting bone breakdown, is teriparatide, which is given as an injection to patients with a history of fractures or those who are at high risk for them.

Calcitonin, available in oral or nasal spray form, is an older medication used to decrease bone loss. Taken alone, calcitonin is not nearly as effective as bisphosphonates, SERMs, or hormone therapy.

FRAGILITY FRACTURES

Osteoporosis is often called a silent disease because it has no symptoms in its early stage. In fact, bone fracture is often the first indication of osteoporosis. Fractures caused by osteoporosis are typically called fragility fractures—fractures that occur as a result of a relatively minor injury or blow, such as falling from standing height or less. The most common sites of fragility fractures are the vertebrae, hip, wrist, and shoulder. Osteoporosis is a contributing factor in as many as 1.5 million fractures each year.

Fractures of the hip are among the most debilitating and costly consequences of osteoporosis. Among those at greatest risk for hip fracture are women over age 65. Slender, small-boned women may be more prone to such fractures than are large, heavy-boned women. A family history of fractures in later life is another risk factor. Women who have a low dietary intake of calcium, who smoke, or who drink alcohol excessively are also at higher risk, as are those with arthritis or poor balance, coordination, and eyesight.

In women over age 75, the most commonly performed surgery is repair of a hip fracture. And, although modern orthopaedic surgical techniques and care can assist in healing of the bone, most hip fracture patients require extended periods of rehabilitation. Around one of very four people who have an osteoporotic hip fracture need long-term nursing home care, and virtually all these patients need extended assistance from their families or home care providers. Walking aids may be necessary for several months after the injury, and many patients permanently require canes or walkers to move around their homes or outdoors.

Prevention of hip fractures is far less costly, in both financial and human terms, than treatment after the bone is broken. A diet high in calcium and vitamin D, regular exercise, and the correct medications can help prevent weak bones and the possibility of hip fracture.

Paying attention to home safety is also important, especially for older women. Most of these injuries occur as a result of a fall, and most falls occur in the home. AARP recommends taking the following measures to "fall-proof" your surroundings:

+ Remove the clutter, pick up papers or clothes from the ground, move garbage bins under cabinets.
+ Keep living areas well lit.
+ Be aware of your surroundings. Know where your furniture is placed and any stairs or change of entry levels.
+ Clean up any spills.
+ Be sure that your furniture is stable.
+ Use nonslip mats in the bathtub and on shower floors.
+ Secure area rugs with double-faced tape, tacks, or slip-resistant backing.

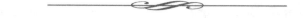

Get the Facts: Menopause Is Nothing to Fear

By Cheryl Ladd, actor, singer, humanitarian, and author of *Token Chick: A Woman's Guide to Golfing with the Boys*

At 46, menopause was the last thing on my mind. I felt young, healthy, and vibrant. When I began experiencing unfamiliar symptoms, including night sweats and mood swings, it never occurred to me that I might be entering menopause.

I did a little research and found out that my symptoms might be related to estrogen loss. I began to work through the first phase of my denial—it was time to admit I was experiencing the onset of menopause.

Even when I started to entertain the notion that these changes might signal menopause, I denied that I needed to speak with someone about it. After all, I was doing everything right. I ate well, exercised, and took a daily calcium supplement—all the things I was supposed to do to protect my health.

I didn't realize that some serious health conditions for women can come on silently, without any noticeable symptoms at all. A woman may have no idea, for instance, that she's developed high blood pressure or elevated cholesterol until a heart attack occurs. Likewise, osteoporosis may not reveal itself until a fracture occurs from a simple fall.

I considered myself informed on health matters and thought I could handle menopause without too much trouble. Only later did I realize that this was another form of denial.

Eventually, my mood swings got to a point that my husband asked me to please speak with the doctor. I was always such an upbeat person, yet I had begun spending time in bed, weeping. It was so unlike me.

People have said menopausal symptoms are in a woman's head, but I know they're real. My doctor helped me understand what was happening to me and what it meant; he explained the various risks posed by estrogen loss. He gave me the information I needed to work with him to develop a health plan that is right for me. When you have this kind of discussion with your doctor, you become part of the team.

When we first talked, my doctor suggested I take a bone mineral density test. I'd been a gymnast and a dancer and had stayed physically active my whole life. I felt my bones were protected by my healthy lifestyle. I was sure I had the bones of a 20-year-old. Imagine my surprise when the results came in that I had already experienced early menopausal bone loss in my left hip!

As a petite, fair woman I knew I was at risk for osteoporosis, but I was not aware that the estrogen loss of menopause increased that risk.

I found menopause to be an unnerving, confusing time and was dismayed at the lack of clear, straightforward information available until I started speaking with my doctor. With information like I received from my doctor, all women can celebrate menopause as the transition to a new phase in their lives and make it a less fearful time, no matter what treatment option they decide is right for them.

(Reprinted with permission by Cheryl Ladd)

What Is Osteoarthritis?

Osteoarthritis (OA) develops when the cartilage covering the bone ends gradually wears away. For these reasons, OA is sometimes called "wear-and-tear" disease. In many cases, bone growths, or spurs, develop in the joints. Athletes may develop OA at a young age, particularly due to injuries of the knee that subsequently promote wear and tear of the joint. In OA, the joints become inflamed and swollen, and continued use of the joint is painful. Osteoarthritis is often more painful in weight-bearing joints such as the knee, hip, and spine than it is in the wrist, elbow, and shoulder joints.

Arthritis affects each person differently. It may progress quickly or slowly. Occasionally, the disease progresses rapidly to the point where the patient is disabled within a few years of the onset of joint pain. Far more commonly, however, the disease progresses over years or even decades. One national survey found that 59 percent of people in the United States age 65 years or older reported arthritis or chronic joint symptoms. Osteoarthritis is significantly more prevalent in women than in men, and the prevalence in all joints and all populations increases dramatically with age.

RISK FACTORS

Osteoarthritis has a strong genetic connection, but there are other risk factors as well that can increase one's risk of developing OA. One of them, as noted above, is female sex. Others include:

- ◆ Obesity. Generally, the more weight a person carries, the greater the pressure is on weight-bearing joints (hip and knee) of the body.
- ◆ Aging. As people age, cartilage normally is less able to repair itself.
- ◆ Nutrition. Calcium and vitamins C and D are needed to build strong bones. Investigators are researching whether an insufficiency of these vitamins may contribute to developing OA in later life.
- ◆ Presence of other diseases and hereditary conditions that affect bones and connective tissues. These include unusual medical problems such as Ehlers-Danlos syndrome, bone dysplasia, and Charcot's joint.
- ◆ Injury or deformity in a joint. There is an increased risk of developing OA in a joint that is not properly aligned or in one that has been injured.

◆ Occupational factors. People who engage in repetitive tasks may overwork their joints and overtire muscles that protect the joints, which increases the risk of OA in that joint.

SYMPTOMS

The following symptoms may signal osteoarthritis:

◆ steady or occasional pain in a joint,
◆ joint stiffness on getting up in the morning or after sitting for a long time,
◆ swelling or tenderness in a joint, and
◆ a feeling of crunching or the sound of bone rubbing on bone.

DIAGNOSIS

Diagnosing osteoarthritis typically includes evaluating symptoms, a physical examination, and x-rays, which show the extent of damage to the joint. Blood tests and other laboratory tests may help determine the type of arthritis.

TREATMENT

Most women with arthritis can continue to perform normal activities of daily living. Exercise programs, anti-inflammatory drugs, and weight reduction for those who are obese can help reduce pain and stiffness and improve function. The goals of treatment are to provide pain relief, increase motion, and improve strength, thus slowing the progression of the arthritis. Treatment includes exercise, medications, surgery, and using assistive devices:

◆ Exercise. Exercise has many benefits. It can help keep your body strong and limber, expand your range of motion, and help control weight. Exercises that many women find helpful include strength exercise, aerobic exercises, range-of-motion activities, and neck and back strength exercises. Moderate exercise such as regular walking can keep the body supple and reduce joint pain and stiffness. Many people also find yoga helpful. Check with your doctor or physical therapist to design a plan that helps strength your body without taxing it too much.
◆ Medications. A wide range of medications can be used to relieve the pain and inflammation of arthritis. Some are available over the counter; others require a doctor's prescription. Each medication has advantages and disadvantages, and it is important to

work with your doctor and health care team to choose the one that is best for you.

Acetaminophen may be used to control mild-to-moderate arthritis pain and is often the first medication recommended. It does not relieve the inflammation, however. Instructions on the medication bottle need to be followed to avoid problems. People who drink alcohol should discuss the use of acetominophen with their physician, as they may be at higher risk for liver damage.

A large class of drugs, called nonsteroidal anti-inflammatory drugs (NSAIDs) is widely used to relieve both the pain and inflammation of arthritis. The older NSAIDs include aspirin, ibuprofen, and naproxen. These drugs, available over the counter, are known to produce gastrointestinal side effects. In some cases, these side effects are limited to minor discomfort, but they may include gastric bleeding. It is important not to exceed the recommended doses and to take these drugs with food or milk to minimize their risk of side effects. These drugs should not be taken for more than 10 days, unless advised to do so by a doctor. If one NSAID causes stomach irritation, you might switch to another one. Another possibility is to combine the NSAID with a drug that protects your stomach lining.

Introduced in 1998, COX-II inhibitors are the newest class of NSAIDs. Compared with older NSAIDs, their chief advantage is that they do not produce gastrointestinal (GI) side effects. They are more expensive, but there is no evidence that they reduce pain and inflammation any better than over-the-counter (OTC) products, and they became the subject of considerable concern in late 2004 and early 2005, prompting the FDA to recommend limiting the use of both of these drugs. The controversy over COX-II inhibitors drew wide media attention and caused great confusion among patients. The best course of action is to work with your physician to determine what drug works best—and is safest—for you.

The current concern over drug safety has prompted many patients to explore other treatment options. For example, liquid cortisone, injected into the joint, may help relieve pain and swelling temporarily. Topical pain relievers are also an option; some contain salicylate, a chemical related to aspirin. Another class of products are the counterirritants, which cause hot or cold feelings that temporarily mask the pain. Finally, some products contain capsaicin, the active ingredient in hot peppers; they work by interfering in the process by which the nerves send pain signals to the brain.

For persons with moderate arthritis of the knee, injections of material to improve the joint fluid may improve pain. These materials, termed hyaluronic acid supplements, are injected into the knee once a week for three to six weeks. These injections are considered a second line of treatment after oral medications. If an individual's pain is not improved with medication such as acetominophen or an NSAID, or if they cannot tolerate NSAIDs because of GI problems, they may be a candidate for a series of hyaluronic acid injections.

Well before the risks associated with COX-II inhibitors came to public attention, many people were turning to alternative therapies for relief of arthritis. One such therapy is acupuncture, which has been shown to reduce knee pain and improve function for people with osteoarthritis when used in conjunction with medical therapy. In one study, people who received acupuncture (the study group) had a 40 percent decrease in pain and a nearly 40 percent increase in function, compared to people who received sham treatment (the control group).

Many people with osteoarthritis find relief by taking glucosamine and chondroitin, two natural substances sold as dietary supplements. Laboratory tests have found that both of these products can make the cartilage healthier and perhaps even repair it. Large-scale trials of effectiveness are ongoing.

If you are interested in using these or any other complementary medicines, be sure to talk with your physician first. Herbal supplements may interact with prescription or OTC medications. For example, glucosamine is a type of sugar, and if you take it and have diabetes, you will need to monitor your blood sugar levels more frequently. Additionally, if you are allergic to shellfish, you need to be aware that glucosamine is extracted from shellfish. Chondroitin may interact with blood-thinning drugs.

The effectiveness of many other alternative approaches to arthritis pain relief, including wearing magnetic bracelets, has not been proved in scientific studies.

♦ Assistive Devices. Canes, crutches, walkers, or splints may help relieve the stress and strain on arthritic joints. Learning how to perform daily activities in a way that is less stressful to painful joints also may be helpful. Certain exercises and physical therapy (such as heat treatments) may decrease stiffness and strengthen the muscles around the joint.

♦ Surgery. When medicines, injections, and other therapies are no longer effective in controlling pain and restoring function, surgery may be appropriate. Different types of operations that may help a person with arthritis include:

- operations to realign a joint (osteotomy) and take stress off the worn region of the joint;
- fusing the joint (arthrodesis) to make it stiff and unable to move (and thus pain-free); and
- joint replacement (arthroplasty). Joint-replacement surgery can often provide dramatic pain relief and restore joint function in persons with severe OA. During this procedure, an orthopaedic surgeon replaces the diseased joint with an implant made of metal, ceramic, plastic, or a combination of these. Like a healthy joint, the artificial one also has smooth, gliding surfaces. A total joint replacement can usually enable a person with severe arthritis in the hip or the knee to walk without pain or stiffness. The physician and patient choose the type of surgery by taking into account the type of arthritis, its severity, and the patient's physical condition.

The decision about when to replace a diseased joint is also based on a number of factors, including the degree of disability, lifestyle, age, and the patient's ability to withstand the risks of surgery. Many patients try to postpone surgery as long as they can, and for many years, physicians, too, recommended delaying the procedure in patients over age 60. There is, however, increasing evidence that waiting too long can make the procedure more complicated, because more bone and cartilage may already be worn away. Increased age puts a patient at greater risk after surgery, and a patient who has been debilitated by arthritis for an extended period may find recovery more prolonged. Reflecting this growing body of evidence, in 2004, a National Institutes of Health consensus panel reported its conclusion that people with less pain and better function before knee replacement do better following surgery than those who were more impaired before surgery.

Joint replacement surgery of the hip and knee may now be done with less invasive techniques. These procedures focus on less injury to the skin, muscles, and tendons and may promote faster recovery. Evidence to date shows no clear difference in outcomes one year following surgery between patients whose surgery is performed using a minimally invasive versus traditional approach. It may be more difficult to put in the implants through a smaller incision, and this may compromise how long the joint lasts. Individuals considering joint replacement surgery should discuss the surgical options with their surgeon.

Sport and Exercise Injuries

Exercise is essential for development and maintenance of bone mass, yet few Americans get the amount of exercise recommended by the U.S. Surgeon General, and inactivity is more than twice as common among women as it is among men. Women of color, women older than age 40, and women without a college education have the lowest levels of participation in leisure-time physical activity.

But there is also some good news: Although women in general, and particularly older women, do not get sufficient exercise, the number of girls and women participating in organized sports has been on the rise. Participation of women in sports has increased dramatically since Title IX of the Education Amendments Act was enacted in 1972. In addition, job opportunities that require high levels of fitness have been opened to women. Women now account for more than one-third of all college athletes and recent United States Olympic team members.

WHAT IS ARTHROSCOPIC SURGERY?

The term, arthroscopic surgery, probably appears more in the sports section of your daily newspaper than in the health section, because many athletes undergo these procedures. The word comes from the Greek root words, *arthron* and *skopos*; in the literal translation "to look at the joint." During arthroscopic surgery, the orthopaedist inserts a long, thin metal tube into a small incision made near the joint. Inside the tube are coated-glass fibers and a series of magnifying lenses. The fibers carry light into the joint and relay a magnified image that is projected onto a video screen or that can be viewed through an eyepiece. One major advantage of arthroscopic surgery is that it requires only a small incision. Before this technique, surgeons had to make large incisions, and wound healing took much longer. Arthroscopic surgery is performed on an outpatient basis under local anesthesia; it is also used for diagnosis.

WHY YOUR SEX MATTERS

Research on sports injuries indicates that injury patterns generally are sport-specific, not sex or gender-specific. There are exceptions, however. Knee injuries and stress fractures of the vertebrae, pelvis, and hip and pelvic floor dysfunction, for example, affect women in greater proportion than they do men.

The reasons for differences in injury rate are the topic of ongoing research. There are distinct differences between the male and female physique that may be at the base of some of the differences in injury rates. For example, women have more body fat and less lean body mass than men; this is a natural consequence of increased estrogen in women and androgen in men. Although men and women have comparable lower-body strength, females have less upper-body strength, even after undergoing training and adjusting for differences in weight and size. Among the most significant male/female differences from the point of view of injury is different alignment of the lower body; women have a wider pelvis, their knees are in greater valgus (knock-kneed position), and their feet are more pronated (rolled in), all factors that may contribute to the disproportionate number of knee injuries in women. Issues of particular concern relating to women's musculoskeletal health and sports and exercise are highlighted below.

WHAT IS FEMALE ATHLETIC TRIAD?

Far too often, female athletes mistakenly think that a childlike body and extremely low weight are essential for excellence in sports. Given this widespread belief, it is not surprising that a high proportion of female athletes suffer from eating disorders such as anorexia and bulimia. Poor eating habits, in turn, lead to a group of health problems that has been called the female athletic triad:

♦ abnormal eating habits, such as crash diets and binge eating;
♦ menstrual dysfunction (athletic amenorrhea) caused by poor nutrition, low calorie intake, high energy demands, physical and emotional stress, or a low percentage of body fat; and
♦ osteoporosis: the low estrogen levels associated with amenorrhea interrupt the body's bone-building processes and weaken the skeleton, making the bones more likely to break. A woman with such bone deterioration during adolescence may never achieve the peak bone mass that she otherwise would.

At greatest risk are women in demanding sports that also reward physical appearance (for example, figure skating, gymnastics) or improved performance (for example, distance running, rowing). The condition is disturbingly common: up to 20 percent of vigorously exercising women, and half of all female professional ballet dancers, may have amenorrhea. Fashion trends and advertising often encourage all women to try to reach unhealthy weight levels. Some female athletes suffer from low self-esteem or depression and may focus on weight loss because they think they are heavier than they actually are. Others feel pressure to lose weight from athletic coaches or parents.

The condition may be difficult to diagnose; one of the early symptoms may be a stress fracture. The best treatment for this syndrome is prevention. Girls or women who already have the condition may benefit from counseling as well as the guidance of a physician and dietitian. Parents and coaches should be on the alert for symptoms of the triad and know how to intervene.

Knee Injuries

The knee is the most commonly injured joint, and the spectrum of such injuries ranges from mild (runner's knee and tendonitis) to severe. Among the most common serious knee injuries is damage to the anterior cruciate ligament (ACL), which keeps the knee stabilized and prevents the leg bone from sliding forward beneath the thigh bone during twisting or pivoting movements. ACL injuries occur most often in people engaging in such sports as soccer, basketball, and volleyball, which require fast stops, starts, and turns. ACL injury rates are two to eight times higher in women than they are in men participating in the same sports. For example, the rate of ACL injuries among female soccer players is four times that of their male counterparts.

Why Your Sex Matters
One reason for the discrepancy is anatomy. In addition, females place more emphasis on their quadriceps muscles than males do, which may partly explain the increased risk of ACL injuries in women. Women also tend to land on a flat foot rather than on their toes, and with less hip and knee flexion, than men do. This can also contribute to the increased injury rate in women. Differences in training, neuromuscular response, and hormonal response may also play a role.

Treatment
Treatment of ACL injuries requires rehabilitation to restore range of motion, strength, and balance. Women who do not participate in sports that require jumping, cutting, or pivoting, or women who plan to stop competing, may decide to follow a nonsurgical approach. However, women who intend to continue in sports, particularly those that involve jumping, cutting, or pivoting, are typically offered surgery. The goal of surgery is to improve stability and reduce the risk of future injuries. Research demonstrates similar outcomes in male and female patients. Following surgery, patients must undergo a lengthy rehabilitation program to restore the joint's strength and mobility, and they may have to

wear a knee brace. It may be six months to a year before they can return to their sport.

Prevention
To prevent ACL injuries women should try to:

- land safely, on the ball of the foot, then rock back to the middle to gain balance;
- pivot in a crouched, rather than an upright, position;
- stop gently, using three little steps, rather than one big one; and
- do routine exercises to strengthen the legs and keep the knee joint flexible, such as leg presses and squats.

SHOULDER AND ARM INJURIES

Shoulder and arm injuries are common in athletes of both sexes, and the proportions of men and women who sustain such injuries do not differ as much as do the proportions of athletes developing leg injuries. Rotator cuff tears are a common source of shoulder pain, especially in women over age 40. Such tears may be the result of a single, traumatic event, although they are more commonly associated simply with overuse over the years. At particular risk are women who participate in sports such as baseball, tennis, weight lifting, and rowing. Shoulder dislocation may occur when the shoulder is struck by a strong force that pulls the arm in an extreme direction, for example, during a fall or in sports.

STRESS FRACTURE

A stress fracture, sometimes called a fatigue fracture, is a tiny crack or cracks in the surface of the bone. It is caused by repetitive stress, such as that associated with frequent bending. The most common sites for stress fractures are in the lower leg and foot. Stress fractures in one of the bones of the back, a condition called spondylosis, is a common cause of back pain in athletes. It occurs most often in sports that are dominated by females, such as dancing and figure skating, but it is also common among gymnasts. Females may be more at risk for a stress injury to the bone because of their hormones and anatomic and sex factors. Treatment options include bracing and surgery.

FROZEN SHOULDER

Frozen shoulder is the common name for adhesive capsulitis, a condition characterized by shoulder pain and a gradually reduced range of motion.

Approximately 70 percent of patients with adhesive capsulitis are women, and 20–30 percent of those affected subsequently have adhesive capsulitis develop in the opposite shoulder as well. It is most common in people between ages 40 and 60. Risk factors include diabetes, thyroid disease, trauma, stroke, prolonged immobilization, and heart attack.

The cause of frozen shoulder is not known. It develops when an inflammation leads to a tightening of the space between the capsule and ball of the arm bone, where it fits into the shoulder joint. The disease has three stages: freezing, frozen, and thawing. The freezing stage lasts between 10 and 36 weeks and is characterized by the most severe pain. The frozen stage lasts between four and 12 months. Pain decreases gradually, but range of motion generally remains limited. The thawing phase is marked by a gradual return of motion and may last as little as 12 months or for years.

Treatment generally involves rest, use of anti-inflammatory agents such as ibuprofen to relieve pain, and gentle range-of-motion exercises. Corticosteroid injections or muscle relaxants may be prescribed for patients with severe pain. Surgery is recommended only if the condition does not resolve after several months.

Carpal Tunnel Syndrome

The carpal tunnel is a narrow passageway of ligaments and bones at the base of the hand. Inside the carpal tunnel is the median nerve, which carries nerve impulses to the thumb and fingers. If the carpal tunnel becomes irritated, it may swell and press on the median nerve. The result may be pain, weakness, numbness, or a burning or tingling sensation in the hand and wrist, and these sensations may radiate up the arm. This condition is called carpal tunnel syndrome (CTS). The dominant hand usually develops the condition first.

Why Your Sex Matters
Women are three times as likely to develop CTS as are men. One reason may be that their carpal tunnels are narrower. Although young women are especially prone to CTS during pregnancy, the condition is generally more prevalent in middle-age and older women People who engage in repetitive, assembly line-type tasks are more likely to develop CTS than are people who do not do such work. Heavy use of a computer keyboard does not necessarily increase a person's risk of CTS.

Treatment involves resting the affected hand and wrist for at least two weeks and using NSAIDs such as aspirin or ibuprofen. CTS surgery is recommended only if symptoms continue for at least six months.

There are no clear-cut rules for preventing CTS. Avoiding repetitive stress, taking breaks, and making adjustments in the work environment may help.

FOOT PROBLEMS

Some foot problems affect women more than they do men; one reason is that narrow, high-heel shoes worn by some women can push together the toes and irritate the nerves of the feet.

Morton's neuroma is a thickening of the nerve between two toes. It is caused by repeated irritation, and usually only one foot is affected. The key symptom is pain in the ball of the foot that may radiate to the toes. The pain gets worse during physical activity and resolves when the shoes are removed or the foot is massaged. Customized shoe inserts may help relieve this problem.

A bunion is a bony knob that forms at the base of the big toe. It is far and away a woman's condition—only one patient in 10 is a man. A bunionette is a similar protrusion on the opposite side of the foot, near the base of the little toe. Although bunions tend to run in families, their main cause is tight shoes, particularly high heels that force the toes forward. Left untreated, the bunion may force the big toe inward, moving weight to the inner part of the foot and causing the arch to collapse. Arthritis of the toe may develop. Surgery is recommended if simpler measures, such as wearing appropriate shoes and using arch supports, are not effective.

Musculoskeletal Health during Pregnancy

The changes in a woman's body that accompany pregnancy, coupled with the strain of carrying a growing fetus, put stress on a woman's musculoskeletal system. Back and wrist pain and leg cramps are among the most frequent complaints.

More than two of every three pregnant women complain of back pain at some point. Low back pain rates increase with advancing maternal age; such pain is also higher in women who have already given birth and in those who have had such back pain during previous pregnancies. As the uterus enlarges, it moves the body's center of gravity forward, causing an increase in the normal curve of the spine. This puts stress on the joints and ligaments of the lower back. In addition, hormones produced during pregnancy cause the pelvic ligaments to loosen and the joints to open. This, too, can cause pain. Back pain can be particularly severe if a woman gains more than the recommended amount of weight during pregnancy.

To avoid pain, women should avoid standing, wear comfortable shoes, sit in chairs that provide firm support, and sleep on a firm mattress. Changing position often can also help, as can scheduled periods of rest, with the feet elevated to flex the hips and decrease spinal curving. Sitting pelvic-tilt exercises and aquatic exercises have been shown to decrease pain.

Wrist pain may occur because of swelling, leading to CTS. Another condition that may involve this area is de Quervain's tenosynovitis, an inflammation of the tendons of the back of the wrist. Leg cramps, particularly at night, are another common symptom during pregnancy. Such cramps may sometimes signal a calcium deficiency—a possibility of which your doctor should be aware.

Exercise during Pregnancy

Provided that appropriate precautions are taken, exercising during pregnancy has many health benefits for women. Those who engaged in regular exercise before becoming pregnant should continue to do so. For women who have not yet adopted a regular exercise routine, this may be an excellent time to begin. In addition to providing musculoskeletal benefits, regular exercise is beneficial for the cardiovascular system and helps prevent excessive weight gain. Both the mother and fetus benefit from exercise during pregnancy. Women who exercise regularly during pregnancy may have shorter labors and less need for surgical delivery. There is also evidence that beginning a moderate plan of weight-bearing exercise early in pregnancy can enhance fetal growth.

The American College of Obstetricians and Gynecologists (ACOG) recommends that all women of childbearing age exercise moderately for 30 minutes on most days. While recognizing the overall benefits of a well-planned exercise regime that is monitored by a physician, ACOG also cautions that vigorous exercise should be avoided, or at least strongly curtailed, in certain women. For example, women at high risk for preterm delivery or who have had second- or third-trimester bleeding should not engage in aerobic exercise, while women who are excessively obese, have poorly controlled hypertension, or are heavy smokers, among other factors, should engage in vigorous exercise only to a limited extent. Each pregnant woman's overall health, as well as each potential exercise activity, should be evaluated for its benefits and risks.

Guidelines for Exercise during Pregnancy

♦ Do not exercise on your back after the first trimester of pregnancy, and avoid prolonged periods of motionless standing.

- Stop if you become fatigued; do not exercise to exhaustion.
- As your pregnancy progresses, modify your exercise activity; for example, you may switch from weight-bearing exercise such as jogging to nonweight-bearing exercise such as using a stationary bicycle or swimming.
- Make sure you drink enough water and wear appropriate clothing so that you do not become too hot. Make sure that the room in which you exercise is an appropriate temperature and has adequate air circulation.
- Be aware of nutritional requirements. Pregnancy alone requires an extra 300 calories a day; additional caloric intake depends on the length and intensity of your exercise routine.

Conclusion

A strong musculoskeletal system is key to a healthy, active life for all girls and women—for a toddler who has just learned to walk, the adolescent girl who is captain of her school soccer team, the 50-year-old grandmother who is nearing menopause, and the 85-year-old great-grandmother who wants to maintain her independence as long as she can.

Some aspects of musculoskeletal health depend on heredity and are beyond an individual woman's control. Moreover, innate differences in biology mean that a greater proportion of women than men develop some musculoskeletal disorders. Nonetheless, women can do many things to ensure optimal bone health; two of the most important are proper diet and exercise. Once a bone disease develops, a woman can, with the help of her primary care physician, orthopaedist, and other members of the health team, take steps to ease pain, prevent progression of disease, and maintain an active lifestyle.

Meanwhile, given the medical community's renewed commitment to research and the advent of new medications and diagnostic techniques, it is likely that today's toddlers and adolescents will find it far easier to maintain bone health throughout their lives.

—Laura L. Tosi, MD

Table 1. Bone Health: How Men and Women Differ

A comprehensive, multinational report from the World Health Organization reveals the following:

Osteoarthritis (OA) is a loss of joint cartilage that leads to pain and loss of function. It can occur in any joint, but is most common in the hip. Worldwide, OA affects 9.6 percent of men and 18 percent of women over age 60. The incidence of OA is higher in women than in men at virtually every stage of life.

Osteoporosis (OP) is a disease characterized by low bone mass, deterioration of bone tissue, and increases in bone fragility and susceptibility to fracture. The general prevalence of OA at age 50 is 5 percent for women and 2.4 percent for men; by age 85, the percentages rise to 50 percent and 20 percent, respectively. Other estimates place the risk much higher: on the basis of WHO diagnostic criteria, 54 percent of postmenopausal white women in the northern parts of the United States have OP.

Fragility fractures, defined as fractures occurring in people age 40 and older that occur following low-energy trauma (for example, falling from a standing position) are a direct reflection of OP. More than half of women age 50 experience a fracture at some point in their lives—a far higher proportion than men. For example, in 1990, of the 1.66 million reported hip fractures worldwide, 1.19 million were in women and only 463,000 in men. The incidence of vertebra deformities among people between age 50 and 79 is 1 percent per year among women and 0.6 percent in men. Vertebral fractures often occur spontaneously, in the course of lifting or simply changing positions; only a third of these fractures are associated with a fall. Women have four times as many fractures of the forearm as do men, and women account for three-quarters of fractures of the upper arm.

Lower-back pain is the most common of all musculoskeletal conditions; at any given time, 4–33 percent of the population suffers from it. Back pain, unlike other most common musculoskeletal complaints, is slightly more common in men than it is in women, which may be due to its association with occupational factors such as heavy physical work and lifting.

Table 2. The Bone Health Team

Treatment of bone and muscle disorders is most successful when there is close cooperation among the doctor, patient, and family members. On that team are health care professionals who treat disorders relating to the musculoskeletal system. They include the following physicians and therapists:

Orthopaedic Surgeon or Orthopaedist—a physician with advanced surgical training who specializes in the diagnosis and treatment of musculoskeletal disorders

Physiatrist—a physician who specializes in the evaluation and treatment of musculoskeletal and neurological diseases and conditions to effect rehabilitation of neuromuscular functioning (also called a specialist in physical medicine and rehabilitation)

Rheumatologist—a physician who specializes in internal medicine and has advanced training in rheumatology, which involves diseases of the immune system and the musculoskeletal system, including the joints, muscles, and bones

Physical Therapist—a professional who helps patients return to normal musculoskeletal functioning following illness or injury

Occupational Therapist—a professional who helps patients achieve maximal independence in tasks of daily living after injury or illness

Licensed Acupuncture Therapist—an individual who reduces pain and improves functioning by inserting fine needles into the skin at various points in the body

Your primary care physician is part of your bone health team. Psychologists, social workers, dietitians, and nurse educators, as well as medical specialists such as neurologists and radiologists, may also be part of the team.

CHAPTER 7

The Brain and Degenerative Diseases

Women and men think differently. There is nothing new or earth-shattering about that statement, but research has shown in recent years that the differences go beyond socialization and hormones. There are structural, biological variations between the brains of women and men that account for many differences. We can see them in everyday life, from how men and women relate to driving directions to the degree to which each sex remembers people's faces.

This section provides an overview of sex differences in the brain, from how we relate to the world to degenerative brain disorders. Research is rapidly revealing the brain's secrets, but we continue to have many more questions than answers about how the brain functions and the root causes of its disturbances and deteriorations.

Why Your Sex Matters

STRUCTURAL DIFFERENCES IN THE BRAIN

Basic scientific research indicates that males may have more neurons than females in the cerebral cortex, the gray matter that covers the majority of the brain's surface. Although women have fewer neurons in the cerebral cortex, certain anatomical characteristics of female brains may allow for more connections among nerve cells. In addition, women generally have more gray matter overall. Men generally have more white matter (which transfers information between distant regions). This provides weight to the argument that women and men have equal intellectual capacities, although their brains may go about accomplishing tasks in different ways.

There is an emerging consensus among researchers that human evolution has created two different types of brains designed for equal intellectual performance. By pinpointing the respective intelligence centers of women's and men's brains, researchers have not only quashed questions about intelligence disparities, but are making discoveries that may aid research on dementia and other cognitive impairment diseases of the brain. Such discoveries might help explain why boys are more prone to mental retardation and learning problems than are girls. Some of the theories being explored are that male fetuses require maintenance of more nerve cells in the cerebral cortex than do female fetuses, or that early damage to the male developing brain can result in higher losses of needed neurons.

As the brain ages, the amount of tissue mass declines and the amount of fluid increases. This effect is less severe in women than it is in men, suggesting that women are somewhat less vulnerable to age-related changes in mental abilities. However, women are more prone to dementia than men. We do not yet know the reasons for these sex differences, but one therory is connected to the gray-white matter balance described above. Men have more neurons in the brain than women, but women's fewer neurons handle a larger number of connections, so any time a woman loses a single neuron, she loses more connections than would a man who loses a single neuron. Dementia is discussed more later in this chapter.

LANGUAGE DIFFERENCES

Although men and women have been shown to process some language tasks similarly, there are significant sex differences in other aspects of language processing that scientists are beginning to explore more fully. For example, imaging studies of the living brain indicate that neurons on both sides of the brain in women may be activated when they are listening, while neurons on only one side of men's brains may be activated. Men and women appear to process single words similarly, but in the interpretation of whole sentences, women use both sides of the brain while men use only one side. Additional research is needed to confirm this finding and determine what it means for how women and men use language.

SPATIAL INFORMATION DIFFERENCES

Men and women process spatial information differently. For example, women appear to rely on landmarks to navigate their environment, whereas men tend to use compass directions.

In an imaging study, men were found to activate a distributed system of different brain regions on both sides of the brain while performing a spatial task. Women, however, activated these regions only on the right side of the brain.

MEMORY DIFFERENCES

Some functions of memory appear to be different in males and females. Higher rates of blood flow in certain portions of the brain are associated with increased memory of verbal tasks in women, but not in men. Compared to men, women have been shown to be better at remembering faces.

The differences outlined here are useful for understanding and recognizing that conflicts between the sexes—between partners or spouses and among friends and siblings—are often not the result of intentional antagonism, but the fruit of basic biology. When women complain that men do not listen appropriately or do not remember certain things, a lack of concern or lack of interest may not be the culprit. The same could be said of a man's frustration, whether real or imagined, over a woman's driving habits. At a physical level, the brains of women and men are wired differently. While understanding these differences may not eliminate certain problems, it can foster more patience and acceptance.

What Are Degenerative Brain Disorders?

As some people age, it is normal to experience minor declines in memory and the ability to learn new and complex information. Major changes are not normal, however, and are often the sign of a degenerative condition that needs immediate medical attention.

Because women generally live longer than men, degenerative brain disorders—which typically strike later in life—are of serious concern to them. A recent major study, part of the Women's Health Initiative (WHI) and reported in the *Journal of the American Medical Association* in 2003, showed that women age 65 and older taking combination hormone therapy (estrogen plus progestin) had twice the rate of dementia than women who did not take the medication. An estrogen–only phase of the WHI was stopped in June 2004 when data showed that women on estrogen-only therapy also had a slightly greater dementia risk. The WHI results indicate combination hormone therapy could cause an additional twenty-three cases of dementia per 10,000 women per year, while estrogen-only hormone therapy could trigger an additional twelve cases. The increase of dementia cases by estrogen-only therapy was not statistically significant, but even a small increase is cause for concern when evaluating a treatment being used to prevent disease in otherwise healthy individuals. Also, a European study has shown women who are obese throughout life are more likely to lose brain tissue, which is one of the first indications that a person will develop dementia. For these reasons, women should monitor their health closely and discuss any concerns with their health care providers.

What Is Dementia?

Dementia is used to describe a decline in brain function. Changes in memory, personality, or behavior are frequent signs of dementia. Dementia makes it hard for a person to perform routine, daily tasks. A person with dementia may ask the same questions repeatedly or get lost in familiar places. This person often cannot follow directions; is disoriented about time, people, or places; and may neglect personal safety, hygiene, or nutrition.

Dementia is not a normal part of aging, and some forms of dementia can be improved with treatment. Some treatable conditions can cause dementia, including high fever, dehydration, vitamin deficiency, poor nutrition, bad reactions to medicines, thyroid problems, or a minor head injury. These conditions are serious and should be treated by a doctor as soon as possible. Sometimes dementia gets worse and cannot be cured.

Several disorders, including Huntington's disease and Parkinson's disease, are linked to dementia. The two most common causes of dementia are discussed below. Any persistent changes in memory, personality, or behavior should be checked out by a physician.

WHAT IS ALZHEIMER'S DISEASE?

Alzheimer's disease is the most common cause of dementia. There is currently no cure. Nearly half of all people over age 85 are estimated to have Alzheimer's disease, and 10 percent over age 65 have it. It is the eighth leading cause of death for women in the United States, and several studies have shown that women are at higher risk for developing the disease than men.

Forgetfulness is a common first sign of Alzheimer's. As the disease progresses, language, reasoning, and comprehension are affected, eventually to the point where people cannot take care of themselves. Individuals live an average of eight years after the onset of symptoms, but some live as long as 20 years or more.

The cause of Alzheimer's is unknown, but the disease involves the development of plaques and tangles in the brain's gray matter that interrupt the transmission of information within the brain. As a result, nerve cells in the brain eventually die, triggering the loss of functionality. The damage to the brain from Alzheimer's appears to be more severe in women. However, men with the disease have a higher risk of mortality related to the disease itself, such as the severity of dementia and episodes of delirium. Death among women with Alzheimer's is often connected to malnutrition and the inability to perform the tasks of daily living.

DIAGNOSIS

Right now, Alzheimer's can only be diagnosed definitively by examining the brain after death. Doctors can make a probable diagnosis of the disease, however, that is roughly 90 percent accurate, according to the National Institute on Aging.

TREATMENT

There are some drugs available to improve the brain's functioning, but there is no evidence that they can slow the underlying progression of the disease. No prevention for the disease exists, but the Alzheimer's Association recommends that people stay as physically and mentally active as possible.

Developing new treatments for Alzheimer's disease is an active area of research, according to the National Institutes of Health. Scientists are testing a number of drugs to see if they prevent Alzheimer's disease, slow the disease, or help reduce behavioral symptoms.

Medicines already used to help reduce the risk of heart disease may help lower the chances of developing Alzheimer's disease as well or may slow its progression. Clinical trials of drugs known as statins, which lower cholesterol, have begun to determine if they might help slow down the progression of Alzheimer's.

In other studies, scientists are tracking the health of Alzheimer's patients to see if they exhibit any signs or conditions distinct from the general population that may give clues to the origins and progression of the disease. For example, research has shown that people with Alzheimer's often have higher levels of the amino acid, homocysteine, in their blood. Folic acid and vitamins B6 and B12 can reduce levels of homocysteine in the blood, and scientists are looking to see whether these substances can also slow rates of mental decline.

WHAT IS VASCULAR DEMENTIA?

Vascular dementia, the second most common type of dementia after Alzheimer's, occurs when the arteries that supply blood to the brain narrow or become blocked. Symptoms can strike quickly, often following a stroke, but they also can develop gradually. These symptoms are similar to those of other forms of dementia, described above, making them hard to distinguish from signs of Alzheimer's.

Risk factors for vascular dementia center on:

♦ advanced age (over age 65),
♦ high blood pressure (hypertension),
♦ heart disease, and
♦ diabetes.

Smoking, being overweight, having elevated cholesterol levels, and having a family history of heart problems can also increase your risk for stroke, which is a primary trigger of vascular dementia. Small or mini-strokes, which often go undetected, are a frequent cause of vascular dementia. The effect of these small strokes can very slight, but they can worsen over time. As more blood vessels in the brain are blocked, the mental decline associated with dementia can increase. Temporary loss of vision, speech, or strength or brief episodes of numbness are warning signs of small strokes and should be taken seriously.

Vascular dementia can affect an individual's thinking, language, walking, bladder control, and vision. It commonly begins between ages 60 and 75 and affects men more often than women. Because they live longer, however, women need to be aware of the warning signs of vascular dementia as they age; some aspects of dementia can be prevented with appropriate medical treatment, such as reducing high blood pressure.

What Is Parkinson's Disease?

Parkinson's disease is the second most common degenerative brain disease after Alzheimer's. Parkinson's is a chronic, progressive disease that results from the death or injury of nerve cells (substantia nigra) in the midbrain. These cells allow the brain to communicate with itself and coordinate the body's movement; without them, the body's movement becomes somewhat unregulated.

As with other degenerative diseases, Parkinson's symptoms can sometimes be mistaken as common signs of aging. There are four key symptoms of Parkinson's:

♦ tremors (shaking of a leg or arm when it is at rest);
♦ slowed physical movement;
♦ stiffness or rigidity in the arms, legs, or trunk; and
♦ poor balance.

When two of these symptoms are present at the same time, especially if they occur more prominently on one side of the body than the other, Parkinson's is the likely diagnosis. Initial symptoms are usually mild and begin on one side of the body and can spread to the other side of the body over time.

RISK FACTORS

There is a family history of Parkinson disease in 5–10 percent of patients. At any age, men are 1.5 times more likely than women to get Parkinson's disease. It is not clear why men are affected more often, but some researchers believe men are exposed to environmental toxins more frequently that can trigger the disease.

TREATMENT AND MANAGEMENT

The progression of the disease varies from patient to patient. As symptoms worsen, patients often have trouble with routine tasks because of tremors and reduced mobility. As symptoms progress, it is important for patients to talk with their physicians, so that optimal treatment can be established. According to the National Parkinson's Foundation, "the goal of treatment is not to abolish symptoms, but rather to help the patient manage their symptoms, function independently, and make the appropriate adjustments to a chronic illness. The illness will not go away, but management of its symptoms can be successful in reducing disability or other handicap."

Although Parkinson's affects more men, the gender gap may close in the future. Environmental exposures, such as exposure to pesticides, have been linked to Parkinson's disease. Women now work in a wider variety of professions than ever—military service, for example—and their environmental exposure more closely parallels men's exposure than it has in the past.

—RICHARD SCHMITZ, MA, AND MARTIN S. RUSINOWITZ, MD

CHAPTER 8

Cancer

Bladder Cancer

WHAT IS BLADDER CANCER?

Bladder cancer is the fifth most common cancer of Americans and the eighth most common cancer of American women (fourth among men). More than 60,000 new cases of bladder cancer will be diagnosed in the United States this year, and more than 13,000 individuals will die from metastatic disease (cancer that has spread beyond the confines of its site of origin). Although this is equal to the annual number of deaths from either ovarian or rectal cancer, most American women know too little about bladder cancer.

Bladder cancer is a malignant tumor arising from the lining cells of the urinary tract, a system that includes the kidneys, the ureters (tubes carrying urine from the kidneys to the bladder), the bladder (an oval container of fluid wrapped with a thick cover of muscle and fat) located in the pelvis, and the first part of the urethra (the tube that carries urine from the bladder to the outside world). The normal cells that line this system are called transitional cells, and cancers arising from these cells are referred to as transitional cell cancers or carcinomas (another word for cancer). See the figure on the next page that demonstrates the normal location and structure of the upper and lower urinary tract in the female (A) and male (B).

Bladder cancer occurs in two clinically significant forms: superficial and invasive. The former is more common and accounts for approximately 75 percent of all cases diagnosed. Superficial cancers tend to recur after treatment but do not typically spread beyond the bladder. Invasive tumors are less common but are much more dangerous. These tumors spread early in their development and cause almost all of the deaths attributed to bladder cancer.

RISK FACTORS

Cigarette smoking is the leading cause of bladder cancer and may account for 30 percent of the bladder cancers found in women. Exposure to

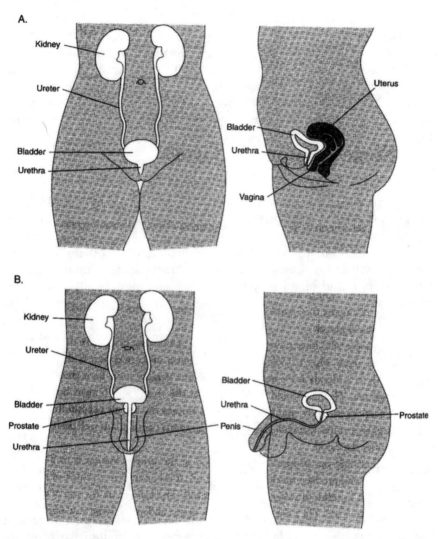

The normal location and structure of the upper and lower urinary tract in the female (A) and male (B).

secondhand smoke may also increase the risk of bladder cancer. In addition, exposure to certain industrial chemicals and environmental toxins may increase the risk of this type of cancer. Firefighters, hairdressers, truck drivers, painters, printers, and individuals working in the automotive, tire, rubber, chemical, petroleum, textile, dye, and aluminum industries may be at increased risk of bladder cancer.

Symptoms

The most common symptom of bladder cancer is hematuria (blood in the urine). Hematuria can sometimes be seen (gross hematuria), although it is usually detected by a physician during routine analysis of urine that looks clear to the naked eye (microscopic hematuria). Most bleeding associated with bladder cancer is painless; however, about 30 percent of bladder cancer patients experience "irritative voiding symptoms," such as burning, frequent urination, or sensation of incomplete emptying.

Why Your Sex Matters

Most physicians learn something about bladder cancer in medical school, but few ever treat patients with this disease. Physicians in family practice and internal medicine may associate irritative voiding symptoms with urinary tract infection in women and not immediately think that these symptoms may reflect the presence of a urinary tract tumor. Although urinary tract infection and bladder dysfunction are common problems of aging women, unexplained blood in the urine of a female patient, particularly when not associated with a proven infection, requires the attention of a urologist (a specialized surgeon with training in the diagnosis and treatment of urinary tract disease) and a complete evaluation.

Diagnosis

Once a patient has been referred to a urologist, a routine set of tests is performed to evaluate the urinary tract and explain signs and symptoms that may reflect the presence of a urinary tract cancer. Urologists check the urine for the presence of infection, and they examine the lining of the bladder with a small scope introduced into the bladder through the urethra (cystoscope) and often order radiologic studies (x-rays) of the urinary tract to search for tumors or other abnormalities. Usually discovered at the time of cystoscopy, bladder tumors appear as small growths resembling seaweed or small bushes. Invasive tumors look solid and can grow very large, creeping through the muscle of the bladder wall and eventually escaping into the tissues that surround the bladder. To diagnose a bladder tumor, the urologist removes part or all of the tumor with a special knife attached to the end of the cystoscope and sends the tissue for evaluation by a pathologist. The pathologist in turn examines the cells of the tumor under the microscope to determine if the growth is a cancer.

If cancer is identified in the biopsy, the pathologist attempts to determine if muscle tissue, representing the tissue underneath the tumor, is involved. Determining the location and extent of a tumor is called staging.

Patients often confuse grading and staging. Grade refers to the appearance of cells under the microscope. Low-grade tumor cells look similar to normal cells; high-grade cells share very few characteristics of normal cells. Invasive bladder tumors are almost always composed of high-grade tumor cells. Low-stage tumors (stage I or II) are confined to the organ of origin; high-stage tumors (stages III and IV) have moved from the bladder to the tissue surrounding the bladder or to other organs (liver, lung, bones, or lymph nodes). As you might expect, the extent of a tumor (the stage) is a good—though not perfect—indication of an individual patient's chance of survival: the lower the stage, the better the chances are of cure. Once a tumor is diagnosed, the patient and urologist must confer about treatment. Superficial tumors are treated differently from invasive bladder cancers.

TREATMENT

Superficial bladder tumors are treated by simple removal using a specifically modified cystoscope. The tumor is removed transurethrally (transurethral resection, or TUR, "scraped out"), and the area where the tumor arose usually is cauterized (heated to a high temperature using an electrical current). High-grade superficial tumors are often treated with TUR and followed with medication to reduce the risk of tumor recurrence. Fortunately, most superficial tumors are low-grade, and these cancers have a 30 percent relapse rate. Higher-grade superficial tumors recur more frequently, in about 70 percent of cases. Superficial bladder cancer is really a chronic (lifelong) illness that requires constant surveillance and frequent treatment to control.

Invasive bladder cancer is most commonly treated by either partial or complete removal of the bladder and some surrounding organs. In women, this operation can remove not only the bladder and urethra, but also the uterus, ovaries, fallopian tubes, and part of the vagina. Surgeons have recently developed methods for reconstructing the lower urinary tract, including creating a new bladder using a piece of the patient's small intestine. In women of childbearing age, it is not always necessary to remove the uterus and ovaries, even if reconstruction is performed.

An alternative to bladder removal is bladder preservation. For some patients with invasive tumors, removing the bladder is not necessary. Instead, after a complete TUR, during which all visible signs of tumor are removed, the patient is treated with systemic chemotherapy and radiation therapy to the bladder. This approach preserves the bladder and eradicates the cancer in approximately 40 percent of appropriately selected patients. This is still considered a relatively unusual therapy and should be administered by a multidisciplinary team composed of a urologist, medical oncologist, and radiation oncologist.

SCREENING/PREVENTION

Screening for bladder cancer is not currently recommended by the National Institutes of Health (NIH), the American Cancer Society, or the American Urologic Association. Tools for population-based screening have not been developed, but molecular tests are currently being evaluated in clinical trials. These tests can be used successfully to test urine for the presence of cells and cellular components (DNA, protein, enzymes). The most effective preventive measures are not smoking and maintaining a healthy lifestyle and diet.

WHY YOUR SEX MATTERS

Historically, bladder cancer has been considered a disease of older Caucasian men. Three-quarters of bladder cancer patients are male. Yet women are more likely to present with more advanced tumors than men and have a worse prognosis than men at almost every stage of the disease. This is particularly true for African American women. This disparity can be explained by the fact that women and their physicians tend to ignore the most basic symptom of bladder cancer—blood in the urine. Although there may be many reasons for this, it is likely that most women associate hematuria with menstruation or menopause. In many cases, physicians may misdiagnose this symptom initially as postmenopausal bleeding, simple cystitis, or a urinary tract infection. As a result, a bladder cancer diagnosis can be missed for a year or more. Awareness, coupled with insistence on prompt appropriate evaluation and treatment, may change this outcome.

—STEPHANIE SHAPIRO; DIANE ZIPURSKY QUALE;
AND MARK P. SCHOENBERG, MD, FACS

What Is Breast Cancer?

Like all parts of your body, the cells in your breasts usually grow and rest in cycles. The periods of growth and rest in each cell are controlled by genes in the cell's nucleus. When your genes are in good working order, they keep cell growth under control. But when your genes develop an abnormality, they sometimes lose their ability to control this cycle. Breast cancer results from an uncontrolled growth of breast cells.

There are many forms of breast cancer, all of which have differing prognoses. The most common forms are:

♦ ductal carcinoma in-situ—noninvasive breast cancer, where the abnormal breast cells are confined to the milk ducts, and
♦ invasive ductal carcinoma—a cancer that begins in the milk ducts and invades into the normal surrounding breast tissue, and
♦ invasive lobular carcinoma—a cancer that begins in the milk-making part of the breast and invades into the normal surrounding breast tissue.

Two other types—including tubular carcinoma and mucinous carcinoma—which represent 1–2 percent of all breast cancers, have favorable prognoses. Other, rarer types of breast cancer include inflammatory breast cancer, Paget's disease of the nipple, and phyllodes tumor.

WHO GETS BREAST CANCER?

It is estimated that more than 211,000 new cases of invasive breast cancer are diagnosed in the United States each year, along with 58,000 new cases of noninvasive breast cancer. Every woman, by virtue of her sex, is at some risk for breast cancer. As you get older, your risk increases. Assuming you live to age 90, your risk of getting breast cancer over your lifetime is about 14 percent. Stated another way, there is an 86 percent chance that you will not get breast cancer.

RISK FACTORS

After being female, the biggest risk for breast cancer is growing older. The longer you live, the higher your risk:

♦ From birth to age 39, one woman in 231 will get breast cancer (less than 0.5 percent risk).
♦ From ages 40 to 49, the chance is one in 68 (1.5 percent risk).
♦ From agest 50 to 59, the chance is one in 37 (2.7 percent risk).
♦ From ages 60 to 69, the chance is one in 26 (nearly 4 percent risk).

Risk increases with age for several reasons, including the wear and tear of living, which increases the chance that a genetic abnormality will develop that your body does not find and fix.

Ethnicity may have an impact on risk. One study that compared breast cancers in Nigeria, Senegal, and North America discovered that women of

African descent are more likely than women of European descent to develop a more virulent form of breast cancer.

Prolonged, uninterrupted exposure to estrogen can increase breast cancer risk. Breast cell growth—both normal and abnormal—is stimulated by the presence of estrogen. This includes estrogen that your body produces normally as well as estrogen you might take in another form. The following risk factors for breast cancer are related to prolonged exposure to estrogen without any breaks or interruptions:

♦ starting menstruation at a young age;

♦ going through menopause at a late age;

♦ taking menopause hormone therapy for more than five years with estrogen alone or with estrogen and progesterone, but most breast cancers that are diagnosed in women on hormone therapy tend to be very early stage and very treatable (your own risk of developing breast cancer may increase by five to 40 percent; if your risk was 10 percent before taking hormone therapy, your risk would increase to less than 15 percent);

♦ never having had a full-term pregnancy;

♦ having a first full-term pregnancy after age 30;

♦ being overweight, which increases the production of estrogen outside the ovaries and adds to the overall level of estrogen in the body;

♦ exposure to estrogens in the environment (such as estrogen fed to fatten beef cattle or the breakdown products of the pesticide, DDT, which mimic the effects of estrogen in the body); and

♦ having more than two alcoholic drinks per week, which can limit your liver's ability to regulate blood estrogen levels.

Smoking may be associated with a small increase in breast cancer risk. Diet also may play a role in your level of risk for breast cancer. Limited, new research suggests that a low-fat diet may help reduce the risk of breast cancer recurrence.

A personal history of breast cancer is a risk factor for breast cancer recurrence or the formation of a new breast cancer. If you have already been diagnosed with breast cancer, your risk of developing it again is higher than if you had never had the disease. The risk is about 1 percent per year, so that over a 10-year period, your risk would be about 10 percent. However, medication is available to help reduce that risk. One new study indicates that measurement by MRI of breast tumor volume—before, during, and after chemotherapy—may help predict the rate of breast cancer recurrence. A history of benign breast disease may also be a risk factor for developing breast cancer.

A family history of breast cancer can have a significant impact on your risk, but does not automatically assume that any case of breast cancer in your family means you are a high-risk candidate. For example, if your grandmother was diagnosed with breast cancer at age 75, this does not mean your risk of the disease is increased. Many cases of postmenopausal breast cancer cannot be attributed to a specific gene mutation. Your grandmother was most likely just one of the one in 15 women in that age bracket who gets breast cancer from the wear and tear of aging.

INHERITED RISK FACTORS

Other patterns of family history may strongly suggest an inherited gene abnormality that is independent of normal aging and is associated with a relatively higher risk of breast cancer. The following signs suggest that there may be an inherited gene abnormality in your family:

♦ having a mother, sister, or daughter with breast or ovarian cancer;
♦ having multiple generations of family members (on either your mother's or your father's side) affected by breast or ovarian cancer;
♦ having relatives who were diagnosed with breast cancer at a young age (usually before menopause and under age 50);
♦ having relatives who had both breasts affected by cancer;
♦ having a man in your family who has had breast cancer; or
♦ coming from an Ashkenazi Jewish family (from Eastern Europe).

You can inherit a breast cancer gene abnormality from your mother or your father. If one of your parents has a gene abnormality, you have a 50 percent chance of inheriting the gene. If you do inherit a gene abnormality, your risk of developing the disease depends on the specific abnormality found, the pattern of its behavior in your family, plus the uniqueness of your own body. The risk of breast cancer in these families ranges greatly—from 40 to 80 percent over the course of a lifetime.

To date, most inherited cases of breast cancer have been associated with two genes: BRCA1, which stands for **BR**east **CA**ncer gene one, and BRCA2, or **BR**east **CA**ncer gene two. These genes usually keep breast cells growing normally and prevent any cancer cell growth. But if these genes contain abnormalities, or mutations, they can be associated with an increased breast cancer risk. Specific abnormalities in the BRCA1 and BRCA2 genes are more commonly found in Ashkenazi Jewish women than they are in women of other ethnic origins. About one in 40 Ashkenazi Jews—with or without breast cancer—has a genetic mutation in BRCA1 or BRCA2.

Despite the increased risk presented by inheriting an abnormal gene, it is important to remember that not every person with an inherited BRCA1 or BRCA2 abnormality develops cancer. The risks associated with BRCA1 and BRCA2 mutations may be affected by:

◆ lifestyle and environmental factors,
◆ how well other genes work with BRCA1 and BRCA2 to protect the body against cancer, and
◆ the particular abnormality and how it affects the proteins in the body that are supposed to suppress cancer.

Also, many people mistakenly believe that the cancers caused by inherited genetic abnormalities are more aggressive than other cancers. In fact, recent evidence suggests that a woman with an abnormal gene who develops breast or ovarian cancer may have a less aggressive form of the disease than women without an abnormal gene.

Most women who get breast cancer do not have an inherited abnormal breast cancer gene. These abnormalities probably account for only 10 percent of all breast cancers. However, women with an abnormal breast cancer gene have up to an 85 percent risk of developing breast cancer by age 70. These women also are at increased risk of developing ovarian cancer.

GENETIC TESTING

Identifying BRCA1 and BRCA2 has led to new techniques for detecting and treating breast cancer and lowering the risk for the disease. There are both advantages and disadvantages of seeking genetic testing if you have a family member with a known breast cancer gene mutation.

The advantages include:

◆ If your test result is normal, your genetic counselor can tell you with greater certainty that you have the same relatively low risk of developing breast or ovarian cancer as women in the general population. Routine screening for breast cancer is still important for you, however, as it is for all women.
◆ If your test result is abnormal, closely monitoring the health of your breasts and ovaries can help find a cancer in its earliest stage, when it is most treatable and curable. In addition, you may want to consider:

- taking medication that could reduce your risk of developing breast cancer;
- making lifestyle and family planning changes or decisions to help improve your odds;
- participating in a clinical trial on breast cancer prevention to see whether other drugs are effective; or
- preventive surgical removal of your breasts, ovaries, or both before cancer has an opportunity to form.

- If your test result is abnormal and you develop cancer, knowing you have a genetic abnormality will give you more information on which to base your treatment decisions.

The disadvantages of genetic testing include:

- Normal test results do not guarantee healthy genes.
- For some women, an abnormal test result can trigger anxiety, depression, or anger. Even though the result does not mean that a woman will definitely get breast cancer, many women with an abnormal gene assume they will. If you think knowing the information may be too hard for you emotionally, consider not having genetic testing until more is known about how to beat the disease.
- If you learn that you have passed on an abnormal gene to your children, you may feel guilty and worried.
- It is not yet clear exactly what you should or should not do once you get your genetic test results. We still do not know the most effective ways to prevent breast cancer. For example, removing the breasts and ovaries to lower cancer risk may not get rid of every breast- and ovary-related cell. Even after such surgery, a woman with an abnormal breast cancer gene must be monitored regularly; cancer may show up in nearby tissues and organs.
- You may worry about discrimination in getting insurance coverage or employment based on your genetic information.
- Genetic testing may not answer all of your questions. In families with an abnormal breast cancer gene, other factors that are not yet understood may contribute to high risk.

SYMPTOMS AND DIAGNOSIS

Breast cancer can exist without symptoms, which is why screening is so important. If there are early signs of breast cancer, the most common are:

- a single, firm, and most often painless lump;
- swelling and unusual appearance of a portion of the skin on the breast or underarm;
- inversion of the breast nipple or the nipple developing a rash, a change in skin texture, or having a bloody or other discharge other than breast milk; and
- part of the breast surface becoming depressed.

The earlier breast cancer is found and diagnosed, the better are your chances of beating it. Screening tests—including breast self-exam and mammography—look for signs of disease in women without symptoms; they should be part of every healthy woman's routine.

A newer form of mammography is digital, incorporating modern electronics and computers into x-ray mammography methods. Instead of acquiring an image on film, it is collected electronically and can be stored directly into a computer. Because there is no film developing and the image comes up instantaneously on the computer monitor, the study tends to be faster. Research indicates digital mammography may be better for women with dense breasts or who are younger than age 50 or are perimenopausal. Diagnostic tests (such as magnetic resonance imaging [MRI], blood tests, or bone scans) become part of the picture when breast cancer is suspected or has been diagnosed.

A diagnosis of cancer must be proven by the presence of cancer cells as seen under a microscope. This is why a biopsy—a very small operation that removes tissue from an area of concern in the body—is required to get the cells for microscopic analysis. Various techniques are used to biopsy tissue:

- **Needle biopsy** of palpable lesions is the least invasive and can be done in the doctor's office, with results often available in 24 hours. The surgeon obtains material for microscopic analysis using a needle with a hollow center. New technologies are helping to improve the effectiveness of needle biopsy. In some cases, a technique called needle localization guides biopsy of a non-palpable lesion (a mass that cannot be felt) that was detected by mammography. This procedure is often done prior to surgical biopsy. MRI guided, vacuum-assisted biopsy can be provided under local rather than general anesthesia, is less painful, and allows the doctor to assess more tissue more quickly.
- **Stereotactic needle biopsy** (core biopsy) removes multiple pieces of a lesion. If the lesion cannot be felt, the needle is guided to the area of concern with the help of mammography or ultra-

sound. If a lesion is found only by MRI, then needle biopsy may be guided by that technique. If a lesion is seen on ultrasound, then the biopsy may be done using ultrasound guidance.

♦ **Incisional biopsy** is more like regular surgery—it involves removing a small piece of tissue for sectioning and examination. Often, incisional biopsies are done when needle biopsies are inconclusive or if the lump, mammographic change, or suspicious rash is too extensive or too big to be removed easily.

♦ **Excisional biopsy** is the most involved kind of biopsy. It attempts to remove the entire suspicious lump of tissue from the breast. This is the surest way to establish the diagnosis without winding up with a false negative. Removing the entire lump also provides you some peace of mind. Both incisional and excisional biopsies can be done in an outpatient center or hospital, using local anesthesia.

There are constant improvements in biopsies; for example, newer instruments exist that allow same-day turnaround for breast and other biopsies.

After an initial diagnosis, many tests may be conducted to help determine the best treatment. These tests are designed to determine whether the cancer is invasive and whether lymph nodes are involved and, if so, how many. Other critical factors include the size, tumor grade, and hormone receptor status of the tumor.

TREATMENT

In recent years, there has been an explosion of life-saving treatment advances against breast cancer. Instead of only one or two options, today there is a large—and sometimes overwhelming—menu of treatment choices that fight the complex mix of cells in each individual cancer. You will need to work closely with your doctor to determine which is best for you. The options include surgery, radiation, hormonal (antiestrogen) therapy, and/or chemotherapy. You also need to stay current with research news about potential breast cancer vaccines, genetic therapies, and other innovations in treating breast cancer.

RISK REDUCTION

Since some risk factors for cancer are beyond your control, risk reduction measures focus on those factors you can control and on ensuring early diagnosis. If you smoke, try to stop for good. You should exercise regularly. One large study involving nurses from the entire United States found that breast cancer patients who walk or do other kinds of moderate exercise for three to five hours a week are about 50 percent less likely to die from breast cancer than are women who are less active.

You may be able to minimize your exposure to estrogen by:

♦ limiting consumption to no more than two alcoholic drinks per week or stopping completely;
♦ decreasing the amount of red meat and other sources of animal fat (including dairy fat in cheese, milk, and ice cream) in your diet;
♦ losing weight if you are overweight and maintaining a healthy weight; and
♦ avoiding estrogen-like products if you have already had breast cancer; some soy or herbal supplements have estrogen-like actions.

Finally, stay on top of research news; many scientists are studying risk factors for breast cancer, and many others are exploring new therapies. In addition, research is being done on a class of drugs, called aromatase inhibitors, that are intended to clock formation of estrogen. The theory is that these drugs might reduce breast cancer in certain high-risk women.

—MARISA WEISS, MD

Surviving Colorectal Cancer

By Ruth Bader Ginsburg
Associate Justice, Supreme Court of the United States

In the summer of 1999, I was teaching on the Greek island of Crete. I began having digestive symptoms and was initially diagnosed with acute diverticulitis, a painful condition that occurs when pouches form inside the colon and become infected. I began treatment in Greece, but upon my return to Washington, D.C., my condition was correctly diagnosed as colorectal cancer. I've been told that this misdiagnosis happens fairly often because extensive testing is required to tell the two conditions apart.

My advice—to all near or approaching what the French call a certain age—is to have a colonoscopy. Many women, myself once included, are religious about having periodic Pap tests and mammograms, but do not consider colorectal cancers to be women's diseases. I've learned that colorectal cancer is the third leading cause of death for women. And colorectal cancer is insidious: it often begins and lingers without symptoms, as it did in my case. Early detection can make a huge difference to survival prospects.

Some people shy away because they recall having the examination years ago and found it particularly unpleasant, as I did when I first had a colonoscopy in the 1980s. I can assure these people that the current procedure is not nearly as awful, and scientists continue to discover ways of improving the tests.

Cancer is a dreadful disease. The surgery, chemotherapy, and radiation are not easy to bear physically and may generate anxiety for people. My family and I were greatly helped by caring doctors and nurses who helped alleviate our fears by telling us what we needed to know as the treatment progressed. Because I knew what to expect, I was able to schedule my therapy around the Court's calendar, missing no days that term.

For me, work was the best balm. It also was helpful to hear from people who had had similar surgery and postoperative therapy, people who are alive years later and feeling fine.

Medical science has made enormous progress since my husband had cancer in 1958. In those days we had not yet heard the word, chemotherapy. Even so, part of today's treatment seems to me more of an experience-based art than an exact science. And one must make choices. In my case, one choice was whether to undergo daily radiation with simultaneous chemotherapy infusion for several weeks. Did I need all or any of it? Or did I not? What were the ups and downs, the pluses and minuses, short and long term? The doctors I consulted were not altogether unanimous in their responses. Much as I wished I could have been given crisp, unqualified right answers, ultimately I had to decide. It helped to be fully informed before I did so.

I was fortunate to be treated at a hospital with accomplished nurses and doctors who are also caring people. A reminder of this is my graduation certificate from the hardest course I have ever taken, which hangs in a prominent place in my chambers at the Court. It reads:

On February 29, 2000, Justice Ginsburg graduated from the Washington Hospital Center Department of Strange Events and even Stranger People. Let all who read this know we could not dampen the spirit nor stifle the sense of humor no matter how hard we tried—and boy did we try. We graduate you with respect and love.

The certificate is signed by the four able, good-humored radiology technicians who attended to me daily during six long weeks.

I began with a piece of advice, and I'll end this story with equally true counsel: there is nothing like a cancer bout to make one relish the joys of being alive. It is as though a special, zestful spice seasons my work and days. Each thing I do comes with a heightened appreciation that I am able to do it.

(Reprinted with permission by Justice Ruth Bader Ginsburg)

Colorectal Cancer

WHAT IS COLORECTAL CANCER?

Colorectal cancer (CRC) is the third most common cancer in women, causing 11 percent of new cancer cases and 10 percent of cancer deaths. From 1996 to 2000 slightly more men than women in the United States developed and died from colorectal cancer, with the rates highest among African Americans. During this same period, it was calculated that one in 17 men and one in 18 women would develop invasive (advanced) colorectal cancer. During 1998–2000 the incidence of CRC declined 3 percent per year, likely due in part to early detection of CRC and removal of precancerous lesions. In addition, during the last 15 years there has been a 1.7 percent per year decline in death from colorectal cancer due to a decreasing incidence rate and better survival, a result in part of detecting less advanced cancer.

RISK FACTORS

The risk of developing colorectal cancer depends on whether other family members have had intestinal polyps, colorectal cancer, or other associated cancers.

Women with symptoms of bleeding from the bowel, abdominal pain, or constipation not explained by a poor-fiber diet should be evaluated by their doctors and, in most cases, should have a colonoscopy. If symptoms persist or worsen, it is important to make sure the symptoms are taken seriously and that a physician performs a thorough evaluation. In a woman with no symptoms, it is important to screen for precancerous lesions and cancer.

Women are at high risk for developing colorectal cancer and should see a specialist if they have:

- inflammatory bowel disease;
- a family history of colorectal cancer in more than two relatives;

- a parent or child under the age of 50 with colorectal cancer; or
- a family history of cancers of other intestinal tract organs, brain, or urinary tract.

A family history of polyps also increases the risk of CRC and polyps in an individual. Screening for all of these individuals may start at a very young age.

In an average-risk individual with no family history of cancer or polyps, screening should start at age 50, preferably with a colonoscopy. If no polyps are found, this procedure should be repeated every 10 years.

In an individual with a first-degree relative (parent or child) or two second-degree relatives (grandparents, aunts, or uncles) with colorectal cancer or adenomas (a benign tumor of glandular tissue), screening should begin at age 40 or 10 years before the first cancer or polyp was detected in the relative, if he or she was younger than 40 at the time. If nothing is found, screening should be repeated in five to 10 years, depending on the family history.

SPECIAL RISK FACTORS FOR WOMEN

Asymptomatic women with previous reproductive tract cancers require special consideration for CRC screening. Endometrial cancer and ovarian cancer increase the risk of CRC. When uterine cancer is diagnosed before age 50, the risk of CRC is over three times higher. Ovarian cancer increases the risk for CRC if diagnosed before age 65 and especially before age 50, when it increases the risk more than three and a half times. However, cervical cancer does not increase the risk for CRC.

The effect of breast cancer on the risk of a woman developing colorectal cancer or adenomatous polyps is controversial. Two reviews in 1994 and a recent study based on review of data from a large population from 1974 to 1995 determined that there was no increased risk of CRC in women with breast cancer overall, and in fact, there was a reduction in rectal cancer, most prominent among African American women. In contrast, a clinical expert panel concluded in 1998 that the increased risk of CRC in a woman with a breast cancer history was similar to that in a person having a first-degree relative with CRC. Recent studies of patients with BRCA, a gene that increases the risk of breast cancer, did not find an increase in associated CRC.

Forty percent of women with hereditary nonpolyposis colorectal cancer (HNPCC), a genetic condition associated with a high risk of colorectal cancer and other cancers, develop endometrial cancer (cancer of the uterus). The family history will help the physician identify this condition, which requires early and more frequent screening. Women with ovarian or endometrial cancer diagnosed before age 50 and who do not have

HNPCC, should have a colonoscopy every three to five years. At this time it is recommended that women who have had an ovarian or endometrial cancer, diagnosed at older than age 50 without HNPCC and those women who have had a personal history of breast cancer should undergo average-risk CRC screening if there are no other reasons for increased screening.

DIAGNOSIS AND SCREENING

The theory behind colorectal cancer screening is that:

♦ cancers discovered at an early stage when they are more curable decrease the mortality rate due to colorectal cancer, and
♦ removal of precancerous lesions decreases the risk of colorectal cancer.

Colorectal cancer is the result of several sequential changes in the DNA in the lining of the colon (the mucosa). These changes result in a loss of control of cell growth, leading to development of a cancer. In an individual over age 50 it is estimated that it takes at least 10 years for changes to occur that result in a colorectal cancer. Such cancers come from adenomatous polyps.

Several strategies exist for CRC screening, including checking for blood in the stool or visualizing the bowel by flexible sigmoidoscopy, colonoscopy, or by an x-ray technique. Fecal occult blood testing (FOBT) (checking for blood in the stool), screening flexible sigmoidoscopy directly, and colonoscopy indirectly have all been shown to reduce mortality from CRC in the total population. Annual FOBT usually detects only one in four cancers.

Flexible sigmoidoscopy is an endoscope that is inserted into the rectum and advanced into the left side of the colon, usually about two feet. Because of its length, only one-third to one-half of the colon is viewed; cancers and premalignant polyps beyond its reach are missed. Because one usually only takes enemas before the test, the visualized colon may not be clean, and more polyps or cancers may be missed. Flexible sigmoidoscopy has been shown to save lives from cancers found in the part of the colon reached by the flexible sigmoidoscope. However, about 50 percent of people with advanced premalignant polyps (the kind that are likely to turn into cancer soon) have no polyps or cancer within the reach of the flexible sigmoidoscope, and people with cancers on the right side of the colon frequently have normal sigmoidoscopy examinations.

A recent study showed that flexible sigmoidoscopy missed twice as many (two-thirds) cancers in women than in men (one-third of the cancers). Therefore colonoscopy, a test with an endoscope that visualizes the whole colon, is the best test for seeing and removing premalignant polyps or finding early cancer in women.

Virtual colonoscopy (the use of x-rays and computers to produce two- and three-dimensional images of the colon), which currently uses laxatives to clean out the colon, is being evaluated to determine if it is as accurate as a standard colonoscopy. Stool tests to detect genetic material that is associated with changes in precancerous or cancerous tumors are not available for the general public and need further testing. Studies have shown that barium enema misses too many polyps/cancers. At this time the best test for screening is a colonoscopy, during which polyps can be removed.

SCREENING CHALLENGES

Adherence to CRC screening guidelines in the United States is poor for men and women. In 1997 a study of more than 9,000 individuals found that only 21 percent of women and 18 percent of men had completed fecal occult blood testing during the preceding year, and 27 percent of women and 35 percent of men had undergone sigmoidoscopy during the preceding five years. In studies reported in 2003, the rate of FOBT done within the previous two years was reported to be 18–24 percent, and sigmoidoscopy or colonoscopy to be 33 percent. Just over 40 percent of the 16,000 women in the Women's Health Initiative were screened for CRC by sigmoidoscopy or colonoscopy. It is encouraging that progress has been made in CRC screening, but we still have a long way to go to achieve near 100 percent compliance.

PREVENTION

Numerous factors have been found to influence the risk of developing colorectal cancer in women. Factors that increase the overall risk for CRC are cigarette smoking (for longer than 35 years) and obesity. Removal of the gallbladder increases the risk for cancers on the right side of the colon only. Recent studies have shown that neither fiber nor vitamin E appears to change the incidence of colorectal cancer in women.

Numerous factors have been found as well to decrease the risk of colorectal cancer. In the Nurses' Health Study, women had a significant reduction in risk of CRC after 20 years of consistent aspirin use, taking only four to six aspirins per week. In addition, after 15 years of ingestion of a multivitamin containing folate, women had a decreased risk for all colon cancers except rectal cancers. Although there are numerous substances in the multivitamins, folate was thought to be the one most responsible for this reduction in CRC. Calcium has been shown to decrease both the risk of adenomas and CRC. In the Calcium Polyp Prevention Study, subjects taking 1,200 mg of supplemental calcium per day had a 20 percent reduction in their risk of developing new adenomas over four years. Women taking 1,250 mg of calcium per day had a reduced rate of left-sided colon cancer than did women taking less than 500 mg of calcium per day when the dietary calcium intake was less than or equal to 700 mg per day. Several studies, including the Women's Health Initiative, have shown hormone therapy to be beneficial in reducing colorectal cancer. It is not known whether survival rates are affected by hormone therapy

Exercise is important in reducing colorectal cancer, regardless of a woman's weight. Women who participate in high-energy activity for a significant amount of time every week have about half the relative risk of colon cancer than do those women who participate in almost no activity.

—JACQUELINE L. WOLF, MD

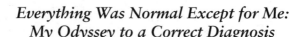

Everything Was Normal Except for Me:
My Odyssey to a Correct Diagnosis

By Fran Drescher, actor, producer, writer, director, and author of ***Enter Whining*** **and** ***Cancer Schmancer***

Women need to understand gynecological cancers and the tests that can help detect them. We should know what's out there. We should be in control. Never be passive when it comes to comes to your health. Open a mouth! Nobody knows your body as well as you do.

It took forever—more than two years and eight doctors—before one of them decided to give me a D&C, which stands for dilatation and curettage, whatever the hell that is. Basically, it's when they scrape tissue from the uterus for biopsy. In the end, this was the only test I needed to find my cancer. Because I was atypical for contracting uterine cancer, at each turn in the road I kept being steered in the wrong direction.

Why was I experiencing strange bleeding and cramping in the middle of my cycle? All I needed was a simple panty liner and I could easily ignore it. But it was becoming chronic, so after a few cycles I decided to call Doctor #1, the gynecologist I'd been seeing for years. "What do you

make of my midmonth staining?" I asked. "You're probably peri-menopausal. It's the precursor to menopause and a common symptom in middle-aged women." Middlewhat?

The staining and cramping persisted, and it made me feel embarrassed and inadequate. If I was truly perimenopausal as Doctor #1 suggested, that meant I was getting old. I hated that idea. So, while I pretended to be the picture of health to the outside world, I secretly decided to see another gynecologist. His exam was pretty typical: stirrups, pelvic, and Pap.

I seemed to be bruising really easily. On the show I was doing a lot of physical comedy, and for a time I blamed it on that, but after a while the bruises were so big and ugly they couldn't be considered normal. I was also beginning to notice a change in my stool. And I ain't talking bar stools, either! So I decided to call my internist, Doctor #3. He checked my heart and lungs. He looked in my ears, my eyes, and my nose. He felt my abdomen, even checked my reflexes. My pulse, normal . . . blood pressure, normal . . . everything normal. As for the midmonth staining, he sided with Doctor #1's conclusion that I was at the threshold of per-imenopause. Regarding my stool changing, he connected it to my diet, and told me I was "eating too much spinach."

So I decided to see a hematologist, Doctor #4, to check out my blood. While I was there I thought he could check out my hormone levels too. I was still afraid of the black-and-blue marks all over my legs and arms, though Doctor #3 didn't see it as a problem. None of my doctors, even the hematologist, seemed particularly worried about my symptoms. I only kept pursuing more doctors because I wanted something that could be fixed. I didn't want to accept that I was perimenopausal and be stuck with that forever. It somehow didn't feel right.

When my armpit felt swollen and sore, I feared that whatever it was had gotten into my lymphatic system. So I made an appointment with Doctor #5, an oncologist and breast specialist. Doctor #5 read my mam-mogram and told me my breasts were unusually dense for my age. "You have the tits of an eighteen-year-old." Well, if that didn't make my whole day. I didn't walk out. I floated. It pacified me for the moment, but the truth is, I still left without a diagnosis.

I decided to go back to Doctor #1. I brought her up to date on the other four doctors I'd seen since my last visit with her. She ordered some blood tests as well as an ultrasound. She did a Pap test and a pelvic exam. Same battery of tests, and again, everything normal. "Well, you're too young for a D&C," she said matter of factly. And like an idiot, even though it was just a stupid test, I was flattered to be too young for it. The only thing that ever showed up was an elevated FSH (follicle-stimulating hormone) level, which is the messenger hormone in the brain that tells the progesterone it's time to kick in. It seemed safe to assume I was experiencing lower-than-normal progesterone. Doctor #1 once again held firm on the perimenopausal theory and prescribed progesterone pills.

When I called Doctor #1 and told her the progesterone didn't seem to be making much of a difference, she said, "Double the dose and see if that works." So I did. Unfortunately I was having a horrible reaction to the double dose of progesterone—something I didn't realize until it was almost too late . . . If I'd had mood swings before, now I was completely jumping out of my skin. I really felt insane and had no coping mechanisms. I felt like I was capable of murdering someone or killing myself. I called Doctor #1 and described my extreme reaction to the pills. Without skipping a beat, she said, "Well, why don't you try half the dosage and see how you feel?" I'd started by taking one pill in the first place, before doubling it to two in the second place! Jeez, what was she thinking?

I now began to experience a nagging leg pain. It was mostly in my left leg and occurred mostly at night. I tried lying with pillows under my legs, wearing socks, rubbing Ben Gay, using a heating pad, and even filling hot water bottles. Sexy, huh? But nothing, and I mean nothing, worked. So I made an appointment with a vascular specialist, Doctor #6. I mean the leg thing was the worst symptom of all. I felt like a trapped wild animal. If I didn't get help soon, I was gonna chew my leg off! Doctor #6 used a wand that looked like an ultrasound and scanned my arterial system for any blockages. But once again the test showed nothing. "You probably have night cramps. No one knows why we get them, but they're very common. I've been told tonic water helps." That's when I called the neurologist, Doctor #7. He requested an MRI (magnetic resonance imaging) of the hip and leg area. RLS (restless leg syndrome) was the closest thing to a diagnosis I ever got. No connection was made between my leg pain and my other symptoms.

I just wanted to feel good again. I wanted to have sex without cramps. The longer I went without a diagnosis, the worse I felt and the more I feared that when they figured out what it was, it wouldn't be caught in time. Perhaps Doctor #8 would help me once and for all. She told me my symptoms did not indicate cancer but rather a perimenopausal hormone imbalance. "Birth control pills are the way to go!" she exclaimed with great confidence.

The birth control pills weren't giving me the irritability I'd felt from the progesterone, but it was suddenly making me bleed 24/7, and my leg cramps were bothering me more than ever. Annoyed and disappointed, I said, "This can't be the right treatment for me!" [Doctor #8] said "just as a precautionary measure," she'd do a D&C to scrape some tissue from the uterus for biopsy.

It seemed like any other day, but it wasn't. The phone rang. It was my gynecologist. "You have adenocarcinoma. I'm very surprised myself."

Now, in the time I was experiencing symptoms and searching for a diagnosis, I'd never once picked up the phone and reached out to [my sister], an experienced nurse who is married to a doctor. "I'd also feel better if the surgeon did her own biopsy. I always like it when the surgeon starts fresh with her own tests."

My sister was now in full medical mode. Though [the surgeon] felt the second biopsy wasn't necessary, she wanted to gain my trust by accommodating my sister's request. [Afterwards] she said, "I'm glad we listened to your sister because the second biopsy shows a more advanced cancer than the first. I'm going to want to do a radical hysterectomy."

Although getting cancer was probably the worst thing that ever happened to me (did I say "probably"?), there have been so many wonderful silver linings too. I know my loved ones better, and I know how to live my life more completely. That's my real triumph.

(From *Cancer Schmancer* by Fran Drescher.
Copyright © 2002 by Fran Drescher. By permission of Warner Books, Inc.)

Gynecological Cancers

WHAT IS UTERINE CANCER?

Cancer of the uterus is the most common malignancy of the female reproductive system. In 2004, there were approximately 40,320 new cases of and 7,090 deaths from uterine cancer.

There are different types of uterine cancer. The most common form is endometrial cancer, which arises from the inner glandular lining of the uterus. Less common are uterine sarcomas, which arise from the smooth muscle of the uterus and account for only 3 percent of all uterine cancer.

Uterine fibroids, also called myomas, are extremely common, benign, smooth muscle tumors of the uterus. Approximately 25 percent of reproductive age women may have this condition. Many women with uterine fibroids worry about the possibility of undiagnosed uterine cancer, but extensive data have demonstrated that uterine fibroids very rarely become cancerous (less than 0.2 percent), and most can be safely followed without treatment.

Risk Factors
The risk of endometrial cancer increases when a woman is exposed to excess estrogen without the opposing effects of another hormone called progesterone. The following is a list of risk factors:

◆ obesity;
◆ frequent irregular cycles without ovulation (for example, women with polycystic ovarian syndrome, one of the leading causes of female infertility);
◆ estrogen replacement therapy without progesterone;
◆ tamoxifen therapy (most often used in breast cancer patients, it can promote estrogen-like effects on the uterine lining);
◆ low number of full-term pregnancies;
◆ diabetes; and
◆ hypertension.

A history of oral contraceptive use most likely decreases the risk.

Symptoms and Diagnosis
Abnormal bleeding is the classic symptom that brings women with uterine cancers to their doctors for initial evaluation. These symptoms should prompt a timely work-up:

◆ in postmenopausal women not on hormone therapy, any amount of vaginal bleeding
◆ in premenopausal women (especially older than age 35 or with history of irregular cycles)

  • abnormally heavy or prolonged menses, or
  • bleeding between menses.

The vast majority of women with such presentations will be found to have benign conditions responsible for their symptoms. However, uterine cancer must be ruled out.

The first step in diagnosing uterine cancer is an endometrial biopsy, a simple office procedure that takes less than 30 seconds to perform and is more than 90 percent accurate. Pelvic ultrasound and dilation and curettage (D&C) are other diagnostic tools that may be useful in certain cases.

Treatment
Fortunately, more than 70 percent of uterine cancers are diagnosed in the early stages, when surgery is frequently curative. Patients with more advanced or metastatic disease (cancer that has spread outside the uterus) usually require radiation therapy and/or chemotherapy. Evaluation by a gynecologic oncologist is recommended in such cases.

What Is Ovarian Cancer?

Ovarian cancer is the fifth most common cancer in women, with approximately 25,000 new cases and 16,000 fatalities per year. It is the leading cause of death from gynecologic malignancies. More than 90 percent of ovarian cancers arise from the epithelial lining of the ovaries. The disease usually spreads by "exfoliating" into the abdominal cavity, where it forms multiple diffuse tumor nodules.

Risk Factors
A woman's lifetime risk of developing ovarian cancer is approximately one in 70. However, this risk is strongly dependent on age. The risk that an ovarian cyst is malignant increases as a woman ages. In premenopausal women with an ovarian cyst, the risk of malignancy is 13 percent, compared to 45 percent in postmenopausal women.

Factors that influence the number of times a woman ovulates in her lifetime can alter ovarian cancer risk. Theoretically, the surface epithelium of the ovaries is damaged and undergoes subsequent repair with each ovulation. Spontaneous mutations that occur during this reparative process can then lead to the emergence of cancerous cells. Predisposing factors include:

 ♦ early onset of menses,
 ♦ late onset of menopause,
 ♦ history of infertility, and
 ♦ use of talc powder.

Protective factors include

 ♦ increased childbearing—having one full-term pregnancy reduces risk by 30 percent;
 ♦ history of oral contraceptive use—five years or more can reduce risk by more than 50 percent; and
 ♦ tubal ligation.

Genetics
The majority of ovarian cancers occur in women without a strong family history or genetic predisposition. However, up to 10 percent occur in women with genetic or hereditary factors that greatly increase their risk of ovarian, as well as other (breast, endometrial, colon) cancers. The most well-known genetic factors associated with ovarian cancer are in mutations of the BRCA1 and BRCA2 genes. Certain ethnic groups, such as those of Ashkenazi Jewish decent, have a much higher chance of carrying these mutations than does the general population. Scientists have recently discovered a possible role for changes in a gene to the most deadly ovarian cancers.

Hereditary nonpolyposis colorectal cancer (HNPCC) is another hereditary syndrome with genetic mutations that can increase the risk of colon, endometrial, and ovarian cancer. Surgical removal of the ovaries before the disease can develop can reduce risk by 90 percent in high-risk women, but it does not eliminate the risk completely, as cancer can arise in the surrounding tissue.

Symptoms
Early-stage ovarian cancer usually causes no symptoms. Even in more advanced stages, symptoms tend to be nonspecific and include:

- abdominal discomfort or bloating,
- nausea,
- decreased appetite or energy, and
- changes in bowel or urinary habits.

Patients and their physicians frequently overlook these symptoms, leading to delays in diagnosis.

Diagnosis
A diagnosis of ovarian cancer is usually strongly suspected after pelvic and/or abdominal tumors with stereotypical characteristics are seen on radiologic imaging (ultrasound and/or CT scan). The definitive diagnosis is confirmed after a biopsy is examined at the time of or after surgery. There is currently no good screening test for ovarian cancer. Screening with ultrasound and a blood marker called CA-125 have shown disappointing results because of the high rate of false positives and false negatives. The primary use of CA-125 is to follow the effects of treatment. A new technique looking at certain patterns of proteins in the blood (proteomics) is in the early phases of development, but it may offer a sensitive mode of screening for ovarian cancer in the future.

Treatment

The first step in treating ovarian cancer is surgery to remove as much tumor as possible. Studies have shown improved survival if such surgery is performed by a trained gynecological oncologist. Chemotherapy is usually necessary in all but the very early stages. Development of new chemotherapeutic drugs has significantly improved survival in recent years, and clinical trials are ongoing to identify better drug combinations. New biological treatments are also in the pipeline and offer significant promise for the future treatment of ovarian cancer.

WHAT IS CERVICAL CANCER?

The widespread use of Pap smear screening has dramatically reduced the incidence of invasive cervical cancer in Western industrialized countries; however, cervical cancer continues to be a major cause of cancer death in underdeveloped countries. The American Cancer Society estimated approximately 10,000 new cases of cervical cancer in the United States, with about 3,900 deaths in 2004.

Risk Factors

Cervical cancer usually progresses from precancerous lesions over the course of many years. It is one of the few malignancies with a known cause—the human papillomavirus (HPV). There are many different strains of HPV; only certain high-risk subtypes (for example, 16, 18, 31) can lead to precancerous and cancerous lesions. Increased risk is seen with:

- first intercourse at a younger age,
- higher number of sexual partners,
- smoking, and
- use of oral contraceptives.

Screening

The advent of the liquid-based Pap smear in recent years has increased the sensitivity and detection rate of premalignant cervical lesions. The American College of Obstetricians and Gynecologists currently recommends starting Pap screening approximately three years after initiation of sexual activity or at age 21. After three negative screens, the frequency can be decreased in low-risk women. Pap smear combined with HPV typing is a recommended option for women older than age 30. If a women is negative for both, a repeat screen is not necessary for at least three years.

Symptoms
The goal of cervical cancer screening is to identify and treat disease at its early stages, when most patients have no symptoms and treatment can be curative. More advanced stages can present with abnormal vaginal bleeding, bleeding after intercourse, persistent vaginal discharge, or pain.

Treatment
Pre-malignant and very early stage disease can frequently be treated with a fertility-preserving procedure, such as a loop electrosurgical excision procedure (LEEP) or cone that removes a small portion of the cervix. Small, early-stage disease may be cured by a radical hysterectomy (extensive surgery that usually involves removal of the uterus, surrounding tissues, and upper vagina). Large-volume or advanced-stage disease usually requires radiation with chemotherapy.

OTHER GYNECOLOGIC MALIGNANCIES

Vulvar and vaginal cancer occur much less commonly, with an estimated annual incidence in the United States of approximately one per 3,900 women and one per 2,100, respectively. Risk of these malignancies tends to increase with age. Any abnormal vulvar or vaginal lesions should be evaluated by a qualified gynecologist and biopsies performed if there is any suspicion of malignancy.

Gestational trophoblastic disease (involving benign to malignant placental cells) comprises a group of malignancies associated with one in every 1,000 pregnancies in the United States. Effective chemotherapies make these cases highly curable, with a survival rate of close to 100 percent.

—M. ZHANG; RUTH B. LATHI, MD;
AND LINDA C. GIUDICE, MD, PhD

Kidney Cancer

WHAT IS KIDNEY CANCER?

The American Cancer Society estimates that there will be about 36,160 new cases of kidney cancer (22,490 in men and 13,670 in women) in the United States in 2005, and about 12,660 people (8,020 men and 4,640 women) will die from this disease. For reasons that are not clear, the rate of people developing kidney cancer increased slightly in the 1990s, but the increase seems to be leveling off.

And the good news is that the death rate appears to be dropping slightly as well. The five-year survival rate is about 60 percent for all people diagnosed with kidney cancer (including tumors that are localized and those that have metastasized). It is about 90 percent for those whose tumor is confined to the kidney, about 60 percent if it has only spread to nearby tissues, and about 9 percent if it has spread to distant sites.

In about 50 percent of cases, the cancer has not spread outside the kidney when it is discovered. In another 25 percent of people, the cancer has grown locally outside the kidney, and in the remaining 25 percent it has spread to other parts of the body such as the lungs or bones.

RISK FACTORS

Kidney cancer develops most often in people over age 50, but no one knows the exact causes of this disease. Studies have found the following risk factors for kidney cancer:

- ◆ smoking—cigarette smoking is a major risk factor. Cigarette smokers are nearly twice as likely as nonsmokers to develop kidney cancer. Cigar smoking also may increase the risk of this disease.
- ◆ obesity
- ◆ high blood pressure
- ◆ sedentary lifestyle
- ◆ long-term dialysis
- ◆ Von Hippel-Lindau (VHL) syndrome, a rare disease that runs in some families
- ◆ environment—some people have a higher risk of getting kidney cancer because they come in contact with certain chemicals or substances in their workplace. Coke oven workers in the iron and steel industry are at risk, and workers exposed to asbestos or cadmium may be at risk as well.

WHY YOUR SEX MATTERS

Males are more likely than females to be diagnosed with kidney cancer. Each year in the United States, about 20,000 men and 12,000 women learn they have kidney cancer.

SYMPTOMS

Like most other kidney diseases, kidney cancer often has no symptoms until it has reached an advanced stage. Routine medical checkups are the best way to catch kidney cancer early. Common symptoms of kidney cancer can include:

◆ blood in the urine (making the urine slightly rusty to deep red),
◆ pain in the side that does not go away,
◆ a lump or mass in the side or the abdomen,
◆ weight loss,
◆ fever, and
◆ feeling very tired or having a general feeling of poor health.

Most often, these symptoms do not mean cancer. An infection, cyst, or another problem can cause the same symptoms.

DIAGNOSIS

You doctor will perform a physical exam, ask for blood and urine tests, and may use one or more of the following to diagnose kidney cancer:

◆ Intravenous pyelogram (IVP)—Your doctor injects dye into a vein in the arm. The dye travels through the body and collects in the kidneys, which the dye reveals on x-rays. A series of x-rays then tracks the dye as it moves through the kidneys to the ureters and bladder. Because of the high amounts of radiation, pregnant women should not have an IVP. People suffering from chronic kidney disease or kidney failure also should not take the test as it may worsen kidney function.
◆ CT scan—An x-ray machine linked to a computer takes a series of detailed pictures of the kidneys. You may receive an injection of dye so the kidneys show up clearly in the pictures.
◆ Ultrasound test—The ultrasound waves bounce off the kidneys, and a computer uses the echoes to create a picture, called a sonogram.
◆ Biopsy—A biopsy is removal of tissue to look for cancer cells. The doctor inserts a thin needle through the skin into the kidney to remove a small amount of tissue. A pathologist, a doctor who diagnoses disease by studying cells and tissues under a microscope, then looks for cancer cells in the tissue.
◆ Surgery—In most cases, based on the results of the CT scan, ultrasound, and x-rays, the doctor has enough information to recommend surgery to remove part or all of the kidney. A pathologist makes the final diagnosis.

TREATMENT

Kidney cancer can be treated with surgery, radiation, biological therapy, or chemotherapy. Doctors are beginning to combine chemotherapy with new treatments, such as stem cell transplantation, which allows a patient to be treated with high doses of drugs. The high doses destroy both cancer cells and normal blood cells in the bone marrow. Later, the patient receives healthy stem cells from a donor, and new blood cells eventually develop from the transplanted stem cells. Other approaches are also under study; for example, researchers are studying cancer vaccines that help the immune system find and attack kidney cancer cells.

— MICHAEL SPIGLER, CHES

Lung Cancer

WHAT IS LUNG CANCER?

Lung cancer is the leading cause of cancer deaths in the United States. Most people do not realize it, but since 1987, more women have died each year of lung cancer than of breast cancer. It is responsible for about 25 percent of all cancer-related deaths in women in the United States. In the last decade, U.S. women have almost caught up with U.S. men in the number of diagnoses per year. In fact, the U.S. ranks number one in the world in lung cancer incidence in women. Currently, of the approximate 172,000 new cases of lung cancer this year in the U.S., 47 percent will be in women.

Lung cancer is often referred to as one of the "deadly cancers" because, until recently, the number of new diagnoses almost equaled the number of people who die from the disease every year. However, if lung cancer is detected early, it can be treated successfully. With early detection, people survive as long as those with almost any other cancer. Recent studies in the United States and Japan show that more than 96 percent of people who have early-stage lung cancer (when the tumor is still very small and has not spread) live at least eight years after their diagnosis. Other cancer survival rates are based on a five-year survival.

There are two major types of lung cancer: small-cell lung cancer and non-small-cell lung cancer. Most people are diagnosed with non-small-cell lung cancer (NSCLC), of which there are several types. The most common type in women is adenocarcinoma; the most common type of NSCLC in men is squamous cell carcinoma. Each year a small number of people are diagnosed with another type called large or giant-cell carcinoma. There are four stages of non-small-cell lung cancer, I to IV. Stage I is early stage and Stage IV is late stage.

Only about 10 to 15 percent of people develop small-cell lung cancer. It is staged the same as non-small-cell lung cancer. Small-cell lung cancer grows quickly and spreads rapidly, even though it is sometimes diagnosed when only one tumor is visible. Because of these characteristics, small-cell lung cancer is usually treated with chemotherapy rather than surgery.

RISK FACTORS

Tobacco use (smoking) is the direct cause of about 80 percent of lung cancers. U.S. men began smoking in large numbers during World War II, when the military began providing free cigarettes to soldiers—as it continued to do until just recently. Since many American women took up the habit after World War II, and especially in the 1950s and '60s, the number of lung cancer cases in women has trailed behind those in men. For the past several decades, however, the number of women diagnosed with lung cancer has risen steadily. The good news is that, in the last decade, the number of new cases in men has leveled off and actually seems to be dropping, and the number of new cases in women also seems to be leveling off.

Former smokers are at risk as well. Currently, more than half of those diagnosed with lung cancer every year are former smokers, because adults hear the message to quit smoking and eventually do. But cancerous cells have already started developing, and most lung cancers grow very slowly. Former smokers may be diagnosed 10–20 years or more after they quit smoking.

If you have a 20 "pack year" history of smoking, you have a 20 "pack year" risk of developing lung cancer. "Pack years" equal the packs per day times the number of years smoking. So one pack a day for 20 years or two packs a day for 10 years equals a 20 "pack-year" risk. It is important that you talk to your doctor about your risk. The chance that you will be diagnosed with lung cancer does decrease eventually, but any former smoker will always have a higher risk than a person who has never been a smoker. And recent research indicates that women are more than twice as likely than men to develop lung cancer after the same number of "pack years."

If you are one of the almost 50 million people in the United States who smoke, *quit*! Smoking is not only a major health risk for lung cancer, but it can also put you at risk for many other types of cancer, heart disease, stroke, and other diseases. Studies have shown that secondhand smoke can put children at greater risk for developing asthma, upper respiratory tract infections like bronchitis, and ear infections that can cause serious hearing loss. Smoking during pregnancy can cause serious problems, including low birth weight in the baby.

We are only beginning to understand the negative effects of passive smoke on others. A woman does not have to smoke to develop lung cancer. Somewhere between 10 and 15 percent of lung cancers in the United States develop in people who have never smoked. Exposure to second-hand smoke puts a woman at risk for lung cancer. In the past decade, about 40 percent of the lung cancer cases diagnosed in Japanese women are thought to be due to exposure to passive smoke in their homes, because for many years almost all Japanese men smoked. For reasons we are not sure of, women seem to be more sensitive to the cancer-causing effects of tobacco than men. Fortunately for Japanese women and men, only about 50 percent of men in Japan are still currently smoking. Sadly, like their American counterparts, more Japanese women, like women in the rest of the world, are now smokers, themselves.

Smoking marijuana also increases your risk for lung cancer, especially if you also smoke cigarettes.

We all know that some people who do not smoke develop lung cancer. Air pollutants can cause this cancer as well. One of the most common pollutant is the radon found in the soil in some parts of the country. If you live in an area where there is radon, use a home test kit to see if it is present in your home, especially in a basement area. Mitigation systems can lower the level to an acceptable federal standard. Asbestos is also a common cause of lung cancer, as are diesel exhaust and laboratory or manufacturing chemicals. If you work or live in an environment where you are exposed to any of these air pollutants, talk to your doctor about your risk.

The other major risk factor for developing lung cancer is your family genetics. We do not quite understand the exact level of risk. One hopes these questions will be answered in the next decade, as many genetic studies are completed in which researchers are looking at the genetics of families where many members developed lung cancer. Researchers are also looking at the genetics of people with no family history of lung cancer who have developed the disease.

If someone in your family (parent, sibling, other blood-related relative) has had esophageal or head and neck cancer, you are at increased risk for the disease. You are also at increased risk if someone in your family has had breast, prostate, or colorectal cancer, because all these cancers make up a family of cancers derived from the same type of cells.

If you have already been diagnosed with lung cancer, or with another tobacco-related cancer such as esophageal or head and neck cancer, you are at increased risk for developing a second lung cancer. You are also at increased risk for lung cancer if you COPD or other pulmonary disease such as pulmonary fibrosis.

Why Your Sex Matters
Women seem to develop lung cancer at a younger age than men. Most women diagnosed with lung cancer are in their 40s or older. But lung cancer has been diagnosed in teenage women and in women in their 20s and 30s as well. It is not known exactly why most women develop adenocarcinoma, and the number of women developing squamous cell carcinoma seems to be on the rise. One of the possible reasons is obvious; we have different hormones from men; but studies have shown that we also smoke differently from men, and we smoke different types of cigarettes. We also tend to smoke fewer cigarettes per day than men. All of these reasons may influence the type of non-small-cell lung cancer that develops.

SIGNS AND SYMPTOMS OF LUNG CANCER

Common symptoms of lung cancer include:

- shortness of breath;
- fatigue;
- increased amount of coughing or increased sputum production;
- recurring pneumonia;
- pain, especially chest or back pain;
- weakness;
- hoarseness; and
- headache.

The earliest symptom of lung cancer is often a change in your ability to breathe. Many lung cancer patients say that they suddenly began to huff and puff more when they walked up a flight of stairs or tried to walk fast, run, or do aerobics. Often this is ignored because breathing difficulties are frequently cited as a symptom of growing older. But if you are a current or former smoker, and/or someone in your family has lung cancer, it may be worth following up with some tests. The easiest one is a pulmonary function test. Pulmonary function is often lower in people with lung cancer than it is in those without the disease.

Fatigue often accompanies the feeling of breathlessness. If your lungs are not able to function normally it means you are not be getting as much oxygen throughout your body. You will be more tired than usual. Again, we and our healthcare professionals may ignore this symptom or see it as a sign of aging. If fatigue does not go away with rest or reduction of stress, it is wise to see your doctor and discuss possible tests.

Another common early symptom of lung cancer is a cough or cold that does not go away. Some people may be diagnosed with bronchitis or pneumonia several times in a year. If this has happened to you, and antibiotics have not helped or have helped only temporarily, then testing for lung cancer may be appropriate.

Other symptoms include coughing up blood and pain or weakness in the chest or back and sometimes in the arms or legs. If a tumor is large or has spread to other parts of the body, you might become hoarse or have headaches. These symptoms are generally seen when lung cancer is advanced, but that is not always the case.

Why Your Sex Matters
The benefit women may have is that they often pay more attention to the way their bodies feel. Studies have shown that women usually seek a doctor's help earlier than do men. Additional studies show that more women are diagnosed at earlier stage lung cancer than are men. This is part of the reason why women, especially those with early-stage lung cancer, live longer than men after diagnosis of lung cancer.

Diagnosis
There are currently no approved national screening guidelines for the general population or for people at risk for lung cancer. A spiral CT (computed tomography) is the best way for your doctor/s to see whether you have a tumor. It can also show areas in your lungs where emphysema is developing, which is important if you are a smoker. One study revealed that when people who are at risk for emphysema see their CT scans, it facilitates their quitting smoking, and more of these people are able to stay off cigarettes than those who try to quit using other methods.

Some doctors may want to do a chest x-ray, but a study done more than 20 years ago established that this was not an effective way to diagnose lung cancer. Chest x-rays are only effective at finding relatively large tumors, usually larger than 2 cm. Even with newly available computer-assisted detection programs, x-rays can only find nodules about 8 to 10 mm in size with any reliability. Remember, the earlier a lung cancer is found, the better your chances are at having effective therapy.

Another test that might be done is bronchoscopy. In this test a medical specialist inserts a long tube down your throat into your lungs. A small microscope with a camera is inserted through the tube so the doctor can carefully examine the larger bronchi (breathing tubes) in your lungs. The doctor can even remove samples of tissue that she or he suspects might be cancerous.

Other diagnostic measures include coughing up sputum samples from your lungs to check for the presence of cancer cells and the PET (positron emission tomography) scan. The PET scan can detect cancer anywhere in your body, but only if the cancer is about 8 to 10 mm in size.

If you are part of a screening study (see page 145) or have a CT because you are at risk for lung cancer and a nodule is found by CT, it has a good chance of being under 1 cm in size. Some CT-detected nodules or lesions are as small as 2 mm, about the size of a grain of rice. In this case your doctors may suggest waiting one to three months and then performing another CT to see if the nodule grows. If the nodule has not grown, it is probably a scar from a previous infection; if it goes away with antibiotic treatment, then it was a localized infection; if it grows, the next step is a biopsy.

If the nodule is larger, for example, over 10 mm (1 cm, or even larger if it has been detected by other means), then a biopsy should be done right away. If the nodule is located in the center of your chest, the biopsy might be done using the bronchoscope. If it is located in the outer portions of your lungs, then a biopsy might be done by fine-needle aspiration (FNA). To do FNA, the doctor inserts a thin needle through your chest wall into your lung to remove a small piece of the suspected tumor.

Some physicians may want to do a biopsy by opening your chest. This should be done only if the tumor is so large that it could not possibly be benign or non-cancerous. If you have a large tumor (over 1 cm in size), a PET scan is an excellent tool to differentiate between a cancerous and a non-cancerous tumor. At this time you will also have more complete CT scans of your lungs that will include injection of dye into your bloodstream.

Treatments

Treatment and access to treatment for lung cancer have improved considerably over the last few years. Just over a decade ago, less than half of people diagnosed with lung cancer received any treatment at all. Today, almost every patient receives treatment, which may include surgery, chemotherapy, and/or radiation. Treatments also include new medicines that have fewer side effects than standard chemotherapy.

Surgery

Early stage (I and II) lung cancer is usually treated with surgery. Your surgeon will remove either a part of the affected lobe or all of it, depending on the size and location of the nodule. Some older people with heart disease and/or emphysema might not be able to go through open-chest surgery. An option that is used frequently is video-assisted thoracotomy

(VATS) in which three small incisions are made in the chest wall and a portion of a lobe is removed using specialized surgical tools. Non-surgical options, such as radiation or new treatments, such as heat and cold (cryotherapy) that might be in a clinical trial protocol, may be used to destroy the tumor.

Women tend to do better with surgery than men, as evidenced by long-term survival rates. Anyone having surgery for lung cancer will have some difficulty getting used to reduced lung capacity. We normally have five lobes of lung tissue. If even one of these is removed, your ability to get as much oxygen as you could before surgery is reduced. However, many lung cancer survivors get by on just two lobes of lungs and live happy, fulfilled lives. Exercise and good lung health are very important in maintaining the remaining lung tissue at the greatest functionality. People who have been diagnosed with lung cancer should not smoke or have unnecessary exposure to passive smoke or other pulmonary carcinogens.

The major complaint of many women after chest surgery is that the incision scars are often in the same place as their bra, which can be very irritating. If you are to have open-chest surgery, talk to your doctor about where the incision scars will be and whether there are options. If you only have a portion of a lobe removed because you have VATS, you will not have this problem since your scars will be small and strategically located, between the ribs. Studies show that people with early stage lung cancer, especially Stage II, do much better if they have chemotherapy in addition to surgery. If you have early stage lung cancer, be sure to talk to a medical oncologist to discuss additional treatment after surgery.

Chemotherapy
Chemotherapy for lung cancer is used to treat tumors that are more than 1–2 cm in size and when there is a good possibility that the cancer has spread. During surgery, your surgeon will check the lymph nodes in the middle of your chest to see if the cancer has entered the lymph system, or, if your tumor is larger, she or he may do a PET scan to see if this detects cancer in those nodes or in other organs of your body. Chemotherapy for lung cancer is usually a combination of different drugs that work in different ways. This is to ensure the best possible chance of killing as many tumor cells as possible.

Radiation
Radiation may also be used to treat the tumor/s in your lungs or possibly in bones such as ribs or your spine if the cancer has spread there.

Side Effects of Treatment
Both chemotherapy and radiation therapy have improved significantly in the past decade. People who are treated with either therapy now experience far fewer side effects, because many products are now available that help to control them. The most serious side-effect of either chemotherapy or radiation therapy is damage to the bone marrow. This can be life-threatening and your blood cell counts should be monitored carefully. Be sure you talk to your doctors about how they prevent and treat side effects before you begin your treatments.

THE FUTURE OF LUNG CANCER TREATMENT

Some newer, "targeted" drugs, also used to treat lung cancer, stimulate or inhibit a single action of a cell's metabolic pathway. This is very different from the usual chemotherapy drugs that kill every dividing cell in the body. Because the actions of these drugs are targeted, they have far fewer side effects. One drug, gefitinib, seems to work best in women, especially those who have never smoked. Another new produce, erlotinib, will probably be used more in the future since it appears to have fewer side effects and may be more effective. Many targeted therapies are being tested in clinical trials, and most cancers will be treated in the future using these types of drugs.

Even with later-stage lung cancer that is treated without surgery, women do better than men, as shown by better survival rates.

PREVENTION

The best prevention for lung cancer is to never smoke. It is also important to reduce your exposure to passive smoke and to other carcinogens as much as possible. This is especially important for those who have a family member with lung cancer or even a history of cancer in their families.

Studies have shown that eating a diet high in vegetables and fruits is helpful in preventing lung cancer. It is important to eat at least seven servings of varied vegetables and fruits every day, especially if you are at risk.

There have been a number of clinical trials to see if ingesting something can reduce the risk of lung cancer. One study of beta-carotine showed that this vitamin actually increased the risk of lung cancer in people who were current smokers. Other studies have shown no beneficial effect when people at risk drank green tea or took medicines containing retinoids.

Another way to prevent lung cancer is to support national and international laws and treaties that promote clean air and reduce pollution. We must all make sure that our governments enforce those laws that are on the books, and we must actively encourage our lawmakers to make even more stringent laws to prevent air pollution.

EARLY DETECTION

Early detection is sometimes called secondary prevention; but, in fact, if you are detected with lung cancer, you have not prevented it. However, if you have taken advantage of the fact that lung cancer can be detected early, you may prevent your own premature death by this disease.

You are at risk for lung cancer if any of the following is true:

♦ you are a current or former smoker with at least a ten "pack-year" history;
♦ you have a blood relative who has been diagnosed with lung cancer;
♦ you have received chronic exposure to passive smoke during childhood or as an adult; or
♦ you have been exposed to carcinogenic chemicals (radon, asbestos, diesel fuel, etc.) in the workplace.

If you are experiencing any signs or symptoms of lung cancer, you may want to seek help from a specialist. Lung specialists are called pulmonologists. If you have even one of the risk factors for lung cancer and are 40 years old or older or you are experiencing any signs or symptoms, talk to your pulmonologist or primary care doctor and discuss whether you should be screened for lung cancer. Make sure you and your doctor talk about your personal risks.

If you are at risk, or are experiencing signs or symptoms, take advantage of the opportunity to enroll in the one early-detection trial now going on in the United States, the International Early Lung Cancer Action Project (I-ELCAP). If you are in a city where a study is going on, call the hospital where the study is located and talk to the study coordinator about how you might enroll or otherwise have a CT scan. In this study you will receive a low-dose spiral CT exam of your lungs.

If you do not live near a trial site, talk to your pulmonologist or your primary care doctor about any signs or symptoms you may be having or your risk factors. If you and your doctor feel your symptom/s or risks warrant it, she or he can order a CT of your lungs. This should be covered by your medical insurance as long as your doctor lists any signs or symptoms on the report.

The CT scan is the best test for detecting lung cancer. It can find any nodules or tumors when they are much smaller than those that can be seen by chest x-ray. The radiation dose for the low-dose screening CT is about the same as for a chest x-ray. Because the CT scan can find very small nodules, most of which are not cancerous, your doctor should follow the protocol suggested by the I-ELCAP program to help you avoid unnecessary medical procedures. If you have nodules of less than 10 mm, you will probably get a course of antibiotics and have another CT scan in a few months. Both scans should be read by someone who is able to determine if any nodule has grown. This is a very important step and should not be ignored. One of the major benefits of the CT scan is that the nodules can be seen in three dimensions. With a chest x-ray, a tumor can only be seen in two dimensions. Often, growth in these tiny nodules can only be seen by looking at and comparing a nodule in all three dimensions over a period of time. Your doctor can go to the I-ELCAP Web site for more information on the exact protocol. If your lungs are cancer free, it will be important that you continue to have this screen every year in the same way you are screened annually for breast or cervical cancer. This gives you the best chance of finding an early-stage tumor, which can be treated more easily.

If a nodule is found and cancer is suspected because of growth or the appearance of a larger nodule, a biopsy should be done before you and your doctor decide on treatment. You want to be sure that it is, indeed, cancer and what type of cancer it is, so it can be treated appropriately.

Like other cancers, lung cancer is most curable when it is detected early. For most people, waiting for the results of a test can be worrisome, but they are well worth the wait. In the best of circumstances, you will not have lung cancer. But if you are diagnosed with lung cancer, and it is found in an early stage, you will have the greatest opportunity for successful treatment and survival. If you are diagnosed with late-stage lung cancer, perhaps because you or your doctor ignored early signs or symptoms, remember that it can still be treated more successfully than it was in previous times, and new therapies are being tested all the time. One hopes that, within a few years, we will be able to detect minor changes in the blood to find lung cancer before a nodule has a chance to develop. There eventually may be treatments that will kill those cancer cells before they affect quality of life in any way. Remember, the most important thing you can do is quit smoking if you are currently a smoker. And if you are at risk for lung cancer, talk to your doctor about your risks and develop a plan for managing them.

—Peggy McCarthy, MBA, and Michael E. Kalafer, MD

Be Careful What You Hope For

By Rosalind Brannigan

The cancer, the doctors told me, had originated in my brain, my breasts, or my lungs. Let it be my lungs, I prayed, as the prospects of brain or breast cancer were too frightening. I soon learned how wrong I was. I did not know then that the survival rate for lung cancer is only 15 percent.

In November 2003, I broke my arm at my health club and was diagnosed with incurable (stage IV) lung cancer that had metastasized to my shoulder and arm—a big shock for someone who stopped smoking 38 years ago, exercises an hour a day, and has worked in public health for the past 25 years.

At the time of my diagnosis, I was under the care of four highly regarded physicians (an allergist, two ear, nose, and throat specialists, and an internist). My symptoms were hoarseness, complete exhaustion, and severe pain in my arm—the result, I thought, of a sports injury. Two of my physicians had experienced recent sports injuries and were very sympathetic.

Since my diagnosis, I have read extensively about lung cancer and am fully aware of the challenges in diagnosing this disease. However, among the warning signs of lung cancer are the very symptoms I presented to my doctors (some others are chronic cough, shortness of breath, unexplained weight loss, and pain in the chest).

None of these physicians suggested even a chest x-ray, though I reported on all medical forms that my father had died of lung cancer. I had also smoked, as had almost all of my peers, in the early 1960s. But since I had quit smoking decades ago, lung cancer wasn't even on my radar screen in 2003. Lung cancer is not on most women's radar screens, nor, it appears, on those of many physicians.

My treatment involved major surgery to insert a titanium rod from my shoulder to elbow, radiation, and six months of weekly chemotherapy. At one point after surgery and radiation, my left arm had to be wrapped in heavy bandages to combat lymphedema, swelling that occurs because the lymphatic drainage system has been reduced. When asked about this condition, I received sympathetic responses if I said I had bone cancer. If I said I had lung cancer, however, the appalled response invariably was, "Did you smoke?"

In September 2004, three months after the first round of chemotherapy ended, my cancer returned and had metastasized to my liver. I began *weekly chemotherapy sessions again. Shortly thereafter, a test at Massachusetts General Hospital showed that I have the genetic mutation to be a candidate for Iressa (a new targeted therapy that only works for one in ten individuals with advanced lung cancer), which I began taking in October 2004. Five months later, tests showed that all the tumors in my liver are gone, and the tumor in my lung continues to shrink. However, it was announced in December 2004 that the U.S. Food and Drug Administration (FDA) is reviewing Iressa's fast-track approval and may take the drug off the market. At an FDA hearing in March 2005, I presented my results with Iressa and urged the panel to keep it on the market.*

Unfortunately, in April 2005, the metastasized bone cancer in my spine, which had been stable, began to spread, and once again, I received radiation treatment. At times, I feel like a "California brushfire," but I remain relentlessly optimistic that new drugs coming on the market will help extend my life.

For women who quit smoking years ago and think they are not at risk for lung cancer, this should be a wake-up call. They should be alert to the warning signs of lung cancer and see their doctors if they have questions.

(Reprinted with permission of Rosaline Brannigan, MPH, who died while this book was in progress. Ms. Brannigan was vice president of Drug Strategies, a nonprofit research institute, and an advocate for lung cancer patients.)

Oral Cancer

WHAT IS ORAL CANCER?

Oral cancer, sometimes referred to as oral and pharyngeal cancer, includes cancers of the mouth, tongue, and throat. They account for roughly 4 percent of all cancers diagnosed in the United States, yet their survival rate remains one of the lowest of all cancers. The number of new cases has decreased over the past 20 years, and in the past two years, cases have dropped by 5 percent annually. The American Cancer Society estimates that about 29,370 new cases of oral cancer will be diagnosed in the United States in 2005.

WHY YOUR SEX MATTERS

Of these new oral cancer cases, 19,100 will be diagnosed in men and 10, 270 will be diagnosed in women. Although men are diagnosed with these cancers twice as often as women, the rate at which men develop oral cancer is *decreasing*, and the rate at which women develop the disease is *increasing*. In 1950 six men developed oral cancer for every one woman; by 1997 it was approximately two men for every one woman. This may be due to the increase of alcohol and tobacco use among women.

Oral cancer strikes women of all ages, races, and ethnic backgrounds. It is estimated that 7,320 people will die of oral and pharyngeal cancer in 2005: 4,910 men and 2,410 women. For all stages of the disease combined, the five-year relative survival rate is 59 percent. If the cancer is found early, before it has spread to the lymph nodes, the five-year relative survival rate is around 81 percent.

Figure 1 shows the increasing number of adults over age 65 in the U.S. population through 2030. Once they reach age 65, women have an average of 19 years additional years of life. Since the risk of oral cancer increases with advancing age, women need to ask their dentists for an oral cancer examination during their annual dental visits.

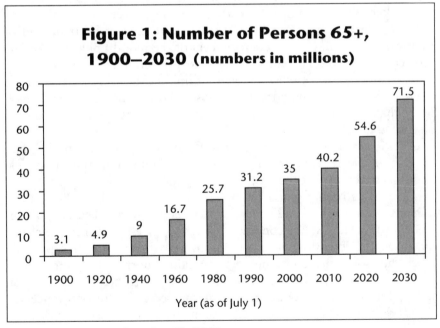

Figure 1: Number of Persons 65+, 1900–2030 (numbers in millions)

Year (as of July 1)

Source: www.aoa.gov/stats/profile/2003

RISK FACTORS

Risk factors associated with an increased risk for oral and pharyngeal cancers include:

♦ advancing age,
♦ use of tobacco (both smoking and smokeless),
♦ alcohol use,
♦ prior history of oral cancer, and
♦ race; African Americans are also at increased risk.

Sun exposure is a risk factor for lip cancer. While some risk factors are known, it is estimated that approximately 25 percent of people who develop oral cancer have no known risk factors, and this number is increasing.

Tobacco and alcohol use are the major risk factors for oral cancers. Approximately 90 percent of people with oral cancers use tobacco. All forms of tobacco use—smokeless/chewing, cigars, and pipes as well as cigarettes—increase the risk for the disease. Smokers are up to six times more likely than nonsmokers to develop oral cancers. Also, about 33 percent of people who continue to smoke after successful treatment of their cancer will develop second cancers of the mouth, pharynx, or larynx, compared to 6 percent of those who stop smoking.

In addition, people who frequently drink alcohol are six times more likely to have oral cancer than are those who do not consume alcohol. More than 75 percent of oral and pharyngeal cancers are associated with alcohol use.

Ultraviolet light is a significant risk factor for lip cancer, and the incidence of lip cancer is decreasing in the United States. One third of people with lip cancer are in occupations with significant sun exposure.

Patients with compromised immune systems have also been shown to be at increased risk of oral and pharyngeal cancer. Vitamin A deficiency, Plummer-Vinson syndrome (a condition consisting of chronic iron deficiency anemia; difficulty swallowing; small, thin growths of tissue that partially block the esophagus; and other less-common abnormalities), and human papillomavirus (HPV) infection also have been suggested as possible risk factors for oral cancer. Other factors that increase risk for oral cancer include organ transplant and subsequent long-term immunosuppression.

SYMPTOMS/DIAGNOSIS

Oral cancer occurs most commonly on the floor of the mouth, the sides of the tongue, or the back of the throat. Pain is often not associated with oral and pharyngeal cancer; possible signs and symptoms of oral and pharyngeal cancer include:

♦ mouth sore that does not heal or bleeds easily,
♦ lump or bump in mouth or neck,
♦ red or white patch in mouth,
♦ sore throat or throat problems, and
♦ difficulty chewing.

Hoarseness or difficulty swallowing can also be symptoms of oral cancer. Hoarseness unrelated to a cold, allergies, or other upper respiratory infection should be evaluated by a physician. Swallowing difficulties should also be evaluated by your physician or dentist.

Often the red or white patch in the mouth that signals cancer does not hurt. For this reason, it may be easy to ignore or forget. However, all sores in the mouth—whether they hurt or not—should heal within two weeks. Examine your mouth every day when you brush your teeth. Lift up your tongue and look at the floor of your mouth, on the sides or inside of your cheeks, and at the hard and soft palate for any red or white sores. If you notice one, watch it to be sure that it heals in 10–14 days.

For those parts of your mouth that are difficult for you to see at home (the back of your throat), a regular dental checkup is necessary, with an examination of the entire oral cavity to find oral and pharyngeal cancers early, when they are most treatable. A recent public awareness campaign conducted by the American Dental Association focused on the need for a regular oral cancer screening exam for early detection of oral cancer.

TREATMENT

Treatment of oral cancer, which usually includes surgery and radiation therapy, depends of the type of cell causing the cancer. Limiting exposure to risk factors such as sunlight, excessive use of alcohol, and all forms of tobacco use may decrease your risk for oral cancer.

PREVENTIVE STRATEGIES

Major actions you can take to prevent oral and pharyngeal cancer include:

♦ limiting or quitting alcohol use,
♦ limiting or quitting tobacco use,
♦ avoiding the midday sun,
♦ wearing a wide-brim hat,

♦ using sunscreen, and
♦ eating a healthy diet.

Using a sunscreen on your face and lips is recommended to prevent both skin and lip cancers. Quitting tobacco or alcohol, even after many years of use, lowers the risk for disease. Alcohol and tobacco work together to damage the cells of the mouth: tobacco directly damages the DNA, while alcohol increases the effect or penetration of tobacco damage.

Tobacco cessation is one of the most effective means of decreasing oral cancer risk. However, research on tobacco cessation shows that nicotine patches and gums are less effective in helping women quit tobacco than men. It is not clear what causes this disparity.

The antidepressant, bupropion, has been shown to be effective in women who are trying to stop smoking. Your dentist can be as successful as your physician in helping you quit tobacco use. The literature has demonstrated that it often takes five attempts to quit tobacco use before an individual quits for good. So do not be discouraged if you do not succeed at first. Keep trying. Stopping tobacco use is one of the best things you can do for your oral health as well as your overall health.

—Linda C. Niessen, DMD, MPH, and Denise J. Fedele, DMD, MS

Women and Skin Cancer

What Is Skin Cancer?

How many times have you had a friend tell you, "I have skin cancer"? It is the most common form of cancer in the United States. Many women think of the worst possible scenario when the word, "cancer," is mentioned. However, two types of skin cancer are rarely metastatic and often curable. These types—basal cell carcinoma (BCC) and squamous cell carcinoma (SCC)—make up 95 percent of nonmelanoma skin cancers (meaning they do not develop from moles). BCCs and SCCs can be serious. They can invade muscle, cartilage, and bone, causing significant local destruction, disfigurement, and scarring.

Of the one million nonmelanoma skin cancers diagnosed each year, approximately 175,000 will occur in American women. Worldwide, Australian women have the highest incidence rate. According to the Skin Cancer Foundation, skin cancer takes decades to develop, and the effects of ultraviolet radiation are cumulative. Women who sunbathe for just a few weeks every summer are exposed to a considerable amount of sun, which can lead to skin cancer in vulnerable skin types.

The most lethal form of skin cancer is malignant melanoma. Potentially fatal, malignant melanoma is not very common, but it is the most frequent cancer in women ages 25–29 and the second most common form of cancer in those ages 30–34.

WHO'S AT RISK?

Fitzpatrick's Sun-Reactive Skin types

Skin Type	Skin Color	Tanning Response
Type I	White	Always burn, never tan
Type II	White	Usually burn, tan with difficulty
Type III	White	Sometimes mild burn, tan average
Type IV	Brown	Rarely burn, tan with ease
Type V	Dark brown	Very rarely burn, tan very easily
Type VI	Black	No burn, tan very easily

Women with the least melanin in their skin (blond and blue-eyed) are especially susceptible for developing one or more skin cancers, including melanoma. Skin type is often categorized according to the Fitzpatrick skin type scale, with lower-number skin types more susceptible to developing skin cancer. According to the Skin Cancer Foundation, 80 percent of an individual's lifetime sun exposure occurs before the age of 20.

WHY YOUR SEX MATTERS

Skin cancer can appear anywhere on the body, even on areas that have relatively little sun exposure. According to Perry Robbins, clinical professor of dermatology at New York University School of Medicine and founder of the Skin Cancer Foundation, "over 80 percent of non-melanoma skin cancers appear on the face, head, neck, and back of the hands." High-risk areas for women to develop melanoma include the back of the calves, top of the thighs, abdomen, and chest, because women have less body hair and wear two-piece bathing suits. It is important for women to perform monthly skin exams and visit their dermatologist if they develop a pimple or open sore that does not heal or a mole that looks like it is changing color or size.

Dermatologists frequently diagnose multiple skin cancers on women who have worked summers as lifeguards or are employed as physical education coaches. Women who may have not worked in the sun but have spent many hours sunbathing without sunscreen, or who use baby oil and iodine instead of sunscreen, are also at greater risk. Another major increase to women's risk of developing skin cancer is the growth in popularity over the past two decades, despite public education campaigning, of indoor tanning. Many studies conducted in the United States and Europe confirm that melanomas result from exposure to artificial sunlamps found in most tanning salons. Unfortunately, the same studies indicate that approximately 75 percent of people who use these facilities are women, typically younger than 30. Many states now have restrictive legislation regarding tanning beds.

The consequences of chronic sun exposure to the skin are readily apparent when a woman compares the exposed skin of her face, hands, and neck with areas that are more protected such as the abdomen or buttocks. Women who have not protected their skin experience more deep wrinkles, loss of elasticity (the skin's ability to be stretched and return to its normal shape), coarse/parched skin with areas of thinning and thickening, brown spots, and broken blood vessels. Additionally, precancerous lesions, called actinic keratoses, start appearing as smooth, flat, or slightly raised pink spots that become irregular, scaly, or wartlike. If left untreated these lesions may eventually turn into squamous cell carcinomas.

TREATMENTS

Techniques and medical methods to treat skin cancers vary and may include surgerical excision, Mohs' microsurgery, immunotherapy, topical chemotherapy (5FU) treatments, and photodynamic therapy. Treatments that are more specific for photoaging include dermabrasion, chemical peel, laser treatmens, collagen/filler injection, and plastic surgery. Medications containing retinoids have been proven to reduce fine wrinkling, pore size, and mottled pigmentation; they can also stimulate blood flow to give a more youthful, rosy appearance to the skin. Using retinoids is also thought to prevent new precancerous lesions from developing. Women being treated with a tretinoin product may find it useful to purchase a moisturizer or foundation with a sun protection factor (SPF) added, as their skin may be more sensitive to ultraviolet light. These treatments may not be safe for pregnant women, so check with your doctor first.

Women who are considering treatment for photaging may want to meet first with a board-certified dermatologist and a board-certified plastic surgeon. There are several options for treating sun-damaged skin and combinations of cosmetic treatments, including face-lifts. Women seeking care for precancerous/cancereous lesions should find a board-certified dermatologist to get a second opinion, if necessary. However, it is important to remember that waiting too long can allow a cancer to develop further and, ultimately, result in far more extensive treatment.

OTHER ISSUES FOR WOMEN

Many of the results of photoaging do not pose health threats, but they can have an adverse emotional effect, particularly among women. In a society that values good looks and a youthful appearance, most females do not want to have preventable acquired cosmetic flaws or to look old prematurely. Fortunately, many positive achievements in skin care have occurred since 1979. When sun exposure is limited or completely avoided for a number of years, a new layer of collagen (protein and elastin responsible for the support and elasticity of the skin) appears in the dermis, causing the skin to start appearing younger and more attractive. Besides prevention, a number of safe and effective treatments can contribute significantly in making your skin look young and healthy.

Cosmetic procedures are not for everyone. For some people, wearing attractive clothing and stylish haircuts can boost confidence and self-esteem. Luckily, marvelous camouflage and bleaching products are available for all female skin types with pigmentation problems, unsightly scars, or broken blood vessels. These products can be worn with makeup or alone. A healthful alternative to soaking up the sun is self-tanning products. Newer products are far more effective than the earlier generations of "bronzers," and many formulations are designed specifically for women's skin; some products even incorporate a sunscreen. A new trend of "airbrushing" on a tan looks very natural and lasts for approximately three weeks.

PREVENTING SKIN CANCER AND PROTECTING YOUR SKIN

When French designer Coco Chanel introduced the world to the "suntanned body," she was not aware that by the late 1970s, great strides in skin care were starting to dispel what she once advocated. To prevent or reduce the effects of skin cancer and photoaging, women should avoid the sun around noontime, seek shade whenever available, and wear protective clothing and sunscreens. Improvements in sunscreens and sunblocks have been made, and their production and marketing have become more sophisticated in the last 25 years. Sunscreens are available in a variety of vehicles—gels, lotions, and creams, and with SPFs ranging from 2 to 50 and above. A good sunscreen should provide broad-spectrum protection against ultraviolet (UVA) and ultraviolet B (UVB) light.

Many cosmetics now contain sunscreens, which are also incorporated into fabrics in some lines of clothing. Other measures of prevention include seeing a board-certified dermatologist once a year for a skin exam and every six months if you already have a history of skin cancer or precancerous lesions.

—SUSAN H. WEINKLE, MD, AND HARRIET LIN HALL, ARNP, DNC

CHAPTER 9

Digestive Tract and Liver Diseases

When the bowels are normal, we take them for granted and pay them little attention. However, when bowel function changes and causes pain or results in constipation or diarrhea, many of our waking hours may be devoted to concern over or performance of the bowels. Such focused attention on the bowels often results in frequent consultations with physicians. In the United States, Canada, and Northern Europe, women are more than twice as likely as men to seek the advice of physicians for changes in bowel function. This chapter discusses diseases of the gastrointestinal tract and liver that are more common in or of particular concern to women.

What Is Normal Bowel Function?

Normal bowel function differs from person to person. Frequency of bowel movements from three times a week to two to three times a day is normal. Abnormal bowel function may mean a change in the frequency of stool; a change in the consistency or ease in elimination of the stool; the occurrence of gas, cramping, or pain; or the person's belief that the bowel movements should be different from what they are.

WHY YOUR SEX MATTERS

Women report many changes in bowel function throughout their lives. Reports of variations during the premenstrual period, in pregnancy, and after hysterectomy have inspired clinical and basic research studies on the effect of changes in female sex hormone levels on normal gastrointestinal processes. Two disorders of bowel function—irritable bowel syndrome and intractable constipation—are more common in women than they are in men, lending further support to the possible effect of female hormones on bowel function.

What Is Irritable Bowel Syndrome?

Although definitions vary among physicians, researchers define irritable bowel syndrome (IBS) as at least 12 weeks (not necessarily consecutive) of abdominal discomfort or pain within the past 52 weeks, accompanied by two of the three following features:

- ◆ pain or discomfort not relieved by defecation (bowel movement),
- ◆ onset of pain or discomfort associated with a change in stool frequency, or
- ◆ onset of pain or discomfort associated with a change in stool appearance or form.

Irritable bowel syndrome (IBS) occurs in about 10–20 percent of the population and is twice as common in women as it is in men in the United States and Europe. Overall about 14–25 percent of women have irritable bowel syndrome. The exact incidence is difficult to estimate, because most people with symptoms do not consult a physician. However, people with IBS account for over one of every three visits to gastroenterologists.

Risk Factors

Following an episode of viral or bacterial gastroenteritis, up to one-third of people may develop IBS-like symptoms. Stress exacerbates these symptoms and may be important in its onset. Those who develop IBS are more likely to have stressful life events before and three months after the infection and are more likely to have had anxiety or depression at the time of the infection. Anxiety and depression occur in 42–60 percent and fibromyalgia in 32–70 percent of women with IBS.

Many factors contribute to of the cause of IBS. Patients with IBS experience abnormal sensitivity in the bowel, abnormal movement in the intestines, activation of part of the brain, psychological stress, and abnormalities in the bowel's own nervous system. A subgroup of IBS patients clearly has increased perception of pain when a large volume is present in the rectum. During a normal day some patients with IBS are aware of small bowel contractions. It is thought that many hormones from the gut and brain play a role in symptoms getting worse.

Symptoms

Common symptoms of IBS include:

- ◆ abnormal stool frequency (less than three per week or more than three per day),

- abnormal stool form (lumpy/hard or loose/watery), and
- abnormal stool passage (straining, urgency, feeling of incomplete elimination, passage of mucus, and bloating or feeling of abdominal distension).

Rectal pain, sudden urges to have a bowel movement and, sometimes, accidents with the stool (fecal incontinence) can occur. Respiratory and urinary tract symptoms, such as increased urinary frequency and urgency, are common in patients with IBS.

History that should prompt further testing includes unexplained weight loss, abdominal pain; or diarrhea that awakens one from sleep; fat in the stool; fever; and blood in the stool (except when it actually can be seen to come from a hemorrhoid or local cut in the skin). Onset in old age does occur, but other problems that occur in older women should be excluded before a diagnosis of IBS is made. Medications are a common cause for IBS-like symptoms.

IBS symptoms can vary from person to person and can differ between men and women. Diarrhea and frequent stools are more common in men than women, but they can still occur in up to two-thirds of women. Delayed emptying of the stomach occurs in as many as 30 percent of IBS patients and is more common in women. Constipation with infrequent bowel movements, straining at stool, hard stools, or incomplete elimination of stool occurs in 50 percent of women, and these symptoms are more common in women than in men. Bloating is more common in women with IBS.

Abdominal pain is necessary to diagnose IBS. Distinguishing a gastrointestinal from a gynecologic source of abdominal pain can be difficult, and your doctor may want you to see a gynecologist. Endometriosis (the presence in the abdomen or pelvis of cells lining the uterus) can mimic irritable bowel syndrome. Although IBS is defined by lower abdominal complaints, there is an increased incidence (25–50 percent) of upper gastrointestinal complaints such as reflux and heartburn.

DIAGNOSIS

There is no test for diagnosing IBS. Tests are only useful to make sure that another condition, such as inflammatory bowel disease or colorectal cancer, is not causing the symptoms. All women age 50 or older or any woman with unexplained rectal bleeding should have a colonoscopy (see chapter 8).

If you suffer from bloating, intolerance to lactose (the sugar in milk) should be excluded. In those with lactose intolerance, the onset of bloating with or without abdominal pain may occur several minutes to hours after ingesting a milk product. For diagnosis, maintain a completely lactose-free diet for one to two weeks or have a hydrogen breath test or serial blood glucose level tests after lactose ingestion. Avoidance of lactose-containing foods and medications should help decrease or eliminate gas in a lactose-intolerant individual. Foods with lactose are milk, cream, cheese, butter, whey, casein, lactalbumin, milk solids, yogurt, ice cream, ice milk, and prepared foods that contain these substances. Many lactose-intolerant people tolerate milk products pretreated with lactase or taken with lactase pills and yogurt.

TREATMENT

IBS treatments are directed toward relief of symptoms and stress management. New therapies act on receptors in the gut for serotonin (a substance released by the nerves), which are important for gut motion and function. No one therapy will help all patients. Some people stop having symptoms without therapy, but many women require treatment for their symptoms. Most IBS patients continue to have symptoms intermittently for years.

One of the mainstays of therapy is fiber. The typical American diet is poor in fiber, although a good healthy diet should contain 25–30 grams every day. Changes in diet with the aim of increasing fiber intake to 25–40 grams of fiber should be one of the first treatments undertaken for both constipation and diarrhea, although most studies show that fiber is not helpful for diarrhea. The increased fiber in stool results in increased water in the stool and, therefore, bulkier stool. There are two sources of fiber: insoluble (wheat bran, lignin, methylcellulose, hemicellulose, flax seed, or calcium polycarbophil) and soluble (oat bran, psyllium, gums, guar, or pectin). Bloating and gas are common after ingesting some sources of fiber, but it is difficult to predict which ones will produce no or few side effects in an individual. Patients may tolerate one type of fiber and not others.

Bloating may respond to elimination of foods likely to cause gas. These include beans, brussel sprouts, carrots, celery, onions, apricots, bananas, prunes, raisins, pretzels, and wheat germ. *Beano*, an over-the-counter product containing the enzyme α-galactosidase may help prevent the gas formed from the digestion of beans and peas. Bloating and gas may also be eased by ingesting activated charcoal, simethicone, or enteric-coated peppermint capsules.

Other therapies include

- ◆ Anticholinergic agents: These are the most frequently used medications to treat IBS and may be beneficial for abdominal pain and diarrhea associated with IBS.
- ◆ Antidiarrheal agents for chronic diarrhea or frequent stools.

- Anxiolytics and antidepressants: Anxiolytic medications, including benzodiazepines and barbituates, chlordiazepoxide (Lithium®), lorazepam (Ativan®), and diazepam (Valium®), may help diminish the IBS symptoms associated with stress and anxiety, but there is a risk of dependency with their use. Tricyclic antidepressants may help abdominal pain. Selective serotonin reuptake inhibitors (SSRIs) have been used successfully with IBS by treating symptoms of concurrent anxiety and depression.
- 5-HT3 Aantagonists and 5-HT4 agonists: Two new drugs available for IBS act on the serotonin receptors in the gut. Alosetron (Lotronex®) is effective in a large percentage of women (but not men) with diarrhea-predominant IBS; its major side effect is constipation. It is available only from physicians who have special training in its use. Tegaserod (Zelnorm®) helps constipation and gas and bloating in some women and men.
- Complementary and alternative options: Herbs have been useful in some patients with IBS, and acupuncture treatment is currently being studied.
- Psychological treatments: Psychotherapeutic approaches are often effective in treating IBS either alone or in conjunction with other therapies. These include cognitive behavioral therapy, interpersonal psychotherapy, hypnosis, and stress management.

What Is Intractable Constipation?

Constipation causes much consternation and often results in a significant amount of time spent in trying to produce a bowel movement. Chronic constipation has been reported by 21 percent of women. Patients with severe, intractable constipation of no known origin are predominantly young women age 16–50 who generally have one or fewer bowel movements per week. Their gastrointestinal movement is less than those of normal women or men.

TREATMENT

Treatment is difficult and often meets with limited success. Increased fiber should be the first line of therapy, but fiber alone may not be successful; adequate hydration and exercise are also important.

Avoidance of bowel-stimulating laxatives, which may result in dependence, should be the aim of therapy, but they often need to be used. You should try lactulose, a nonabsorbable sugar, before attempting other treatments, which can include milk of magnesia, magnesium citrate, castor oil, bisacodyl USP (Dulcolax®), senna, cascara sagrada, or polyethylene glycol preparations. However, lactulose may cause intolerable bloating. Herbal teas or the prescription tegaserod may also be helpful.

Menstrual Cycle and Gastrointestinal Function

Menstruating women undergo many physiological changes throughout each cycle. Normal menstruating women often report periods of constipation or diarrhea that seem to fluctuate with their menstrual cycle. Menstruating women complain of more intestinal symptoms shortly before and during early menses, including bloating and abdominal discomfort. Women with IBS may have increased symptoms during their menstrual periods.

With the abrupt fall in levels of female sex hormones after a hysterectomy, most women have no change in their bowel function. However, a small number experience marked constipation requiring therapeutic intervention.

Relationship between Abuse and Pelvic and Abdominal Pain

Abuse is a major epidemic in the United States. Estimates of the incidence of childhood sexual abuse in the United States vary from 15 to 38 percent, and there are two to four times as many abused women as abused men. Physical and sexual abuse not only affect a woman's psychological well-being, but they often result in gynecologic and gastrointestinal symptoms as well. The incidence of sexual abuse appears to be higher in patients with IBS than it is in the general population. A history of abuse is particularly noted in IBS patients with pain as their predominant complaint. It is important to tell your doctor about abuse. Some diagnostic testing, such as endoscopy, may bring back traumatic memories of abuse, and psychological intervention may be of benefit

Pregnancy and Bowel Function

Pregnant women undergo profound changes in anatomy and physiology that affect the gastrointestinal tract and liver. Gastroesophageal reflux disease is common, occurring in more than 80 percent of pregnant women, while peptic ulcer disease is reduced. Many women have changed bowel function. Gallbladder sludge, a pre-gallstone condition, increases, and subsequent gallstone disease is directly related to the number of pregnancies.

Evaluation and treatment of gastrointestinal disease in pregnancy should take into consideration the health of the mother while attempting to achieve an optimal outcome for the baby. The safety of drugs approved for use in pregnancy has been assessed through animal studies, trials in pregnant women, and post marketing studies. Drugs are classed in four categories: those in A and B are considered safe in pregnancy, drugs in category C are generally safe, and category D drugs should be used only if there is a strong clinical indication.

NAUSEA AND VOMITING IN PREGNANCY AND HYPEREMESIS GRAVIDARUM

Nausea and vomiting in pregnancy (NVP) is common, occurring in 50–90 percent of pregnancies. NVP is far more common among women in the first trimester than in the third, with symptoms usually peaking at nine weeks' gestation and decreasing significantly by 18 weeks. Nausea and vomiting occur more frequently in women with multiple fetuses than they do in those with a single fetus. While it is often a troubling condition causing significant distress, numerous studies have shown NVP not to be harmful and even to be associated with lower risks of miscarriage, low birth weight, and delivery before due date.

In contrast to NVP, hyperemesis gravidarum is a serious condition characterized by severe vomiting, which may result in dehydration, weight loss, and the need for nutrition administered through a vein. This condition, which occurs most commonly in the first trimester, tends to occur in patients who are overweight, have had many previous pregnancies, and are pregnant with more than one fetus.

GASTROESOPHAGEAL REFLUX DISEASE IN PREGNANCY

About 40–80 percent of pregnant women experience symptomatic gastroesophageal reflux disease (GERD, or acid reflux). The condition usually begins in the first or second trimester and generally persists throughout pregnancy, with significant improvement following delivery. Symptoms of GERD are similar in pregnant and nonpregnant women and include heartburn, regurgitation, and nausea. Complications of GERD are uncommon in pregnancy.

Initial treatment of acid reflux consists of conservative measures such as avoiding foods and exposures that may provoke reflux symptoms. In particular, women should avoid fatty foods, citrus juices, caffeine, chocolate, peppermint, garlic, onions, alcohol, and smoking. Nighttime reflux symptoms may be alleviated by elevating the head of the bed by six inches and limiting food and fluid intake within four hours of bedtime. When symptoms do not respond to these interventions, a trial of medical therapy is appropriate. Antacids are believed to be safe in pregnancy.

PEPTIC ULCER DISEASE IN PREGNANCY

Many studies suggest a decreased incidence of peptic ulcer disease (PUD) in pregnancy. However, if you have a peptic ulcer while you are pregnant, be assured that the standard therapies are safe. Antacids are commonly used and are felt to be safe in pregnancy. Sucralfate (Carafate®, a class B drug) promotes ulcer healing, and when administered orally, is safe and poses no risk to the fetus. Extensive experience has shown that H2 blockers, such as cimetidine (Tagamet®, Tagamet HB®), famotidine (Pepcid AC®), and ranitidine (Zantac®) are safe and effective in pregnancy. Proton pump inhibitors (Nexium®, Prevacid®, Protomix®, AcipHex®) are very effective in acid suppression by binding to the acid pump. Although such treatments are generally regarded as safe in pregnancy, there are no extensive research findings on their use during this time.

CONSTIPATION IN PREGNANCY

It is commonly believed that constipation is a frequent complaint in pregnancy. However, many studies have failed to show that a majority of pregnant women suffer from constipation. Because of constipation or other intestinal complaints, 70 percent of women modify their diets during pregnancy.

Treatment of constipation in pregnancy should be through changes in diet such as increased fiber intake and adequate liquid consumption. Treatment is similar to that in the nonpregnant woman except for mineral oil, phosphosoda, castor oil, and aloe. Mineral oil should be limited to short periods, because of the possibility of malabsorption of vitamins and nutrients. Phosphosoda, castor oil, and aloe should not be used at all.

IRRITABLE BOWEL SYNDROME IN PREGNANCY

No large study has followed women with IBS through pregnancy to see if their symptoms require the same treatment. Although most IBS medications can be used in pregnancy, tricyclic antidepressant drugs should not be.

THE LIVER AND GALLBLADDER IN PREGNANCY

The liver is affected by the myriad changes that occur in pregnancy. Even in uncomplicated pregnancies, liver function tests may differ from prepregnancy, and gallbladder volume increases while its motility decreases. Some specific abnormalities of the liver can occur during pregnancy, such as intrahepatic cholestasis of pregnancy, characterized by itching, and acute fatty liver of pregnancy, which is very uncommon. (These abnormalities are not discussed here.)

What Is Fecal Incontinence?

The uncontrollable elimination of stool (fecal incontinence) and gas is a relatively common, albeit embarrassing, situation that occurs in 2–15 percent of people. It causes many women to limit their social interactions and, in extreme situations, may even make a person housebound because of anxiety over soiling clothes or creating an offensive odor in public. Fecal incontinence increases with age when the anal sphincter may become weaker. In women, the average age of onset of fecal incontinence is 61.

Up to 35 percent of women develop defects in the anal sphincter after their first vaginal delivery that can result in fecal incontinence, although it is unclear why this minor trauma ultimately has that result.

Diarrhea, diabetes, constipation, laxative use, spinal cord injuries, and hemorrhoids also contribute to incontinence. Numerous studies are available for evaluating incontinence. Improving bowel function by controlling diarrhea or constipation, biofeedback therapy, and/or surgical repair may improve incontinence. New therapies are being tested and developed. For day-to-day assurance, one can wear panty liners or adult diapers.

What Is Inflammatory Bowel Disease?

Inflammatory bowel disease (IBD) is an inflammatory condition of the intestines. The two principal forms are ulcerative colitis (UC) and Crohn's disease. Although Crohn's disease and ulcerative colitis have a similar incidence in men and women, some studies suggest that slightly more men develop ulcerative colitis, and slightly more women develop Crohn's disease. Thus, there are sex differences in some manifestations of IBD.

SYMPTOMS

Ulcerative colitis and Crohn's disease are characterized by abdominal pain, diarrhea, and gastrointestinal bleeding. Many problems occur outside of the gastrointestinal tract (extraintestinal).

WHY YOUR SEX MATTERS

Certain features such as *erythema nodosum* (a red painful rash often on the legs) and eye disease are more likely to occur in women. Primary sclerosing cholangitis (narrowing of the bile ducts) and ankylosing spondylitis (deforming back disease), on the other hand, are more common in men. The reasons for these sex-based differences are unclear.

There are no studies documenting different sex-based response rates to drugs used to treat IBD. In spite of the vast literature on the treatment of IBD, very few studies have been conducted with regard to genetics, natural history of disease, or response to treatment based on sex. Sex can affect body image, result in different disease manifestations, and affect treatment considerations with regard to fertility, pregnancy, and risk of osteoporosis.

Body Image and Sexuality in Inflammatory Bowel Disease
The disease process itself, as well as surgical therapy, can affect body image and sexuality. Loss of basic bodily functions, such as no control of stool elimination or incontinence, can reduce self-esteem and alter body image. Aches or pains in joints (arthritis and arthralgias) can interfere with normal physical activity. Other extraintestinal manifestations of the disease, such as skin problems or connections of the bowel to the skin, can also adversely affect body image. Surgical scars or ostomies (opening of bowel on the skin surface) are perceived as disfiguring and can promote a negative body image.

Medical treatments for IBD can also profoundly affect body image. For example, corticosteroid therapy can result in significant weight gain, swelling, skin changes such as acne, and increased facial hair. In various studies 42 percent of women report that IBD has an adverse impact on the level of satisfaction with their lives, while 15–20 percent of patients report dissatisfaction with their body image.

Women with UC and Crohn's disease may experience pain with intercourse (dyspareunia) that can reduce the frequency and pleasure of sexual intercourse. A study of 50 women with Crohn's disease found that 24 percent of them had infrequent or no sexual intercourse, compared with 4 percent of age-matched women without Crohn's disease. Dyspareunia was reported by 60 percent of women patients and was commonly named as a reason for less frequent sexual intercourse. Continence-sparing surgical techniques, such as ileal pouch anal anastomosis (IPAA), in which the small intestine (ileum) is connected to the anus, have resulted in improved body image and sexuality. Following IPAA, women generally report satisfying sexual relations.

Effect of IBD on Fertility
Peak onset of IBD occurs during the reproductive years. Fertility rates in patients with IBD are comparable to the general population when voluntary childlessness is considered. An exception is when Crohn's disease is active. In Crohn's disease, decreased fertility appears to correlate with increased disease activity and degree of inflammation.

Reports strongly suggest that fertility may decrease after IPAA surgery for ulcerative colitis, although the reasons for this are not clear. One possibility is that blockage of the fallopian tubes or intrapelvic adhesions (scarring) can interfere with normal reproduction. Adhesion-prevention gels and mesh are under investigation to determine if they can improve fertility.

Male Fertility in IBD
Treatment of men with sulfasalazine results in decreased fertility due to decreased sperm counts, sperm motility, and abnormal sperm appearance. Therefore, if pregnancy is planned, men should be change their therapy from sulfasalazine to another drug at least three months before attempting conception.

Effect of IBD on Pregnancy
In remission, women with IBD are likely to have uncomplicated pregnancies without any increase in the risk of miscarriage, low birth weight, or stillbirth or birth abnormalities. Active Crohn's disease, however, is strongly associated with birth defects and pregnancy complications. Women with Crohn's should be very careful to try to get into and maintain remission before and during pregnancy.

Effect of Pregnancy on IBD
Disease activity during pregnancy appears to correlate with disease activity at the time of conception. Pregnancy itself does not increase the rate of symptom relapse. Rates of relapse in pregnant women with ulcerative colitis and Crohn's disease are similar to those in nonpregnant women.

Mode of Delivery and Risk of Perineal Disease
There is much debate on whether the mode of delivery (vaginal versus Cesarean) affects the subsequent risk of perineal disease in patients with Crohn's disease. The concern is that birth trauma or episiotomy may precipitate perineal disease or exacerbate existing disease. While there is general agreement that women with perirectal abscesses or connections between the rectum and vagina should undergo Cesarean section, it is unclear whether all women with perianal fistulae should undergo Cesarean

section. Women with active perianal Crohn's disease or *a* history of severe perianal involvement may be appropriate candidates for Cesarean section rather than vaginal delivery.

Studies suggest that women who have undergone surgery for ulcerative colitis with either an ileostomy or IPAA are likely to have a normal pregnancy and delivery. However, these patients may have up to a 29 percent incidence of stoma-related dysfunction or complications of the IPAA with increased stool frequency and incontinence during pregnancy. Following delivery, ileal pouch function is restored to what is was before conception.

Patients with IPAA are more likely to undergo Cesarean section, possibly because of obstetricians' concern about inducing perineal or pouch injury. Long-term studies, however, reveal that vaginal delivery does not adversely affect subsequent pouch function. In general, vaginal delivery is safe and well tolerated in patients following IPAA. There are no convincing data that vaginal deliveries result in decreased anal sphincter control and incontinence in women who have undergone IPAA.

Medical Management of IBD during Pregnancy

Management of IBD during pregnancy should be guided by the principle that active disease, not treatment, poses the greatest risk to the pregnancy. Studies reveal that medications used by IBD patients for symptomatic relief of diarrhea are safe to use during pregnancy. Oral anti-inflammatory medications such as sulfasalazine and mesalamine are also safe to use during pregnancy.

Corticosteroids are class B drugs. Budesonide (Entocort EC®), a new oral steroid used in patients with Crohn's disease of the ileum or right colon, is classified as a category C drug in pregnancy, since there are no well-controlled studies of it in pregnant women.

Although no large studies exist on the use of immunomodulatory agents such as 6-mercaptopurine, azathioprine (Imuran®), and cyclosporine for treatment of IBD during pregnancy, several case series and a large series in patients with rheumatoid arthritis using the former two medications suggest that they may be used safely in pregnancy. Use of these agents is justified if the patient has active disease unmanaged by other oral or topical agents

Methotrexate is contraindicated in pregnancy because it causes birth defects, including head, face, and limb defects; central nervous system abnormalities; and suppression of bone marrow. At present, we know only a little about the safety of infliximab (Remicade®), an immunomodulatory agent currently used in Crohn's disease. However, more than 100 reports, as well as drug company data, suggest that it may be safe in pregnancy, and it is classified as a class B agent.

Both male and female patients with IBD are at increased risk of osteoporosis because of their underlying disease and medications that may worsen bone loss. Bone mineral density measurements should be obtained in women with IBD to screen for osteopenia and osteoporosis. Women who are at high risk for accelerated bone loss should take preventive measures, such as using steroid-sparing medications and other therapies for osteopenia and osteoporosis.

What Is Acute Diarrhea?

Diarrhea is defined as an increase in daily stool weight (greater than 200 grams), stool liquidity, and unusual stool frequency (more than three incidences a day). Acute diarrhea, or gastroenteritis, is a common, generally self-limited problem that usually requires no specific treatment. Viruses, bacteria and their toxins, and parasites are the most frequent causes of the illness. The specific cause need not be pursued unless the illness lasts for more than seven days, the person has significant rectal bleeding or is extremely ill, or there is an outbreak of many cases that need investigating. The sudden onset of lower abdominal cramping, watery diarrhea, nausea, and vomiting are characteristic.

WHY YOUR SEX MATTERS

Infectious diarrhea affects men and women equally. It is an important topic for women, however, because women frequently take care of their families when they develop diarrhea, and by virtue of doing most of the cooking, they play an important role in preventing food-borne illness.

TREATMENT

Treatment of people with acute diarrhea can be divided into three areas:

- ◆ prevention of disease,
- ◆ general measures of management of diarrhea, and
- ◆ treatment with antibiotics.

PREVENTION

Food-borne pathogens are responsible for 70 percent of diarrheal disease worldwide. Recent trends, such as eating raw oysters and fish and increased consumption of imported fresh fruit and vegetables, increase the risk of food-borne pathogens. Most efforts to decrease the risk of food contamination must be done in the home. A 1995–96 multistate survey found that 50 percent of Americans eat undercooked eggs, 20 percent consume pink hamburgers, and 20 percent do not wash their hands after handling raw meat or chicken. These are all potential sources of infection. Focusing on hygiene, food storage, and preparation can significantly decrease the risk of food-borne illness.

Infected poultry and poultry products are common causes of salmonella and campylobacter infection; unpasteurized milk can cause these and other types of infections, and undercooked beef is an important source of *Escherichia coli* bacteria, which cause diarrhea. Food that is improperly refrigerated may develop preformed toxins (poisons) that can cause disease. Processed meat, such as bologna, may cause listeria infection. Pregnant women who contract listeria or campylobacter are at greater risk of miscarrying.

Viral gastroenteritis is spread from person to person, and therefore is difficult to prevent. Shigellosis has a propensity to spread by person-to-person contact under conditions of poor hygiene; infection with *Entamoeba histolytica* is often by travel, and *Giardia lamblia* can be acquired not only during travel, but also by ingestion of giardia cysts from a contaminated water supply.

The most frequent mode of transmission of *E. histolytica* within the United States is sexual contact or close person-to-person contact with an asymptomatic cyst passer. Up to 33 percent of asymptomatic children in daycare centers carry *G. lamblia*, and in more than half of all traceable outbreaks of Salmonella gastroenteritis, the source is an asymptomatic carrier employed as a food handler. It is estimated that about 0.2 percent of people infected with nontyphoid Salmonella become carriers, and about one-third of nontyphosa carriers have gallstones, and two thirds are female. Treatment with antibiotics is generally unsuccessful; only removal of the gallbladder may be successful in eliminating the nontyphosa strain from its carrier.

Traveler's diarrhea is the acute, watery diarrhea common among travelers to underdeveloped nations. It is recommended that prophylactic antibiotics not be given for routine prevention of traveler's diarrhea. There is evidence showing bismuth subsalicylate is effective in preventing or treating this diarrhea. In one study of travelers in Mexico, diarrhea developed in 23 percent of persons taking four tablespoons of bismuth subsalicylate (the main ingredient in Pepto–Bismol® and similar products) four times a day, compared with 61 percent of persons taking a placebo (or sugar pill).

A big problem of patients with diarrhea is fluid and electrolyte imbalance. For mild diarrhea, two bouillon cubes in water are an excellent source for salt repletion. Various commercially available electrolyte solutions and drinks such as Gatorade, are to a lesser degree, good sources of electrolyte and sugar repletion. For moderate (3–10 percent) dehydration, an oral rehydration solution (ORS) is recommended. With severe dehydration (greater than 10 percent), severe vomiting, or severe gastric distention, intravenous fluid replacement is recommended. More recently, cereal- and rice-based oral rehydration solutions have been shown to be superior to traditional glucose-based ORS. The cereal-and-rice-base ORS decrease stool volume. When the diarrhea is better and you start to resume your normal diet, it may be wise to delay ingesting milk or milk products because lactose intolerance frequently occurs after acute diarrhea.

If you have uncomplicated acute gastroenteritis caused by viruses or bacterial toxins, you can use loperamide(Imodium®), or diphenoxylate (Lomotil®) in small doses or bismuth subsalicylate, which has been shown to reduce symptoms in students with toxigenic *E. coli* infection and volunteers with Norwalk infection. It is given as 30 ml or two tablets every half hour for four hours and, after the first 24 hours, 30 ml or two tablets four times a day. In a trial comparing loperamide and bismuth subsalicylate in traveler's diarrhea, loperamide (8 mg/day) was superior in decreasing the number of stools. Narcotics should rarely be used in people with bacterial infections; and antibiotics are only used for a limited number of bacterial infections.

What Is Gallbladder Disease?

Gallbladder disease is one of the most common gastrointestinal problems in the United States. Between 1988 and 1994, an estimated 6.3 million men and 14.2 million women age 20–74 had gallbladder disease.

Cholesterol gallstones, which account for 80 percent of all gallstones, are caused when cholesterol becomes supersaturated in the bile, followed by crystal formation, aggregation and precipitation of the crystals, and growth into stones.

Risk Factors

The major risk factors for cholesterol gallstones are obesity, large and rapid weight loss, pregnancy, and drugs such as clofibrate, oral contraceptives, estrogen treatment, progestin, ceftriaxone, and octreotide. Other factors are a genetic predisposition and diseases of the last part of the small intestines (terminal ileum). Gallstones develop in approximately 25 percent of obese patients on strict dietary limitation and in up to 50 percent of patients with gastric bypass. Rapid weight loss is an important factor in forming gallstones.

Among women, gallstones occur most frequently in Mexican Americans (28 percent), followed by non-Hispanic whites (16.6 percent), and non-Hispanic blacks (14 percent). Gallstones increase with age and pregnancies. After age 50 their prevalence is as high as 30 percent. The Pima Indians have one of the highest risks of gallstone disease (70 percent in women older 25).

WHY YOUR SEX MATTERS

Pregnancy is a particularly important factor in development of biliary sludge and gallstones. Estrogen during pregnancy causes increased saturation of cholesterol in the bile. The bile is stored in the gallbladder, which has a larger volume and empties more poorly in pregnancy. These factors predispose a woman to gallstones.

Studies have shown that biliary sludge develops in up to 31 percent of women during pregnancy, and new gallstones develop in 2 percent during pregnancy. The risk of developing biliary sludge and gallstones is most pronounced during the second and third trimesters and the first month postpartum, and the risk increases with each pregnancy and is independent of breastfeeding.

Pregnant women with gallstones have a higher frequency of symptoms than do nonpregnant woman; up to a third of pregnant women with gallstones develop pain or biliary colic, ten times more than in nonpregnant women.

SYMPTOMS

Most gallstones are asymptomatic. In an Italian study of 151 people with gallstones, only 12 percent had developed symptoms after two years and 26 percent after 10 years. Three percent had complications after 10 years. These complications included pancreatitis, acute cholecystitis (inflammation of the gallbladder wall), and common bile duct stones. A University of Michigan study of faculty members (almost all men) reported fewer complications than did the Italian study. The most common complication of gallstone disease is acute cholecystitis, which causes abdominal pain, usually in the upper right part of the abdomen, fever, and a high white blood cell count.

DIAGNOSIS

Diagnosis of gallbladder stones is done by an abdominal ultrasound or an oral cholecystogram (a study in which a dye accumulates in the gallbladder and can then be visualized on an x-ray). A HIDA (hepatobiliary iminodiacetic acid) scan helps evaluate acute cholecystitis. To detect gallstones that have fallen into the passageway below the gallbladder, an ERCP (endoscopic retrograde cannulation of the pancreatic duct) or MRCP (an MRI scan) can be done. At the time of the ERCP, stones can be removed from the ducts.

It is often difficult to determine the cause of abdominal pain in pregnancy because of its many causes and the localization of the abdominal organs during this time. The most common procedure for diagnosing gallstones in pregnancy is an abdominal ultrasound. In addition, ERCP and MRCP can be used in pregnancy.

Removal of the gallbladder is usually done by laparascopic cholecystectomy. This procedure is done by making small cuts in the abdomen through which the gallbladder can be surgically removed. Major surgery is rarely needed.

Liver Disease in Women

WHAT IS AUTOIMMUNE HEPATITIS?

As discussed in chapter 5, autoimmune diseases are more prevalent in women than in men. One autoimmune disease is autoimmune hepatitis, an inflammatory condition of the liver. This uncommon disorder accounts for 20 percent of chronic hepatitis in the United States. Four times as many women as men have the disease and the average age of onset of the disease is 20–40. Other autoimmune conditions may occur in association with autoimmune hepatitis, including joint pain or arthritis, skin rashes, inflammation of the thyroid, and Sjögren's syndrome (a condition of decreased tear and saliva production).

Symptoms
Many patients with autoimmune hepatitis are only discovered when liver function test results are found to be elevated. In one-third to three-quarters of patients, the disease presents with no symptoms and may not be obvious until cirrhosis (scarring) of the liver is noted. There may be vague symptoms, such as fatigue, loss of appetite, or discomfort in the upper right side of the abdomen.

Diagnosis
A physical examination often shows an enlarged liver. The diagnosis is often made by an abnormal antinuclear antibody (ANA) and an anti-smooth muscle antibody (ASMA) in the blood. A liver biopsy helps evaluate the disease and determine whether treatment is needed.

Treatment
Treatment, generally with steroids and/or an immunosuppressant drug, is usually reserved for people with severe inflammation on liver biopsy.

WHAT IS PRIMARY BILIARY CIRRHOSIS?

Primary biliary cirrhosis (PBC) is also an autoimmune disease. Instead of affecting primarily the liver cells, as in autoimmune hepatitis, PBC affects the bile ducts (the tubes that carry the bile out of the liver). The bile ducts are progressively destroyed and lead to scarring in the liver and, eventually, cirrhosis.

Risk Factors
The risk of developing PBC is increased 500 times in first-degree relatives. Other autoimmune diseases are also associated with PBC, including thyroid disease, Sjögren's syndrome, and scleroderma as well as arthritis.

Why Your Sex Matters
Ninety percent of PBC cases occur in women, and usually in middle age.

Symptoms
The typical symptom is itching. One of four patients may have no symptoms, and the disease may only be detected by an elevated blood test, called alkaline phosphatase. Rarely do patients present with advanced disease. The liver may be enlarged on examination, but this occurs only in one of four people.

Diagnosis
The diagnosis is made by measuring the antimitochondrial antibody (AMA), which is elevated in all but 5–10 percent of patients with PBC. A liver biopsy confirms the diagnosis and helps determine the severity of the disease.

Treatment
Treatment is with ursodeoxycholic acid, a bile acid, which decreases the itching and appears to improve the outcome of the disease.

Summary

Many conditions of the gastrointestinal tract and liver may be more common in women than in men or may have certain manifestations that are of particular concern to women. Conditions that are more common in women are irritable bowel syndrome, constipation, gallstones, autoimmune hepatitis, and primary biliary cirrhosis. Inflammatory bowel disease has certain manifestations that are experienced by women more often than men.

Common conditions such as intestinal infections, fecal incontinence, and diarrhea are particularly important to women.

During pregnancy, gastrointestinal disease and liver disease may develop. Treatment during pregnancy must take into consideration the safety of medications to the developing fetus.

— JACQUELINE L. WOLF, MD

Note: Brand names are included in this chapter when only one product has been approved by the U.S. Food and Drug Administration (FDA) or when the chemical name is not commonly used; neither the author nor the Society for Women's Health Research is recommending any particular product.

CHAPTER 10

Eye Diseases

This chapter discusses major eye diseases that are more common in women or are of particular concern to women: macular degeneration, cataract formation, glaucoma, and diabetes complications. Another common disease is dry eye syndrome. Most of these diseases affect many women in greater numbers as they become older. In some cases, the higher prevalence of these diseases in women seems to be due to the fact that women live longer than men; in others, the disease process itself may affect women differently or more often.

With the cost of health care continuing to escalate at rapid rates, the value and cost-effectiveness of health treatments are under scrutiny. Recent studies have shown that vision is highly appreciated at all ages and by both sexes, regardless of education level, race, income, or socioeconomic level. We discuss the major eye diseases with the knowledge that their treatments are very cost-effective, even if expensive, because vision is highly valued, felt to be important to our overall quality of life, and a major determinant of productivity and self-sufficiency in an aging population.

What Is Age-Related Macular Degeneration?

Age-related macular degeneration (ARMD) is a degenerative disease affecting the macula, the central portion of the retina that controls central vision. The loss of retinal integrity causes a decrease in central vision; the peripheral fields are not affected, thus preserving some navigating ability. Reading, driving, watching television, and computer work are significantly affected by poorer central vision.

ARMD is the major cause of legal blindness in the United States. It has been estimated to be present in 1.6 percent of all people age 55 and older.

ARMD is known to have two forms: dry (atropic) and wet (exudative or neovascular). Atrophic changes in the deep layer of the retina, called the pigment epithelium, are often present in the former. Deposits of extracellular material, called drusen, may be the first sign of ARMD seen in the retina.

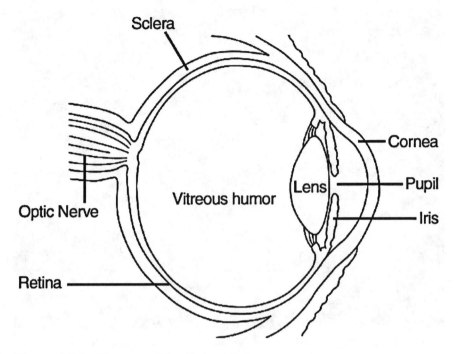

Figure 10.1. Diagram of the Normal Eye
Source: National Eye Institute, U.S. National Institutes of Health

The wet form of macular degeneration is often associated with a relatively rapid decline in central vision over days to weeks rather than years. Once one eye is affected with the wet changes, the other eye has a 10 percent chance of developing similar changes within one year. This rises to a 28 percent chance in three years and 42 percent in five years. This form of ARMD is characterized by new, fragile, small blood vessel growth in the middle layer of the eye, called the choroid. Leaking fluid from these vessels can cause localized detachment of the retina and bleeding into or under the retinal tissue.

RISK FACTORS

Smoking and age have been identified as definite risk factors for ARMD. Although there is not full agreement on these, some other factors are believed to increase the likelihood of ARMD:

- family history of ARMD,
- ethnicity of non-Hispanic whites,

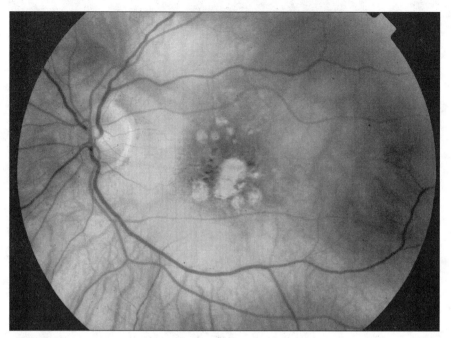

Figure 10.2. Atropic Changes of Age Related Macular Disease

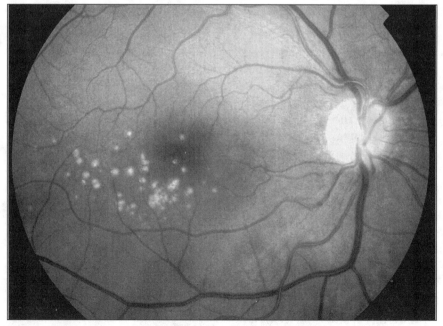

Figure 10.3. Drusen (yellow circles) of Age Related Macular Disease

◆ sunlight,
◆ cataract surgery, and
◆ cardiovascular disease.

WHY YOUR SEX MATTERS

Because aging is a risk factor, more women than men have ARMD. Even when researchers correct for the fact that there are more women than men of advanced age, about 55 percent of all people with ARMD are women.

SYMPTOMS/DIAGNOSIS

The symptoms of ARMD vary with its different forms. Slow advancing central visual loss in one or both eyes is noted with the dry form, and more rapid loss of vision or acute distortion of images is seen when loss is due to hemorrhage into or under the retina. People with ARMD see straight edges, such as door jams or cupboards, as curved; opthalmologists can give patients a tool in a grid pattern (the Amsler grid) to track any changes in this distortion. Recognizing this type of visual distortion can signal the need to consider treatment. Prompt evaluation by the eye physician is necessary when this occurs.

This evaluation includes a dilated eye exam and, often, an intravenous (IV) dye (fluoroscein) study with photographs of the macula.

TREATMENT

Some drug treatments slow the progression of the disease, and new products are in the pipeline that researchers hope will be able to improve eyesight.

Diet has been a topic of interest in the prevention and treatment of ARMD for a long time. The most recent and comprehensive data support use of zinc alone or in combination with antioxidants (vitamins C and E and beta carotene) to reduce the progression of ARMD in persons with macular changes with significant intermediate-size drusen. It should be noted that beta carotene supplementation has been linked to increased risk of lung cancer and, possibly, an increased risk of heart disease and therefore is not recommended for smokers.

Thermal (hot) laser therapy is a long-standing treatment for wet macular degeneration. Laser treatment has been demonstrated to be beneficial in preventing or delaying large losses of visual acuity for at least five years. Among those treated with laser, new blood vessel growth (neovascularization) was observed to reoccur in 26 percent of eyes within five years.

Recently, a new treatment involving an IV injection of a dye in conjunction with use of a cold photo-activating laser has been shown to benefit patients with well-defined neovascularization in treating areas where heat laser cannot be used. Steroids injected into the eye have been found to provide short-term improvement in vision in two-thirds of patients studied. Adverse effects, including infection secondary to the injection, seen in 1 percent of patients, are a concern to be considered with this mode of therapy.

Photodynamic therapy (PDT) is being studied, as are a number of antivascular growth factor molecules. These medicines are usually injected into the eye every four to six weeks. Surgical treatment for ARMD involving either removal of the neovascularization or the hemorrhage beneath the macula or translocation of the macular area of the retina continues to be investigated.

What Is a Cataract?

A cataract is an opacity in the lens of the eye, located just behind the pupil, that causes obstruction of vision and increasing blindness as the lens becomes cloudier and, ultimately, opaque if left untreated. Legal blindness in the United States is a visual level of 20/200, meaning one has the ability to see at 20 feet what a normal person (without a cataract) can see at a distance of 200 feet. With this visual acuity, people can walk and read with the help of low-vision aids. It is estimated that 20.5 million people over age 40 have a cataract in at least one eye; this is expected to rise to 30.1 million by 2020.

Risk Factors

Most cataracts occur in persons over age 60 or in younger persons with associated risk factors for cataract formation, such as:

- sunlight exposure,
- smoking,
- alcohol consumption,
- corticosteroid and other drug therapies,
- low education,
- ocular trauma, chronic inflammation, and
- diabetes.

Effective preventive measures are not well founded. It is believed that ultraviolet light protection and reduced smoking can slow cataract growth. There is some evidence that use of antioxidant vitamins can as well.

WHY YOUR SEX MATTERS

Cataracts affect women in greater numbers as they become older.

SYMPTOMS

Patients with cataracts commonly describe problems with night driving or reading small print or difficulty seeing television or road signs.

TREATMENT

Treatment with microsurgical techniques is indicated when the decreasing vision interferes with daily activities. Cataract surgery often can restore the lost vision and is the most widely performed surgical procedure in the United States.

In this procedure, the lens of the eye is surgically removed, often through a very small incision, and generally replaced with an artificial lens sized to afford good vision with minimal additional correction needed. Surgical advances in treatment of cataracts far outdistance the progress seen in understanding how cataracts are formed and how they can be otherwise treated or prevented.

Surgery is completed on an outpatient basis, and patients can return to usual activities of daily living within days. Often glasses are needed mainly for reading after a short healing period (approximately three weeks). It should be remembered that sometimes the amount of vision regained following cataract surgery is limited due to other eye conditions.

The prognosis after cataract surgery is generally excellent. Without other ocular problems it is expected that most persons have their vision returned to normal or near normal levels.

What Is Glaucoma?

Glaucoma is the leading cause of irreversible blindness in the world. It is estimated that in 2000, primary open-angle glaucoma affected almost 2.25 million people in the United States. This is expected to exceed 3.33 million people in 2020. Glaucoma is the second most common cause of legal blindness, following age-related macular degeneration, and the leading cause of blindness among African Americans.

Glaucoma defines a group of diseases that are generally characterized by increased intraocular pressure in the eye (IOP). Described more accurately, glaucoma is an optic nerve disease in which damage is caused by pressure in the eye greater than the optic nerve can tolerate to stay healthy. Optic nerve damage causes progressive loss of the individual nerve fibers of the eye serving the retina and results initially in loss of peripheral visual field, progressing to central loss, with eventual irreversible loss of total vision if left untreated adequately.

There are five main categories of glaucoma:

- **Primary open-angle glaucoma (POAG),** the most common type of glaucoma, occurs when there is higher-than-normal IOP, yet the opening of the eye's drainage system is normal. This can result in permanent loss of the visual field, with peripheral vision loss occurring first, followed by more central vision. As the pressure in the eye often rises slowly, there are no symptoms or pain to warn of the disease and impending damage to the optic nerve.
- **Secondary glaucoma** refers to elevated pressure in the eye due to other diseases or treatments. Often an accumulation of red or white blood cells or pigment can cause an elevated pressure, as can steroid drug use or an old trauma to the eye.
- **Congenital glaucoma** is an elevation of the intraocular pressure often present at birth or shortly thereafter.
- **Low-tension glaucoma** occurs with normal or low IOP, resulting in optic nerve damage similar to that seen in POAG.
- **Acute angle closure glaucoma** occurs in eyes where an irregularity interferes with the eye's drainage system. When the fluid in the eye cannot drain properly, the pressure rises suddenly; and patients have sudden redness and pain in the eye and cloudy vision, often accompanied by nausea and vomiting.

RISK FACTORS

Risk factors include:

- Age—the incidence of POAG rises with age, making it more prevalent in females.
- Race—POAG is four to five times more prevalent in African Americans.
- Family history—POAG occurs two to three times more often in people with parents or a sibling with visual loss due to glaucoma.
- Other factors—low blood pressure, cardiovascular disease, high blood pressure, diabetes mellitus, nearsightedness, and corticosteroid use are believed to be factors in glaucoma development.

This supports the theory that the disease is really one of poorer blood flow to or through the optic nerve. It is not clear whether glaucoma is due to nerve susceptibility, blood flow, or anatomic or physiologic features of the aqueous fluid drainage system.

SCREENING

The American Academy of Ophthalmology recommends a comprehensive eye exam for everyone over age 40 by a practitioner skilled in assessment of the optic nerve and glaucoma. Those individuals with risk factors for glaucoma should be reevaluated every one to two years, while those without risk factors can be seen every three to five years. African American men and women should be screened periodically between ages 20 and 40 as well.

SYMPTOMS/DIAGNOSIS

POAG is painless with slow pressure rises. Pain in the eye and visual symptoms such as cloudy vision or halos and redness can be seen with very high pressure or an acute rise in the pressure. Many patients do not notice narrowing of peripheral visual fields until the central 10–20 degrees of field are affected, with resulting tunnel vision.

Evaluation for glaucoma entails a complete eye exam during which the IOP is measured and the anatomy of the eye and drainage system is evaluated, as is the health of the optic nerve in the posterior portion of the eye. This is often done with a dilated examination. "Cupping" of the optic nerve identifies damage to the nerve fibers at the head of the nerve within the eye. Visual field test evaluation is needed periodically to assess any change or deterioration in field of vision.

TREATMENT

Treatment options are many and generally include:

+ Stepped drug therapy to reduce the intraocular pressure. A number of drug groups bring down the IOP via different mechanisms of action and may be used concurrently if one or two drugs, usually given in eyedrop form, are not effective.
+ Laser therapy (trabeculoplasty) increases the aqueous flow; more than one treatment per eye is often needed. Peripheral iridotomy is performed with laser to increase the flow with narrow-angled glaucoma.
+ Surgical therapy involves construction of a conjunctival pocket called a bleb to increase the flow or implantation of a prosthetic

drain implant if necessary. Studies of the proper time for surgical intervention are ongoing, but they are not conclusive that early surgery is advantageous.

Long-Term Care

Patients with glaucoma require continued, lifelong monitoring and care, including therapy to bring about a target pressure. It is vital for patients to follow the instructions for eyedrop administration; many eyedrops can be taken once or twice daily.

What Is Diabetic Retinopathy?

Diabetic retinopathy is a complication of diabetes mellitus that results in retinal blood vessel damage and abnormal new blood vessel growth. Retinopathy or retina pathology due to diabetes is a major complication and cause of death morbidity among patients with diabetes.

In patients with type 1 diabetes (diabetes that occurs before age 30 and requires insulin therapy), it is uncommon to see retinopathy changes within the first five years after diagnosis. In type 2 diabetes, where it can be difficult to know precisely when the disease begins, the five-year rule does not apply. In fact, vision problems are sometimes the first sign of type 2 diabetes in older patients.

There are two types of diabetic retinopathy:

♦ Nonproliferative diabetic retinopathy occurs when plasma leaks into the retina, causing the breakdown of small retinal blood vessels. Retinopathy centered within the macular area of the eye, the area of central vision, is known as macular edema.
♦ Proliferative diabetic retinopathy is characterized by the occurrence of abnormal new blood vessels, often in the area of the optic disc. Problems arise when these new vessels break and hemorrhage. Often the blood can be cleared by normal body mechanisms initially over weeks and months, but continued or subsequent bleeding episodes without treatment often result in chronic poor vision.

Symptoms

The major symptom of diabetic retinopathy is a loss in vision. This can occur slowly with either nonproliferative or proliferative retinopathy. Proliferative retinopathy also can cause a sudden loss of vision.

Sudden loss of vision from a blood vessel hemorrhaging into the jelly in the back of the eye is a distressing occurrence to most patients; often causing reduced visual acuity, the blood can settle in the lower part of the eye until it is reabsorbed. With repeated hemorrhages, however, surgery may be needed to clear the hemorrhage and restore vision. If you experience sudden changes in vision, contact your doctor immediately for early care.

TREATMENT

Laser therapy applied to the central macular region can help reduce the swelling or thickening in the macular tissues and return vision or minimize any further decrease in eyesight. Laser photocoagulation, called pan-retinal photocoagulation (PRP), is used to reduce the retina's ability to stimulate new blood vessel growth.

Treatment often is performed in the office over one to three visits and may need to be repeated if new blood vessel growth continues or reoccurs. Vitrectomy, or surgery to remove the vitreous jelly in the posterior portion of the eye, often followed by laser photocoagulation, is sometimes necessary to clear the blood and scar tissue from the eye.

Tight blood glucose control is important to reduce the occurrence and progression of diabetic retinopathy.

SCREENING

Patients with type 1 diabetes should have a complete eye exam by an ophthalmologist within three to five years of being diagnosed and then annually. Patients with type 2 diabetes should have a complete eye exam at the time of diagnosis and at least annually thereafter. The need for closer observation is determined by the presence and severity of retinal changes. Women with diabetes who wish to become pregnant should have an eye exam and be followed throughout their pregnancy and for one year after giving birth, since pregnancy can exacerbate diabetes retinopathy.

Patients with evidence of macular edema or with proliferative retinopathy should be monitored closely by an ophthalmologist experienced in managing retinal complications.

What Is Dry Eye Syndrome?

Dry eye syndrome is a common condition that occurs when the eyes do not produce enough normal tears to keep the eye moist and comfortable or tears evaporate too quickly.

RISK FACTORS

As discussed in chapter 5, dry eyes can be part of some autoimmune diseases. In addition, the condition can occur temporarily as a side effect from medication, contact lens chemicals, and LASIK surgery. Some people find that their dry eyes worsen (or only occur) during the winter because of the drying effects of low humidity outside and dry air inside from central heating. Other environmental, occupational, and lifestyle factors (including allergies, smoke, or prolonged computer use) can aggravate dry eye syndrome.

WHY YOUR SEX MATTERS

Women are three times more likely than men to have dry eye syndrome. As with many other conditions, an additional risk factor for developing dry eyes is aging. For this reason alone, since women live longer than men, dry eye syndrome, which affects as many as 14 million people in the United States, is more common in women. Additionally, women tend to have drier skin than men, so as women age and their bodies produce less oil, including that needed to seal tears, women's tear film evaporates faster. Finally, the underlying cause of evaporative dry eye may be low levels of male hormones. The drop in hormones—both estrogen and androgen—as women age can diminish the quantity and quality of tears. Androgen can also calm inflammation, so its decrease also dilutes any soothing that would otherwise be provided to the inflamed eye and tear glands. Studies have shown that estrogen therapy appears to worsen dry eye.

SYMPTOMS AND DIAGNOSIS

As discussed in chapter 5, symptoms of dry eye syndrome include pain, a burning sensation, itching, light sensitivity, eyelids that stick together, and mucus accumulation in the corners of the eyes on awakening. Some people also have intermittent blurring of vision. Often poor quality tears can result in extra reflex tearing and watery eyes. Mild cases may be self-diagnosed, but anyone with severe dry eye should see a physician, who can perform the tests discussed in chapter 5.

TREATMENT

The main therapy for dry eye syndrome includes artificial tears or ointments containing all the components of normal tears. Preservative free eye drops can help educe redness and irritation of the eyes. Researchers are developing eyedrops containing androgens. A recent new prescription product containing cyclosporine can increase tear production in some people. Decreasing drainage of tears by surgically closing or plugging tear ducts with special plugs can be useful in making eyes more lubricated and comfortable. Decreasing evaporation—through the use of a humidifier or swim or ski goggles—also can offer some relief, particularly during the winter months or when sleeping. Irritation from dry eyes can be made worse by crusty lashes or lids; soaking your closed eyes with warm water followed by daily washing the lashes with baby shampoo or commercially available lid scrubs can help keep the lids free of crusts and minimize infections.

—MELISSA BROWN, MD, MN, MBA

CHAPTER 11

Heart Disease

How the Heart Works

Slightly larger than a clenched fist, the heart is located under the breastbone and slants slightly to the left. It is the hardest working muscle in the body, and its steady beating enables the heart to supply blood to all parts of the body day and night, year after year, nonstop throughout your life. In a 70-year lifetime, an average human heart beats more than 2.5 billion times, pumping approximately one million barrels of blood.

The heart consists of two halves, each of which is divided into two chambers. The upper chambers are called atria; the lower chambers are called ventricles. A fibrous septum separates the atria, and a wall of muscle, called the ventricular septum, separates the left and right ventricles. Valves separate the chambers on each side and regulate the flow of blood through the four chambers and out into the aorta (to the body from the left ventricle) and pulmonary artery (to the lungs from the right ventricle).

Heart valves open and close with each beat of the heart. When functioning correctly, they are like one-way doors and keep blood from flowing backward. As the heart relaxes, blood is pumped from the atria through the valves into the ventricles. Then, with each heartbeat, blood is pumped from the ventricles into the aorta and pulmonary artery. The "lubb-dubb" sound you may think of as your heart beating is the sound of these valves opening and closing.

Blood vessels called veins return blood to the heart, and blood vessels called arteries carry blood away from the heart. The right side of the heart receives blood from the body and pumps the blood through the pulmonary arteries to the lungs to pick up oxygen, turning the blood bright red. The oxygen-rich blood returns to the left side of the heart and is pumped out to the body through the main artery, called the aorta. See Figure 11–1 on next page.

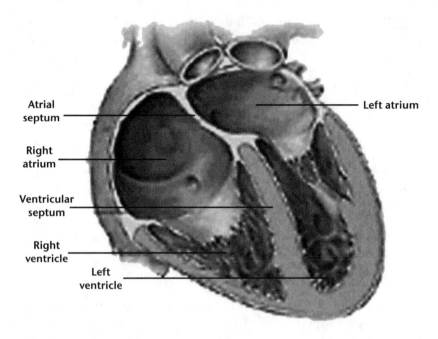

Atrial septum

Right atrium

Ventricular septum

Right ventricle

Left ventricle

Left atrium

Figure 11.1
Source: (U.S. Food and Drug Administration, FDA Heart Health Online)

What Is Hypertension?

Blood pressure is the force of circulating blood against the walls of the arteries in the body. Blood pressure varies during the day and night; it is highest in the morning and lowest at night during sleep. Blood pressure generally increases with activity and decreases with rest. When blood pressure stays elevated, it is called high blood pressure, or hypertension.

Approximately one in four Americans has high blood pressure, according to the American Heart Association, yet nearly a third of them do not know it. Hypertension has no symptoms; it is identified only by measuring with a blood pressure cuff. It is very common in African Americans, who may develop it earlier in life and more often than whites. If left uncontrolled, hypertension can lead to stroke, heart attack, heart failure, kidney damage, blindness, or other conditions. While it cannot be cured once it has developed, high blood pressure can be controlled by lifestyle changes and medications.

Blood pressure is recorded as two numbers: the pressure as the heart beats (systolic) and the pressure as the heart relaxes between beats (diastolic). Both measurements are important. The systolic measurement is written above or before the diastolic number. For example, a blood pressure measurement of 120/80 mmHg (millimeters of mercury) is expressed as "120 over 80."

A normal blood pressure is 120 over 80. A systolic pressure of 120–139 or a diastolic pressure of 80–89 is considered to be prehypertension, which means that you do not have high blood pressure that requires drug treatment now, but you are likely to develop it in the future. Stage 1 hypertension is a systolic pressure of 140–159 or a diastolic pressure of 90–99. Stage 2 hypertension occurs when the systolic pressure is equal to or greater than 160 or the diastolic pressure is equal to or greater than 100. Isolated systolic hypertension (ISH), when the systolic pressure is 140 or more and the diastolic pressure is normal, is the most common form of high blood pressure for older Americans, especially older women.

WHY YOUR SEX MATTERS

Although more men than women have hypertension at younger ages, women develop hypertension at a greater rate than men as they age; it is more common in women older than age 60 than in similarly aged men. More than 75 percent of African American women older than age 75 have hypertension.

Women are more likely than men to be aware that they have hypertension and to seek and receive treatment. Despite that fact, women are less likely to have their blood pressure adequately controlled, according to the National Heart, Lung, and Blood Institute (NHLBI).

RISK FACTORS

Most of the time, when someone develops hypertension, the cause is not known. According to the NHLBI, aging can be considered a risk factor for developing hypertension. Even those who do not have high blood pressure at age 55 face a 90 percent chance of developing it during their lifetime. This is the basis for the recommendation to have blood pressure measured annually. Low levels of physical activity and obesity contribute to developing hypertension.

ADDITIONAL RISKS FACING WOMEN

Pregnancy
Blood pressure changes are common throughout pregnancy, typically decreasing in the second trimester and increasing to prepregnancy levels in

the third trimester. For this reason, blood pressure should be measured each month for the first two trimesters and weekly thereafter if there is concern about hypertension. You should either lie on your side or sit during blood pressure measurements after the 20th week; the enlarged uterus can obstruct blood flow and decrease blood pressure when you lie on your back.

Menopause

It is unclear whether menopause itself is associated with hypertension or if the greater numbers of menopausal women developing hypertension has to do with menopause-related weight gain or simply reflects the increase in hypertension that occurs with aging. A recent study indicated that blood pressure does not increase significantly with menopausal hormone therapy (HT) in most women with or without high blood pressure. Since a few women may experience a rise in blood pressure attributable to estrogen, it is recommended that all women being treated with HT have their blood pressure monitored more frequently.

Oral Contraceptives

A small but definite increase in blood pressure occurs in many women who use oral contraceptives; however, with discontinuation of use, elevated blood pressure typically returns to normal. If you use oral contraceptives, you should have your blood pressure monitored regularly.

TREATMENT

Prehypertension

Currently no antihypertensive drug therapy is indicated for prehypertension, except in patients with chronic kidney disease or diabetes.

Hypertension

Some people can prevent or control high blood pressure by adopting healthier habits, such as:

- eating healthy foods that include fruits, vegetables, and low-fat dairy products;
- cutting down on salt (sodium) in the diet;
- losing excess weight and staying at a healthy weight;
- staying physically active (for example, walking 30 minutes a day); and
- limiting excess alcohol intake.

The most effective lifestyle alterations for women with hypertension are sodium restriction, aerobic exercise, and weight control or loss.

If you follow these guidelines and your blood pressure stays high, your physician usually prescribes one or more drugs to reduce it and keep it below 140/90 (130/80 if you have diabetes or chronic kidney disease). Stage 1 hypertension may be controlled with one drug, but a combination of two or more drugs is generally indicated for stage 2 hypertension. There are several types of medicines, each of which works in a different way, to treat hypertension:

♦ Diuretics, sometimes called water pills, work by helping your kidneys flush excess water and salt from your body and often provide adequate control. Thiazide diuretics may be of particular value for older women because they help retain calcium and are associated with decreased bone loss and decreased risk of hip fracture. However, diuretics may prove a problem in older women with urinary incontinence.

♦ Beta blockers help your heart beat more slowly and with less force.

♦ Angiotensin-converting enzyme (ACE) inhibitors keep your body from making a hormone (angiotensin II) that normally causes blood vessels to constrict.

♦ Angiotensin II receptor blockers (ARBs) are newer blood pressure drugs that protect the blood vessels from angiotensin II.

♦ Calcium channel blockers (CCBs) keep calcium from entering the muscle cells of the heart and blood vessels, causing the blood vessels to dilate.

♦ Alpha blockers reduce nerve impulses that constrict blood vessels.

♦ Alpha-beta blockers reduce nerve impulses to blood vessels the same way alpha blockers do, but they also slow the heartbeat, as beta blockers do.

♦ Nervous system inhibitors relax blood vessels by controlling nerve impulses from the brain, causing blood vessels to dilate.

♦ Vasodilators dilate blood vessels by relaxing the muscle in the vessel walls.

All of the research about medications to treat hypertension indicates that women and men benefit equally from treatment to control elevated blood pressure, and these benefits include significant reduction in stroke and major cardiovascular events, including heart failure.

A Salute to Patient Advocates

By Sharonne N. Hayes, MD, FACC, director, Women's Heart Clinic at Mayo Clinic, and director of the Scientific Advisory Board for WomenHeart: The National Coalition for Women with Heart Disease

Over the more than 20 years that I have practiced medicine, the diagnosis and treatment of heart disease has changed dramatically and immeasurably. Historically, when it came to heart disease, the female sex had been completely ignored. Until a couple of decades ago, women and their doctors were told that, not only did women not get heart disease, but if they did, it wasn't until they were very, very old, and when and if they actually developed heart disease, it was not as serious a condition as it was in men.

While these "facts" were subsequently found to be erroneous, the die had been cast and the damage done. Women with cardiovascular symptoms were ignored. ("It couldn't be her heart!") Women's cardiovascular risk factors were ignored (If she's not at risk for heart disease, why should we treat her risk factors?). Women weren't included in clinical trials related to treatment and prevention of heart disease because they "didn't get heart disease" and were much more "complicated" to study (think hormones!—why do you think they called one of the major risk factor trials MRFIT?).

But now, thanks in large part to the persistence of heart attack survivors and patient advocates, we've started asking evidence-based questions about heart disease, and we're learning about just how wrong we all were. Women are actually more likely than men to die of or have complications from a heart attack, bypass surgery, or coronary artery stenting. This is particularly true in young women with heart disease, who have a two to four times greater risk of dying from a heart attack than a man of the same age.

Women dying, and living, with heart disease have taught this cardiologist quite a few things. I have come to believe that they are the key to erasing the disparities of the past and ensuring the future heart health of our mothers, sisters, and daughters. The efforts of women heart patients are changing the world as we know it.

Each woman heart patient has a story to tell about her personal, and often—because they are still with us—medical, successes. But in my mind, each one also has a story of failure, because they developed heart disease

in the first place, they were misdiagnosed, or their outcomes were poor. Their challenge now is to live each day, to the fullest and in the best health possible. My challenge as a health care provider is to listen to their stories and learn from them, to integrate the vast body of scientific knowledge and apply it appropriately to each patient I see.

Heart disease is also eminently treatable, but the disparities in survival will only be corrected if we get better at earlier diagnosis, and that means knowing the best tests for women. Cardiac diagnostic tests were all designed with men in mind and for men. They were then tested for their accuracy in men. Many of these tests have now been found to be less effective or less accurate in women, or they need to be interpreted differently in women. Patient advocates are helping spur better research in this area.

If we are going to be able to treat women early, when the likelihood of success is greatest, we have to eliminate misdiagnosis, treatment delays, and barriers to care. This means that when a woman has symptoms that suggest heart disease, she needs to "think heart." When she gets to the emergency room or to her doctor's office, her health care providers need to "think heart." We need to make sure we use our proven effective drugs and treatments on women just as promptly, effectively, and intensely as we do on men. Women also need access to good care.

In addition, patient advocates have been spreading the word that heart disease is preventable. More than 80 percent of cardiac events, such as heart attacks, can be prevented if all U.S. women do these "simple" things: exercise at least 30 minutes a day, do not smoke, eat a healthy diet, stay at a normal weight, and have a glass of wine every once in a while. Sound easy? It's not. Only 3 percent of us are actually doing all these things. So, if you think about it, even small changes in the behavior of a small portion of us could have a real impact and save many lives.

So much so, that it's hard to imagine what might be around the next corner. I'm astounded when I look at what I now have to offer my patients from my figurative "little black bag." But the constant, through all of the technical innovations, the genetic sequencing, and the molecular discoveries, has been the relationships I've had with my patients, which have enriched me and taught me more than any of them will probably ever know.

(Reprinted with permission by Sharonne Hayes, MD)

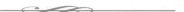

What Is Coronary Heart Disease?

Coronary heart disease (CHD), also known as coronary artery disease, occurs when the blood vessels that supply blood and oxygen to the heart (coronary arteries) narrow, usually resulting from the buildup of fatty and fibrous plaque, known as atherosclerosis. As a result, the flow of blood to the heart muscle decreases and can even stop if the artery becomes obstructed. CHD is the leading cause of death for adult women in the United States; about 250,000 women die from it each year.

WHY YOUR SEX MATTERS

Scientists continue to find important differences in coronary heart disease between women and men. One of the most important differences is that the death rate from CHD is decreasing for men while it is constant or rising for women. Since 1984 more women than men in the United States have died each year from CHD.

Another important difference is that the first signs of CHD tend to appear about 10 or more years later for women than for men. Heart attack, also called myocardial infarction, can occur as much as 20 years later in women. Whether the increase in CHD after menopause is due to hormone lack or to more frequent and increased coronary risk factors is uncertain. Emerging research indicates that menopausal women who have more abdominal fat and higher cholesterol levels, increased blood pressure, or diabetes are at higher risk of CHD because they have more atherosclerosis. But CHD is not a disease only of older women; about 20,000 of the women who die each year from heart attack are younger than age 65, and one-third of them are under 50.

RISK FACTORS

There are a variety of risk factors for developing CHD, some of which can be controlled or modified and others that cannot. Among those that cannot be controlled are aging; family history of CHD; and having had a heart attack, stroke, or transient ischemic attack (TIA or mini-stroke). American Heart Association statistics show that 14 percent of persons who survive a first stroke or heart attack will have another one within a year.

Many factors that increase the risk of developing CHD can be controlled. Prominent among these is smoking, a major risk factor for CHD among women. Women who smoke also have an increased risk for stroke.

Women smokers who use birth control pills have a higher risk of heart attack and stroke than nonsmokers using these pills. Additionally, second-hand smoke—exposure to others' tobacco smoke—increases the risk of CHD for nonsmokers.

Other controllable or treatable conditions that raise the risk for CHD are:

- **High blood cholesterol:** Typically, women's cholesterol levels become higher after age 45, and the bad cholesterol (low-density lipoprotein [LDL]) continues to increase with age. For both men and women, high levels of LDL cholesterol raise the risk of CHD, and high levels of the good cholesterol (high-density lipoprotein [HDL]) lower this risk. Low levels of HDL cholesterol and high triglyceride levels seem to be a stronger risk factor for women than they are for men.

- **High triglyceride levels:** A high level of triglycerides (another blood fat) is often associated with higher levels of total cholesterol and LDL, lower levels of HDL, and increased risk of diabetes. Although scientists are uncertain whether it is a risk factor for CHD by itself, research indicates that it is a stronger risk factor for women than for men, especially when associated with decreased HDL.

- **High blood pressure:** High blood pressure, which is a major risk factor for heart attack and the most important risk factor for stroke, is particularly important for African American women, who are more likely to have hypertension than are Caucasian women. All women have an increased risk of developing high blood pressure if they are obese, have a family history of high blood pressure, are pregnant, take certain types of birth control pills, or have reached menopause.

- **Physical inactivity:** Lack of physical activity is a risk factor for CHD; some studies show that CHD is almost twice as likely to develop in sedentary people as it is in those who are more active. Sedentary lifestyle increases with increased age in women and is more prominent in African American and Mexican American women.

- **Obesity and overweight:** Being overweight can lead to high blood cholesterol levels, high blood pressure, and diabetes and is by itself a risk factor for CHD. Having too much fat, especially in your waist area, increases the likelihood of developing high blood pressure, high blood cholesterol, high triglycerides, diabetes, and CHD. This combination is referred to as the metabolic syndrome.

♦ **Diabetes mellitus:** Women with diabetes have between two to six times the risk of developing CHD and are at much greater risk of having a stroke than are women without diabetes. Having diabetes erases the sex-based protection against CHD seen in women.

The Evidence-Based Guidelines of the American Heart Association for Cardiovascular Disease Prevention in Women highlight goals for a number of lifestyle interventions. Women should not smoke and should avoid environmental tobacco (secondhand smoke) as well. Regarding physical activity, women should get a minimum of 30 minutes of moderate intensity physical activity, such as brisk walking, on most if not all days of the week. This needn't be a nonstop 30-minute bout of exercise; three 10-minute bouts will do as well.

Women who have had a recent cardiac event should participate in a comprehensive exercise and risk-reduction regimen, such as a cardiac rehabilitation or a physician-guided home or community-based program.

A heart-healthy diet is important and should include a large variety of fruits, vegetables, grains, low-fat or non-fat dairy products, fish, legumes, and sources of protein low in saturated fat. Saturated fat intake (found in foods such as dairy products and red meat) should be limited to less than 10 percent of the calories, cholesterol intake to less than 300 mg a day, and women should limit their intake of trans fatty acids such as those found in many processed foods and commercially baked goods. Weight maintenance and reduction can be achieved through an appropriate balance of physical activity, caloric intake, and formal behavioral programs when indicated. The goal is a body mass index of 18.5–24.9 kilograms per meter squared and a waist circumference of less than 35 inches. Omega 3 fatty acid and folic acid supplementation for coronary prevention are suggested only for high-risk women. Depression is considered an important complication of cardiovascular disease in women, and physicians should refer for evaluation and treat when indicated.

Women should "know their numbers," for the major risk factor interventions as well as for the BMI and waist circumference just cited. The box on the next page summarizes the interventions to be used for each risk factor. Optimal blood pressure is less than 120/80 mmHg, which should be achieved through lifestyle approaches. Medication is recommended when blood pressure is in excess of 140/90 mmHg or at lower levels when there is blood pressure-related target organ damage or diabetes.

Major Risk Factor Interventions for Coronary Heart Disease

BLOOD PRESSURE

- Optimal blood pressure of 120/80 mmHg should be maintained initially through lifestyle approaches.
- Pharmacotherapy is indicated when blood pressure is 140/90 mmHg or when it is even lower if there is diabetes or blood pressure-related damage to the kidneys, heart, or brain.

LIPID, LIPOPROTEINS

- Lipids and lipoproteins of LDL under 100 mg/dL, HDL over 50 mg/dL, and triglycerides (TG) under 150 mg/dL should be maintained through lifestyle approaches.
- For lower-risk women, statin therapy is recommended when LDL is in excess of 160 after a trial of lifestyle therapy.
- For intermediate-risk women, statin therapy is recommended when LDL is in excess of 130 after a trial of lifestyle therapy. After LDL control, evaluate for therapy for abnormal HDL, TG levels.
- For high-risk women, statin therapy is recommended, together with lifestyle alterations. In addition, niacin or fibrate therapy should be initiated if HDL and triglyceride values are inappropriate.
- For diabetic women, saturated fat intake should be reduced to less than 7 percent of calories, blood pressure should be less than 120/80 mmHg, and Hgb A1C should be less than 7 percent.

Adapted from table 4 Clinical Recommendations in Mosca et al., "Guide to CVD Prevention in Women," *JACC*, Vol 43, No. 5, 2004.

For lipid numbers, women should know three numbers: optimal levels of bad cholesterol (LDL) should be under 100, good cholesterol (HDL) should be over 50, and triglycerides under 150. The initial methods to attain and maintain these levels are through lifestyle approaches: diet, weight control, and exercise. There are very specific recommendations for medications for women, depending on their level of risk. For high-risk women, those with coronary heart disease or a coronary heart disease risk equivalent or greater than 20 percent chance of having a coronary event in the next 10 years, in addition to a more stringent reduction of saturated fat and cholesterol, statin therapy is recommended together with lifestyle alterations. Also, because low HDL and high triglycerides are an increased risk factor for women, niacin or fibrate therapy should be initiated when these values are inappropriate. For intermediate-risk women, statin therapy is recommended with an LDL level in excess of 130 after a trial of lifestyle therapy. For lower-risk women, statin therapy is recommended with an LDL level greater than 160. The last number to be known is for diabetic patients where lifestyle interventions and medications should be used to achieve near normal hemoglobin A1C, that is less than 7 percent. The A1C measures adequacy of control of blood sugar levels in diabetic patients.

SYMPTOMS AND DIAGNOSIS

There are three main presentations of CHD: angina pectoris, myocardial infarction or heart attack, and sudden cardiac death.

Angina pectoris (from "angina" meaning suffocation, and "pectoris" meaning breast) this means pain, pressure, or discomfort in the chest. Angina is the most common symptom of CHD in women. In general, women with angina tend to be older than men and more often have hypertension, diabetes, and heart failure. Angina is typically precipitated by exertion or emotion and relieved with rest or nitroglycerin. It may be an intermittent pain, uncomfortable pressure, a squeezing sensation, or merely discomfort in the center of the chest. These feelings may also occur in the neck, jaw, back, arms, between the shoulder blades, or downward to the stomach. Many types of chest discomfort and pain are not angina, but are due to muscle or skeletal pain, inflammation, or acid reflux (heartburn). Of course, chest pain can also signal a heart attack. Too often women neglect to have their chest pain symptoms checked out by a physician. It is imperative that women with chest pain have a complete history and physical examination, which should include an assessment of the pain or discomfort, a history of risk factors for coronary heart disease, blood tests, EKG, and other necessary tests, commonly a stress test. Stress tests with or without imaging studies with an echocardiogram or nuclear imaging are most common. X-ray testing for coronary calcium can show that atherosclerosis is present, but it does not define the extent of blockage of the coronary artery.

Women, as well as men, with angina, particularly with an abnormal stress test, often have a coronary angiogram. This is an X-ray examination of the arteries of the heart with injection of contrast material into the arteries that reveals the location and extent of blockage. This can indicate whether balloon angioplasty with or without stenting or coronary artery bypass graft surgery is indicated. Researchers are evaluating the usefulness of a new imaging test, known as magnetic resonance (MR) spectroscopy to define the extent and location of the blockage.

Heart attack occurs when a coronary artery is completely and suddenly blocked. It results in the death of the heart muscle cells supplied by that artery. Although chest pain is the most common symptom of a heart attack for both women and men, women more often have additional symptoms than men, including shortness of breath; fatigue; nausea; and stomach, neck, back, abdomen, or shoulder pain.

Women are more likely to receive an incorrect diagnosis, because the range of symptoms in women differs from what physicians have been taught to think of as typical heart attack symptoms in men. Women also are less likely to receive certain diagnostic tests, such as coronary angiography, even when their need for the tests is the same as a man's, although this difference has decreased over time.

Additionally, women are less likely to recognize their own symptoms as those of a heart attack and often delay seeking emergency treatment. Both of these factors contribute to the fact that women do not receive some lifesaving treatment and appropriate medical management as often or as promptly as men.

Lifesaving interventions can include:

- ◆ coronary thrombolysis, breaking up the blood clot in the coronary artery with drugs;
- ◆ percutaneous transluminal coronary angioplasty (PTCA), in which the narrowed artery is widened with a balloon and often a wire stent (which may or may not be drug eluting) is placed to keep the artery open, or
- ◆ coronary artery bypass graft (CABG) surgery, which places new blood vessels to "bypass" blood flow around clogged arteries.

With a suspected or documented heart attack, you are admitted to a coronary care unit (CCU) in the hospital, where your heart rhythm, EKG, and blood pressure can be monitored and treatments begun. Medicines include aspirin, heparin, a statin drug, a beta blocker drug, and, often, an ACE inhibitor.

Research studies have shown that many of these interventions or treatments pose a greater risk of bleeding in women. But despite the complications of bleeding, women and men benefit equally from thrombolysis (breaking up a clot). Research shows that angioplasty can be as successful for women as it is for men. Women experience more angina after these procedures than men, however, so they more often have a decreased quality of life. The overall hospital death rate for women undergoing CABG surgery is double that for men, but long term, women do as well as or better than men.

TREATMENT FOR HEART ATTACK

People who have had a heart attack can prevent future problems with beta blocking drugs that lessen the workload of the heart by slowing heart rate and decreasing blood pressure. Aspirin or other drugs that "thin" the blood by decreasing the activity of blood platelets prevent new clots from forming. Special blood thinners are needed after angioplasty and stenting, statin drugs lower bad cholesterol, and ACE inhibitors can protect heart function.

Additional Risks for Women with Heart Attack
Women are more likely to die during a hospitalization for a heart attack than are men of the same age group, with the risk greatest for younger women, compared with younger men. This may be because women are more likely to have more than one disorder (called co-morbidities), including diabetes or high blood pressure. Younger women are more likely to be smokers. Also, researchers have discovered that heart attacks appear to be more severe in women than in men, and that women are more likely to have such complications as shock, recurrent chest pain, heart failure, and cardiac rupture. Women are also twice as likely as men to suffer from depression after a heart attack. More research is needed to pinpoint the reasons for these sex differences.

Women are also less likely than men to be prescribed cardiac rehabilitation, a medically supervised program to help patients improve their overall physical and emotional functioning and reduce coronary risk factors. Cardiac rehabilitation programs can include counseling; exercise; and lifestyle and other interventions to reduce risk factors such as high blood pressure, smoking, high blood cholesterol, obesity, and diabetes.

Sudden cardiac death occurs due to life-threatening rhythm disturbances or cardiac arrest. Cardiac arrest may be the first manifestation of coronary heart disease and may occur without any symptoms or warning signs. The incidence of sudden cardiac death in women is increasing, probably due to a number of factors. Fewer women are properly screened and treated for coronary heart disease than men, and there has been a sharp increase in diabetes and obesity among women. Also, because women are less likely than men to recognize symptoms of a heart attack, treatment may be delayed—which raises the risk of sudden cardiac death.

What Is Heart Failure?

Heart failure occurs when your heart loses its ability to pump blood efficiently. It does not mean that your heart has stopped beating, which is referred to as cardiac arrest. Heart failure is usually a chronic, long-term condition, although sometimes it can develop suddenly. There are two kinds of heart failure: systolic, in which the heart pumps poorly, and diastolic, in which the heart relaxes poorly. Heart failure may affect the right side, the left side, or both sides of the heart. In heart failure, many body organs do not receive enough oxygen and nutrients, which damages them and reduces their ability to function properly. In contrast to many other forms of cardiovascular disease that are decreasing in prevalence, the rate of heart failure in the United States has increased in the past two decades.

WHY YOUR SEX MATTERS

Because women live longer than men, more women than men develop heart failure. The outcome of women with heart failure depends a great deal on the cause. Women in one large study tended to do better than men, likely because more women with intact ventricular systolic (pumping) function were included. This raises the question of whether the type of increased mass in the heart ventricle matters to your prognosis. The pattern of increase in ventricular mass differs between women and men; it is more symmetric in women and less so in men. Older women generally have the type of hypertrophy that does not allow the heart to relax well.

A relatively new entity, stress cardiomyopathy, stunning of the heart muscle in response to sudden emotional stress, appears to predominate in women.

RISK FACTORS

The most common causes of heart failure are hypertension and coronary heart disease. Other heart disease, including valvular heart disease, and lung disease can also cause heart failure. Hypertension is a more prominent risk factor for development of heart failure in women than it is in men; however, women who have myocardial infarction are almost twice as likely as their male peers to develop heart failure subsequently.

Women are also at increased risk of developing heart failure if they are overweight, have diabetes, smoke cigarettes, abuse alcohol, or use cocaine. Heart failure becomes more common with advancing age. About 4 percent of women have heart failure at age 70, in contrast to 15 percent at age 85. In general, women who develop heart failure, and particularly older women, are more likely to have had prior hypertension and have preserved pumping function (left ventricular systolic function).

SYMPTOMS AND DIAGNOSIS

If you have heart failure, you may have swelling in your hands or feet and shortness of breath. You may be unable to keep up with your usual activity routine or become easily fatigued. Shortness of breath may occur only during physical activity at first, but it may occur even at rest later. Some people can breathe comfortably only when they are propped up with pillows or sitting upright.

A physical examination may reveal an irregular or a rapid heartbeat, abnormal heart sounds, or heart murmurs. Imaging studies may show that your heart is enlarged and your lungs are congested, and an analysis of your blood may show abnormalities in blood chemistry or liver function. Your doctor may order an echocardiogram (which uses ultrasound waves to make an image of heart function) to differentiate diastolic and systolic heart failure that can be specifically treated and to assess for possible causes for the failure, such as coronary or valvular heart disease.

TREATMENT

Acute heart failure or worsening of heart failure usually requires hospitalization and treatment with oxygen and intravenous medications such as vasodilators and diuretics. Once the condition is under control, your doctor may prescribe medications, including diuretics, ACE inhibitors, angiotensin receptor blockers (ARBs), beta blockers (particularly useful if you have a history of coronary artery disease), aldosterone blockers, and/or digitalis. Studies of beta blockers, ACE inhibitors, and angiotensin receptor blockers show that women seem to benefit as much as men.

Analysis of digitalis treatment has shown that women have a higher death rate than men while taking digitalis; this appears to represent overdosing of the digitalis preparation in women. Finally, calcium channel blocking drugs may have a role in management of diastolic heart failure (a problem with the heart relaxing), but any of these drugs that have a negative impact on ventricular pumping function are contraindicated in patients with systolic heart failure.

Another drug category, aldosterone inhibitors, may improve outcomes in heart failure. A new drug, a nitrate/hydralazine compound, was recently documented to improve heart failure outcomes in African Americans.

For patients unresponsive to medical therapies, newer approaches have included biventricular pacing (with early studies showing comparable improvement in women and men) and cardiac transplantation as a later intervention. Biventricular pacing uses an implantable device to improve the pumping efficiency of the heart. An automatic implanted cardioverter defibrillator (ICD) is used to prevent sudden death from serious arrhythmia in patients with severe systolic heart failure. Women and men who receive cardiac transplantation have comparable survival rates. The sex of a donated heart may make a difference: women seem to do equally well with hearts donated by women or men, while men do better when they receive hearts donated by men.

Your doctor will recommend that you restrict your intake of salt, and if you have systolic heart failure (pumping impairment), you will be advised to limit your fluid intake as well. Once your symptoms are controlled, you should begin low-intensity physical activity. For patients with diastolic heart failure, exercise may also actually improve symptoms.

What Is Valvular Heart Disease?

Valvular heart disease can involve narrowing (stenosis) or inadequate closing (regurgitation) of any of the four heart valves. If you are born with one of these conditions, you have congenital valvular heart disease. The conditions can also develop due to rheumatic heart disease or valve degeneration or infection; then they are considered acquired valvular heart disease. With valve disease, antibiotics are required before dental and many surgical procedures to prevent valve infection (endocarditis) .

Why Your Sex Matters

Two conditions are more common in women than men: mitral valve stenosis and mitral valve prolapse (which occurs in 2–3 percent of the total U.S. population). Although women are more likely to have mitral valve prolapse than men, men typically have more progressive severity of mitral regurgitation and are more likely to require valve repair or replacement. Women typically get aortic valve stenosis at older ages, which may explain why they do less well than men when valve replacement surgery is required.

Symptoms and Diagnosis

If the mitral valve is narrowed, blood flow is restricted from the upper left chamber (atrium) to the lower left chamber (ventricle). The restricted blood flow in mitral valve stenosis leads to an increase in the pressure of blood in the left atrium. Over time, this pressure causes fluid to leak into the lungs. It also can lead to an abnormal heart rhythm (called atrial fibrillation), which further decreases the efficiency of the heart's pumping action. If stenosis is severe, the cardiac output is limited and inadequate blood flow to the body results.

Symptoms of mitral valve stenosis usually take 10–20 years to develop after an episode of acute rheumatic fever and can take as long as 40 years to develop. They include shortness of breath, fatigue or weakness, pounding of the heart (palpitations), and, in severe cases, coughing up blood (because of increased pressure in the lung's blood vessels). Mitral valve stenosis is usually detected by the doctor hearing a heart murmur as blood passes through the narrowed valve; unlike a normal valve, which opens silently, the abnormal valve often makes a snapping sound, and a murmur is caused by turbulent flow as the valve opens to allow blood into the left ventricle. This diagnosis can be confirmed with an echocardiogram.

Mitral valve insufficiency often occurs in association with mitral stenosis in rheumatic heart disease. With the decreased prevalence of rheumatic fever, mitral regurgitation is far more commonly related to endocarditis, degenerative mitral valve disease, coronary heart disease, and mitral valve prolapse. The increased workload of the left ventricle results in progressive left ventricular dilation or an increase in the size of the left ventricular chamber and decreasing ability to exercise at a usual level. Symptoms usually develop gradually and include difficult, labored, uncomfortable breathing (dyspnea); an inability to breathe easily unless one is sitting up (orthopnea); or episodes of respiratory distress that awaken patients from sleep (paroxysmal nocturnal dyspnea). Mitral valve insufficiency is usually diagnosed during a physical examination and confirmed by echocardiography.

If the aortic valve narrows, it is difficult for blood to flow through the valve, increasing the amount of work the heart has to do and causing the left ventricle to malfunction, resulting in reduced blood supply to the heart muscle and body. Chest pain, as well as heart failure and syncope (fainting), can occur. With mild or moderate cases, you most likely will not have any symptoms of aortic valve stenosis or aortic valve insufficiency. However, severe cases can result in shortness of breath, inability to exercise at a usual level, dizziness, or syncope. Exertion might also bring on chest pain or palpitations.

TREATMENT

There is no medical treatment to reverse valve stenosis or regurgitation, but drug therapy can help maintain normal ventricular function. Although many believe that aortic stenosis with calcium deposition in the valve is an atherosclerotic disease, and one study suggested that statins may decrease calcium deposition, a recent research study showed no benefit of statins. A large percentage of elderly people have excess calcium in their aortic valve that can prevent the valve from opening adequately. Because there is currently no medical treatment, heart surgery to replace the valve is the only treatment for aortic stenosis.

If the valve stenosis or regurgitation is severe, you may require surgery to repair or replace the valve. If you are older than 40 or 45, your doctor will order a coronary angiogram to assess whether you also have significant coronary disease requiring CABG surgery at the same time. If you are planning on future pregnancies, bioprosthetic (tissue) valves are more commonly used than mechanical ones because the mechanical ones require anticoagulation therapy, which can pose bleeding and other risks to you and the fetus. Anticoagulant drugs are also associated with increased numbers of abortions and stillbirths. Bioprosthetic valves do not last as long and require reoperation after several years.

Ideally, even in the absence of symptoms, surgical correction of significant valve disease should be performed before there is progressive left ventricular dysfunction.

Pregnancy and Heart Disease

Women with many forms of heart disease can safely tolerate pregnancy, and most women with heart disease who have safely tolerated a pregnancy can tolerate normal labor and delivery. However, because of the major cardiovascular changes during a normal pregnancy, women with heart disease should be evaluated prepregnancy to determine the safety of a pregnancy and should be advised of any specific interventions that should be undertaken before pregnancy.

Circulating blood volume increases about 40 percent during pregnancy, with a comparable increase in cardiac output. Because the plasma volume increases to a greater extent than do red cells, there is relative anemia during pregnancy.

Peripartum cardiomyopathy is a rare disorder (about one in 3,000–4,000 pregnancies in industrialized countries) in which a weakened, enlarged heart is diagnosed in the last months of pregnancy or within five months after delivery. It may occur in childbearing women of any age, but it is most common after age 30. Other risk factors include obesity, multiple pregnancies, and a history of hypertension or preeclampsia. Because symptoms include fatigue and swelling of the ankles, which can occur even without heart disease in late pregnancy, this condition can be challenging to diagnose correctly. It typically presents as increased fatigue and shortness of breath. During a physical examination, your doctor looks for increased jugular venous pressure, lung rales, a third heart sound, often a lower left sternal border or apical systolic murmur, and edema. If you have peripartum cardiomyopathy, you will be prescribed diuretics, vasodilator therapy, digitalis, and possibly anticoagulants. You should not use ACE inhibitors or angiotensin receptor blocker medications before your baby is delivered.

About half of women with peripartum cardiomyopathy recover in about six months. Others remain stable or deteriorate, either gradually or rapidly. If the condition worsens rapidly, you may be a candidate for a heart transplant. With recovery comes the question of developing the condition during repeat pregnancies; about 20 percent of women who recover from this condition develop it again in a later pregnancy. If you do not recover fully and your heart remains enlarged, a future pregnancy will likely result in progression to more severe heart failure. Most doctors counsel women whose left ventricular function has not returned to normal to avoid future pregnancies. Even with recovery, pregnancy may pose a risk.

HYPERTENSION

About 5 percent of all pregnancies are complicated by hypertension, including those of women who have hypertension before getting pregnant; when hypertension is present before the 20th week of pregnancy, it is assumed to be due to preexisting hypertension. Pregnancy-induced hypertension usually develops after the 20th week and typically resolves within a week or two after delivery. This is diagnosed when the systolic pressure increases at least 30 millimeters or the diastolic pressure increases at least 15 millimeters over levels early in pregnancy. As many as 25 percent of women may have pregnancy-induced hypertension with the first pregnancy, and 10 percent may have it with a subsequent pregnancy. If you develop pregnancy-related hypertension, fetal monitoring is important, as are measures of your kidney function, uric acid, platelet count, and protein in your urine. Also, your doctor should monitor your blood pressure after delivery to ensure that the hypertension does not continue.

Generally, hypertension in pregnancy is treated if the blood pressure is in excess of 140/90 or 140/100 after the first trimester. Salt restriction is not recommended as it may decrease blood volume and decrease blood flow to the uterus. Diuretics are typically not recommended as they may also decrease blood volume. The most commonly used antihypertensive drug during pregnancy is alpha-methyldopa, which has a long record of safety with no adverse effects on the mother or fetus. More recently, beta blocking drugs have been shown to be safe and effective in blood pressure control during pregnancy. Alpha-beta blockers are occasionally used as well. ACE inhibitors should not be used during pregnancy because of their association with spontaneous abortion and fetal abnormalities. If you were using ACE inhibitors when you became pregnant, your baby is not likely to have any related birth defects if you stopped taking the medication before the second trimester.

Pre-eclampsia, defined as pregnancy-induced hypertension associated with increased protein in the urine (proteinuria), is responsible for a sizeable proportion of all maternal deaths and can adversely affect both you and your fetus. It affects the placenta, and it can affect the kidney, liver, and brain. Pre-eclampsia is a leading cause of fetal complications, including low birth weight, premature birth, and stillbirth. Symptoms may include headaches, visual symptoms, and, at times, pain in the upper abdomen. When pre-eclampsia causes seizures, the condition is known as eclampsia—the second leading cause of maternal death in the United States. Symptoms in addition to seizures may include nausea and vomiting. If you develop eclampsia, your doctor will administer antihypertensive and seizure medications intravenously and deliver the baby quickly.

Pre-eclampsia is more common in a first pregnancy, in women with five or more pregnancies, twin pregnancies, women who have had pre-eclampsia before, and women under age 20 and over age 35. A number of studies suggest an increase in African American and Asian American women and in women of lower socioeconomic status. Familial factors also seem important. Mothers, but not mothers-in-law, of pre-eclamptic women are more likely to have had pre-eclampsia; similarly daughters, but not daughters-in-law, of women who had pre-eclampsia are more likely to develop it.

Heart Failure/Transplant

In general, if your heart failure has been successfully treated, you should be able to have a safe pregnancy. If you have had a heart transplant, there may be some concerns about immunosuppressive therapy used to prevent rejection of the transplanted heart; studies to date do not show that they cause complications in pregnancy or an increase in birth defects.

Valvular Heart Disease

Mitral valve stenosis is historically the most common form of rheumatic valvular heart disease encountered during pregnancy; the increase in blood volume and increased heart rate that occur with pregnancy may cause symptoms of mitral valve stenosis to appear first during pregnancy. Beta blocking or calcium channel blocking drugs can control arrhythmias. If you have severe stenosis, balloon angioplasty to open the valve can be performed during pregnancy; if a woman with severe mitral stenosis becomes pregnant, she runs the risk of developing heart failure very rapidly. Your baby's health should not be affected by your mitral valve stenosis.

If you have mild to moderate mitral valve regurgitation during pregnancy and previously had no symptoms, pregnancy should pose no problems. In fact, pregnancy will cause a relaxation within the peripheral vascular system and decrease the severity of the regurgitation. Your baby's health should not be affected by your mitral valve regurgitation.

Because of the increase in cardiac output and heart rate during pregnancy, you may first have symptoms of aortic valve stenosis during pregnancy. If the valve narrowing is mild or moderate, your pregnancy and baby's health should not be affected. If you have severe aortic stenosis, your doctor most likely will recommend surgical correction before you become pregnant.

If you have mild to moderate aortic regurgitation during pregnancy and previously had no symptoms, pregnancy should pose no problems, and your baby's health should not be affected. In fact, just as with mitral valve regurgitation, your pregnancy will cause a relaxation within the peripheral vascular system that decreases the severity of the regurgitation.

If you have a bioprosthetic (tissue) valve, you should have its status evaluated before you become pregnant. If you have any type of mechanical valve, the necessary anticoagulation is a risk for bleeding and for fetal abnormalities. Endocarditis (infection of the valve) is of concern for all women with a prosthetic heart valve, who should have antibiotic prophylaxis at the time of either vaginal or Caesarean delivery.

CONGENITAL HEART DISEASE

Women born with severe heart disease generally have a mild condition or have a more severe condition corrected in childhood. For this reason, most adult women who were born with heart disease can become pregnant and carry a baby to delivery safely. There is a 3–16 percent increase in the risk that your baby will be born with a congenital heart disease. However, if your husband has a congenital heart disease, the risk to your baby is still increased over the average, but less so than if you have congenital heart disease. Echocardiography of the fetus can identify congenital heart defects before birth.

Exceptions to this general rule about safe pregnancies are women with pulmonary hypertension, hemodynamically significant valve obstruction, or Marfan's syndrome; doctors generally recommend against pregnancy with these disorders.

Eisenmenger's syndrome, a particular form of severe pulmonary hypertension (high pressure in the lung arteries), is more common in women than it is in men. It results from a large-volume left-to-right shunt within the heart, with the developing pulmonary hypertension subsequently reversing the shunt to a right-to-left shunt with cyanosis, reflecting low oxygen levels in the blood in general circulation. Normal changes that occur during pregnancy, particularly the increase in blood volume, can put greater stress on a woman's heart. If cyanotic congenital heart disease has been corrected, and the woman is no longer symptomatic, pregnancy is well tolerated.

In Marfan's syndrome, the chemical makeup of connective tissue is abnormal, causing these tissues to be abnormal. Connective tissue provides substance and support to tendons, ligaments, blood vessel walls, cartilage, heart valves, and many other structures. The walls of the major arteries are weakened; the weakened aorta wall often stretches, increasing the size of the aorta. The aortic wall can tear, and blood can leak through the tear into the aortic wall, separating its layers (dissection), a life-threatening problem. Another problem that may occur if the aortic wall weakens is that an aneurysm may form. Women with this severe problem require beta blocker therapy even if their blood pressure is normal. During pregnancy (and especially during delivery), stress on the aorta's walls greatly increases the risk of dissection or rupture. That is why pregnancy is not advised for women with Marfan's syndrome who also have a dilated aorta. Even following valve replacement and aortic root dilatation correction, pregnancy poses an increased risk. There is a 50–50 risk of the baby inheriting the syndrome.

Coarctation of the aorta, a narrowing of the aorta between the branches to the upper body and the branches to the lower body alone or as part of Marfan's syndrome, constitutes increased risk during pregnancy. Typically, coarctation is corrected in childhood.

Women with highly complex lesions, such as pulmonary atresia, transposition of the great arteries, have often had complex and multiple corrective procedures and may present problems during pregnancy, The extent of the problems is not well appreciated, since these highly complex surgical procedures have evolved over time and relatively few women have undergone pregnancy with each of the surgical procedures.

What Are Rhythm Disturbances?

The heart generates electrical impulses, which travel through the conduction system of the heart and cause the heart muscle to contract in a coordinated fashion. If the electrical signal does not function properly, your heart's pumping is affected.

WHY YOUR SEX MATTERS

Supraventricular tachycardias (increased-rate abnormal rhythms originating in the upper heart chambers) tend to be more common in women. Women are two to three times more likely to develop the serious ventricular arrhythmia, torsade de pointes, than are men. Additionally, drug-induced prolongation of the QT interval and the resultant torsade de pointes and sudden death is more common than in men. There should be careful monitoring of the QT interval in women taking drugs known to produce prolongation of the QT interval, prominent among which are the antihistamine, terfenadine; the antipsychotic, haloperidol; and the anti-infective, erythromycin.

SYMPTOMS

ost common symptom of most rhythm disturbances is palpitations, rtbeat sensations that feel like pounding or racing. Some people de- ribe their hearts as skipping beats. If you have ventricular arrhythmia, you may also experience extreme lightheadedness or a loss of consciousness; in very severe cases, sudden death can occur.

TREATMENT

If palpitations are your only symptom, and premature beats occur without any cardiovascular disease, most likely you do not need any treatment. If you have severe symptoms, your doctor may prescribe a low dose of beta blocking drugs.

Supraventricular tachycardia is a rapid heart rhythm that can disturb the normal ventricular muscle contraction. Although in the past medical therapies were used in patients with symptomatic supraventricular tachycardias, now they are most often treated with the highly successful nonsurgical procedure known as radiofrequency ablation after a second or third episode of arrhythmia. In this procedure, your doctor guides a catheter with an electrode at its tip to the place in your heart where the electrical signals stimulate the abnormal heart rhythm. Then mild, painless radiofrequency energy (similar to microwave heat) destroys a very small amount of heart cells (about one-fifth of an inch) to stop the extra impulses that cause the rapid heartbeats. There is a comparable success rate for women and men, although women tend to be more symptomatic and have received a longer period of antiarrhythmic drug treatment before being referred for ablation.

Atrial fibrillation is a very fast, uncontrolled heart rhythm that occurs when the upper chambers of the heart (the atria) beat rapidly and irregularly. As we age, we are more likely to develop atrial fibrillation, which is also associated with valvular heart disease, hypertension, coronary heart disease, and heart failure. Atrial fibrillation can be managed by medications for rate or rhythm control. Current data suggest that both strategies require anticoagulant therapy, and the therapy does not differ by sex.

The most common ventricular arrhythmias are premature ventricular beats that often occur in the absence of heart disease and require no treatment. The most serious arrhythmia occurring in the ventricles is torsade de pointes, literally meaning twisting of points. This can cause sudden death. The basis for this is an ECG abnormality—an increase in the QT interval of the ECG—either inherited or due to drugs or blood chemistry abnormalities. Based on a number of clinical trials, drug therapy has been less successful than implantable cardiac defibrillators (ICDs) in preventing sudden death due to this arrhythmia. ICDs are currently recommended for both women and men with left ventricular dysfunction due to coronary and noncoronary heart disease to prevent life-threatening rhythms.

Women and Heart Disease

By Representative Julia Carson (D-IN), the first woman and the first African American Indianapolis, Indiana, has sent to Congress and the sponsor and leading advocate for the "Bringing America Home Act," designed to end homelessness in the United States

When I first ran for Congress in 1997, I was so tired that I often wondered how I could keep going. I had been having chest discomfort on top of the exhaustion and thought I had heart trouble, but as happens with many women patients, my physician missed it. Following the election, I went straight to the emergency room after a lunch meeting one day, because I was out of stamina. They ran tests and called a cardiovascular surgeon. I found out that I needed double bypass heart surgery five days before I was scheduled to take office. I took the oath of office in my hospital room.

Most people don't realize it, but heart disease is the number one killer of all women, and heart disease death rates are 35 percent higher for African American women than for white women. Stroke rates are 71 percent greater. All too often, symptoms of heart disease in women are missed, and we've lost a lot of women because of it.

You just can't ignore the symptoms and risk factors. I've learned that one reason African Americans are more likely than Caucasians to have a heart attack and die from it, is that we tend to have more risk factors co-existing at the same time. I'm diabetic and have high blood pressure, two big risk factors. So, if you're at risk, make sure you have any symptoms checked out. Don't let doctors or anyone else dismiss you before you think you've had a thorough examination.

I've also learned that you have to make sure you are receiving the right treatment. African American women are less likely than white

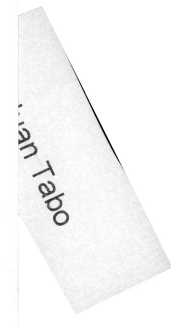

women to be prescribed medicine for their high blood pressure or high cholesterol. I have been prescribed a number of drugs, and I take them every day. I've changed my eating habits, and I make sure I get lots of exercise, mostly walking to and from my office to committee meetings and to the House chamber for votes.

Researchers are beginning to recognize that women experience heart disease differently from men, but more research is needed. And African Americans, both men and women, are not included in clinical studies on heart disease in sufficient numbers. My final message is that you consider what role you can take in helping scientists learn about heart disease and women, especially African American women.

(Repinted with permission of Representative Julia Carson (D-IN))

Special Considerations for Women

APPETITE-SUPPRESSING (ANORECTIC) DRUGS

With the progressive epidemic of obesity, prescription drugs were used increasingly as appetite-suppressing agents, with the greatest prevalence of this drug use in the 1990s. Major concerns subsequently developed with the use of combination appetite suppressant fenfluramine and phentermine (fen-phen). Although each of these drugs individually received FDA approval, combination therapy did not. Both agents were withdrawn from the market in 1997 because of their association with valvular heart disease and with pulmonary hypertension.

Earlier evidence of pulmonary hypertension (elevated pressure in the lung blood vessels) with appetite suppressants had been available with other anorectic drugs used in Europe. A European study of pulmonary hypertension showed that women were more likely than men to have used appetite suppressants, and women with pulmonary hypertension were much more likely to have taken anorectic drugs, with increased duration of use associated with more pulmonary hypertension. Management of these patients is the same as for primary pulmonary hypertension, with anticoagulant therapy, oxygen, diuretics, vasodilator drugs. Pulmonary hypertension rarely regresses.

Early reports suggested abnormalities of the cardiac valves with use of these drugs. Initial reports about these women showed that a few had severe valve regurgitation requiring surgery. The true prevalence of valve disease is not known, since most of the women had not had earlier echocardiographic examination of their heart valves. The current estimate is that 4–9 percent of women using these drugs have aortic or mitral valve regurgitation, with the occurrence increasing with longer use. Follow-up of these women showed that, following diagnosis, the valvular disease either stabilized or regressed with time. Guidelines of the American College of Cardiology for management of patients who have used these anorectic drugs are that the drugs be discontinued and the patients be evaluated by echocardiogram, with repeat echocardiography and clinical examination as follow-up. In those with valvular regurgitation, endocarditis prophylaxis is indicated.

Depression and Heart Disease

Because depression is highly prevalent in women, researchers have examined the relationship between depression and cardiovascular disease. Women with coronary heart disease are more vulnerable to depression than are men, and depression may be a stronger predictor of cardiovascular disease in women. The recently released American Heart Association Evidence-Based Guidelines on Heart Disease Prevention for Women recommended that women with coronary events be assessed for depression and referred for therapy if warranted. In a recent study, depression was particularly prominent among young women with coronary heart disease.

A recent national NHLBI study of cognitive behavioral therapy and medications to treat depression and social isolation in patients following myocardial infarction failed to show benefits. However, a subset analysis of this study suggests there are potential benefits from antidepressant therapy, particularly with selective serotonin reuptake inhibitors (SSRIs), for people after myocardial infarction.

—Nanette K. Wenger, MD, FACC, FAHA, MACP

CHAPTER 12

Kidney Disease

What Do the Kidneys Do?

Kidneys are bean-shaped organs, each about the size of your fist, located near the middle of your back, just below the rib cage. Your kidneys filter the blood in your body, each day removing about two quarts of waste products and excess water, which becomes urine that flows to your bladder for storage until later disposal. Wastes in your blood are products of the normal breakdown of food you eat and from your normal body functions.

The actual filtering occurs in tiny units inside your kidneys, called nephrons. Every kidney has about a million nephrons consisting of tiny blood vessels intertwined with urine-disposing tubes, called tubules. The tubules receive a combination of waste materials and chemicals that your body can still use. Healthy kidneys return the right amount of chemicals back to your bloodstream for return to your body.

In addition to removing wastes, your kidneys release three important hormones:

- erythropoietin, or EPO, which stimulates your body to produce more red blood cells;
- renin, which regulates blood pressure; and
- calcitrol, the active form of vitamin D, which helps maintain calcium for bones and for normal chemical balance in the body.

What Is Kidney Disease?

Kidney disease is America's ninth leading cause of death. More than 10 million Americans have kidney problems, including kidney stones and polycystic kidney disease (PKD). Many people also have chronic kidney disease (CKD), which can lead to kidney failure. Kidney failure occurs when damage to the kidneys has progressed to the point where they no longer function properly and cannot eliminate excess fluid and waste from your blood. More than 7.4 million adults over age 20 have chronic kidney disease, and nearly 80,000 people die from kidney failure each year. The major causes of kidney failure are diabetes and high blood pressure.

What Is a Kidney Stone?

A kidney stone is a solid piece of material that forms in the kidney out of substances in the urine. A stone may stay in the kidney or break loose and travel down the urinary tract. A small stone may pass out of the body without causing much pain. A larger stone may get stuck in a ureter (the tube that connects your kidneys and bladder), the bladder, or the urethra (the tube in your body that urine leaves from). A large stone can block the flow of urine and cause great pain. Small stones also can cause severe pain, from ureteral contraction.

There are four major types of kidney stones:

- The most common type of stone contains calcium. Calcium not needed by the bones and muscles must be removed by the kidneys. In most people, the kidneys flush out extra calcium with the rest of the urine. People who have calcium stones keep the calcium in their kidneys. The calcium then joins other waste products to form a stone. Calcium stones cam be either calcium oxalate or calcium phosphate.
- A struvite stone may form after an infection in the urinary system. These stones contain magnesium and the waste product, ammonia.
- A uric acid stone may form when there is too much acid in the urine. If you tend to form uric acid stones, you may need to cut back on how much meat (protein) you eat.
- The fourth type of kidney stone is called a cystine stone, which is very rare. Cystine is one of the building blocks that make up muscles, nerves, and other parts of the body. The disease that causes cystine stones usually runs in families.

RISK FACTORS

Kidney stones seem to be more prevalent in some patients than in others. Therefore, a patient who has had a kidney stone in the past is more likely to develop stones again.

SYMPTOMS AND DIAGNOSIS

Pain in the area surrounding your kidneys may be caused by kidney stones. The symptoms that warrant a visit to your doctor include:

- extreme pain in your back or side that does not go away,
- blood in your urine,
- fever and chills,
- vomiting,
- urine that smells bad or looks cloudy,
- a burning feeling when you urinate, or
- inability to urinate or urinating much less than normal.

Kidney stones are sometimes found accidentally during routine x-rays or sonograms. If a doctor suspects a kidney stone, she or he may order one of those tests, an abdominal/pelvic CT scan, or an intravenous pyelogram (IVP). During an IVP, your doctor injects dye into a vein in the arm. The dye travels through the body and collects in the kidneys. A series of x-rays then tracks the dye as it moves through the kidneys to the ureters and bladder. People suffering from chronic kidney disease or kidney failure should not take the test as it may worsen kidney failure.

WHY YOUR SEX MATTERS

Kidney stones are more common in men. If a stone is suspected in a pregnant woman, she should not have an IVP, because of the high amounts of radiation involved, which could damage the fetus.

TREATMENT

Drinking plenty of water (two to three quarts a day) can help move the stone along. Most kidney stones pass out of the body without help from a doctor, but sometimes a stone will not go away or becomes too large to pass easily out of your body. There are a number of methods your doctor can use to get rid of the stone:

- **Shock waves** (extracorporeal shock wave lithotripsy): Your doctor uses a machine to send ultrasonic shock waves directly to the kidney stone. The shock waves break a large stone into small stones that pass through your urinary system with your urine. This method does not require surgery. Two types of shock wave machines exist: with one machine, you sit in a tub of water during treatment; the other is used while you lie on an operating table.

♦ **Tunnel surgery** (or percutaneous nephrolithotomy): In this method, the doctor makes a small cut into the patient's back and forms a narrow tunnel through the skin to the stone inside the kidney. With a special device placed in the tunnel, the doctor finds the stone and removes it.

♦ **Ureteroscope:** A ureteroscope looks like a long wire or tube that your doctor inserts into your urethra. The wire or tube then passes up through the bladder and is directed to the ureter. The ureteroscope has a camera that lets the doctor see the stone, and a cage is used to catch the stone and pull it out.

PREVENTION

You can help avoid kidney stones by trying to drink plenty of water every day (enough to make at least two quarts of urine every 24 hours). You can also drink ginger ale, lemon-lime sodas, and fruit juices, although water is best. If you have already had a kidney stone, you should limit your coffee, tea, and cola to one or two cups a day, because the caffeine in these drinks may cause you to lose fluid too quickly. You should avoid mega-dosing on certain vitamins, especially vitamin C, which can increase your chances of developing a stone. Also, depending on the type of stone you had, your doctor may ask you to eat more of some foods and cut back on others or give you medicines to prevent calcium and uric acid stones.

What Is Polycystic Kidney Disease?

More than 600,000 Americans have polycystic kidney disease (PKD), a genetic, life-threatening disease in which numerous cysts grow in the kidneys. These fluid-filled cysts can slowly overtake the kidneys, reducing kidney function and leading to kidney failure. There are two major inherited forms and one noninherited form:

♦ **Autosomal dominant PKD** is the most common inherited form. Symptoms usually develop between age 30 and 40, but they can begin earlier, even in childhood. About 90 percent of all polycystic kidney disease cases are autosomal dominant PKD.

♦ **Autosomal recessive PKD** is a rare, inherited form. Symptoms usually begin in the earliest months of life, even in the womb.

♦ **Acquired cystic kidney disease (ACKD)** shows up along with long-term kidney problems, especially in patients who have kidney failure and who have been on dialysis for a long time. This form tends to occur in later years of life and is not inherited.

WHY YOUR SEX MATTERS

PKD is an inherited disorder, passed from one generation to the next by an affected parent. Each child of a parent with the gene that causes the disease has a 50 percent chance of inheriting it. Scientists also have discovered that approximately 10 percent of people with PKD became affected through spontaneous mutation, not through inheritance. The condition affects men and women equally. There are, however, important treatment distinctions. The two common methods of venal grafts for dialysis patients are the PTFE graft and the AV fistula. Women seem to experience fewer complications than do men with PTFE grafts, whereas men have fewer problems with the AV fistula.

SYMPTOMS AND DIAGNOSIS

The symptoms of PKD include pain in the back and lower sides, headaches, urinary tract infections, unexplained high blood pressure, blood in the urine, and cysts in the kidneys and other organs. Polycystic kidney disease can cause cysts in the liver and problems in other organs, such as the heart, and blood vessels in the brain. These complications help doctors tell it apart from the usually harmless simple cysts that often form in the kidneys in later life. Your doctor will use the following to find out if you have PKD:

♦ ultrasound (a test using sound waves to make an image) of kidney cysts,
♦ ultrasound of cysts in other organs, and
♦ family medical history.

TREATMENT

There is no cure for PKD. Treatments include medicine and surgery to reduce pain, antibiotics to cure infections, and dialysis or transplantation if the kidneys fail. When polycystic kidney disease causes kidneys to fail, which usually happens only after many years, the patient requires dialysis or a kidney transplant. About 60 percent of people with the major type of polycystic kidney disease end up with kidney failure.

What Is Chronic Kidney Disease?

About 20 million Americans have chronic kidney disease (CKD). Nearly 20 million more have CKD and do not know it. CKD can lead to kidney failure (also known as end-stage renal disease, or ESRD). This year, more than 100,000 people will be diagnosed with kidney failure. Roughly one in three African Americans is affected and one in eight Hispanic Americans.

RISK FACTORS

The risk factors and causes of chronic kidney disease and kidney failure are diabetes and high blood pressure (hypertension), both of which can do extensive damage to the tiny filters in the kidneys.

WHY YOUR SEX MATTERS

The number of Americans with CKD is growing at a steady and alarming rate; however, the rates of patients who progress into kidney failure (ESRD) have begun to slow in recent years. This can probably be attributed to earlier detection of CKD, although more prevention strategies can still be applied. While men have higher rates of CKD and kidney failure, the rates for women continue to grow at the same pace as men's.

SYMPTOMS/DIAGNOSIS

CKD in its early stages has no symptoms, so people may not know they have it until they are nearing kidney failure. Also, many people have either diabetes or hypertension without knowing it. People who have high blood pressure, diabetes, or a family history of kidney failure should ask their doctor to test their urine for protein and use their blood test results to calculate their GFR (glomerular filtration rate). The GFR is the best way to determine how well the kidneys are cleaning the blood and will show normal kidney function or place a person in one of five stages of chronic kidney disease, ranging from a slight decrease in kidney function (Stage 1) to kidney failure (Stage 5).

In its later stages, kidney disease may produce such symptoms as lower back pain, increased blood pressure (hypertension is both a cause and a symptom of kidney disease), change in the frequency of urination, coffee-colored urine or blood in the urine, nausea, puffiness (especially around the eyes, and especially in children), and fatigue or listlessness.

TREATMENT

There is no cure for kidney failure. The only treatments available are kidney dialysis or kidney transplantation. There are two types of dialysis: hemodialysis and peritoneal dialysis. Hemodialysis, the more common form, typically involves three to four treatments a week at a dialysis center, and each treatment can last three to four hours. Blood is pumped out of the body for cleansing through an artificial kidney machine and then returned to the body. In peritoneal disease (PD) a catheter is used to fill the abdomen with a cleansing liquid, called dialysate. The walls of the abdominal cavity are lined with a membrane, called the peritoneum, that lets wastes and extra fluid pass from the blood into the dialysate.

There is a serious shortage of donor organs, so the wait for a kidney for transplantation can be years. Transplants can come from a living or deceased donor.

PREVENTION

You can protect yourself against kidney disease or slow the progression of the disease. Diet and lifestyle are key—what is true in the prevention of heart disease is true in the prevention of kidney disease: avoid tobacco products, eat a low-fat diet that includes plenty of fruits and vegetables, drink alcohol in moderation, get regular checkups, and exercise.

SPECIAL ISSUES FOR WOMEN WITH CKD

Menstruation and CKD

When a woman has chronic kidney disease, her menstrual periods tend to be irregular. Once she begins dialysis, her periods may even stop altogether. As kidney function drops below 20 percent of normal, a woman is less likely to conceive because dialysis is not able to perform all of the tasks of the kidneys. The body retains a higher level of waste products than it would with a normal kidney, which can prevent egg production and affect menstruation.

Treatments with erythropoietin (generally given as an injection under the skin one to three times a week) cause about 50 percent of woman on dialysis to get their periods again. This is attributed to the improved hormone levels and the treatment of anemia. Therefore, erythropoietin treatments can increase a woman's fertility, so birth control should be used if a woman is sexually active and does not want to become pregnant.

Sexuality and CKD

Lower hormone levels may cause some women to experience vaginal dryness or painful intercourse. A water-soluble vaginal lubricant can be used to remedy these situations. Side effects of certain medicines and complications from uremia can cause fatigue, menstrual irregularities, and decreased sexual desire. Some medications may also cause hormonal changes, making it difficult for a woman to become aroused or experience an orgasm. Women should discuss these issues with their doctors, as changes in blood pressure medication or taking extra hormones may help the situation. Anemia can also be treated with erythropoietin; however, sometimes the actual dialysis treatment is the cause of fatigue.

Most chronic kidney disease patients find they do not have the same interest in sex. There are emotional, physical, and psychological factors at play that can diminish the sex drive. Getting used to life with a chronic illness and the lifestyle changes that come with it takes time. There can also be stresses related to job, income, and family life to which a woman will have to adjust.

Some women become anxious about changes in their appearance, such as weight loss, or in the case of some peritoneal dialysis patients, weight gain from the sugar in the dialysate, the solution used during dialysis to pull waste products out of the blood. The catheter in the abdomen or fistula in the arm (the access point for hemodialysis patients) may also create anxiety because a woman believes it is unattractive or is afraid it could be damaged. Sharing these feelings with a partner is often the best way to overcome them. It is also rare that anything happens to an access during lovemaking.

Most women need time to adjust to dialysis. They may find their sex drive returns as their energy level increases. It is best to use contraception when being intimate if they do not want to become pregnant. Even if a woman is not having a regular period, she may still be ovulating, making her able to get pregnant.

Pregnancy and CKD
Studies indicate that 1–7 percent of patients on dialysis become pregnant. A national Registry of Pregnancy in Dialysis Patients is maintained to track and study these events and outcomes. About 50 percent of the babies born to women already on dialysis survive. There was evidence that longer dialysis time (more than 20 hours per week) helped improve infant survival. Many of the babies were born premature, which was attributed to high blood pressure. Many CKD patients have high blood pressure, which tends to worsen during pregnancy.

Women with kidney disease who become pregnant should be monitored closely by a high-risk obstetrician and nephrologist; check their blood pressure often; and report any fluid buildup, changes in urination, or symptoms of anemia (for example, coldness, pale skin, shortness of breath).

Menopause and CKD
Women with kidney disease may experience the first signs of menopause at an earlier age. While all menopausal women are at increased risk for developing osteoporosis, this risk is even more critical for those on dialysis or who have had a kidney transplant. Because many women on dialysis tend not to have regular periods, their hormone levels may be compromised before menopause. When kidney failure occurs, dialysis helps to remove wastes from the blood, but it does not replace all of the functions of the kidneys, such as producing hormones. In addition to osteoporosis, lower hormone levels may put women at increased risk for heart disease. Osteoporosis is frequently a complication for those who have a kidney transplant due to the antirejection drugs they must take.

—MICHAEL SPIGLER, CHES

CHAPTER 13

Mental Health and Mental Illnesses

Men and women have different patterns of illness, live different life spans, and respond differently to many medications and other treatments. Understanding sex and gender-based differences is important in approaches to mental health disease prevention, diagnosis, and treatment. Sex is an important variable in the treatment of many psychiatric symptoms and disorders, some—but not all—of which are linked specifically to hormonal changes in women. These diagnoses, treatments, and sex factors are the subject of this chapter.

What Is Mental Health?

Like their bodies, men's and women's brains and minds are mostly alike, but they do differ in some significant ways. These brain differences arise from both our genes and from environmental factors that include family, culture, and experience. There is no neat line between biology and psychology. When our brains undergo change, because of an experience or medication, our thoughts and feelings change as well. When our thoughts and feelings change, as a result of life experience or psychotherapy, our brains undergo change. Culture also interacts with our biology and psychology. For example, different cultures have different traditions about how they understand menopause, and those traditions influence the way symptoms are expressed. We do our best in this chapter to acknowledge cultural differences, but it is not possible to cover them all.

WHY YOUR SEX MATTERS

Sex differences in the brain and the evidence of mental illness on brain scans help to steer research in the most promising directions, but brain scans cannot yet make a diagnosis. Mental disorders are diagnosed on the basis of feelings, thoughts, and behaviors. Therefore, our ideas about normal feelings, thoughts, and behaviors play an important role in our concept of some mental disorders. What we view as normal is often closely related to our gender. For example, we generally expect women to be more passive and dependent than men, and we are more tolerant of men's anger and aggression than we are of women's. When men or women deviate from expected behaviors, even when they are fully able to function and are not troubled by symptoms, there is a tendency to consider them abnormal.

Women's mental and physical symptoms are often taken less seriously than men's. Women who have alcohol problems tend to drink quietly at home rather than getting drunk and violent in a tavern. A belligerent alcoholic man attracts more attention than a depressed and withdrawn woman. Women are more likely to receive prescriptions for psychiatric medications, perhaps because they make more visits to health care providers and suffer more chronic illnesses during their longer life spans. It is important to remember that medication can be used both too often and not often enough. Some prescriptions are written before a thorough diagnosis is made. Alternatively, many people who could benefit from medication are not being treated with it.

MENTAL HEALTH AND WOMEN

Women suffer from depression and anxiety disorders two to three times more often than men. The differences are due to a combination of genetics, hormones, and stressful experiences. Stress is a universal human experience that can be positive *and* negative. Many life changes, like getting married or having a baby, are both stressful and positive. Stress causes changes in our behavior, thoughts, feelings as well as in our body functions: heart rate, digestion, and breathing. Stress that is not overwhelming can be beneficial to our growth and creativity, but stress that is overwhelming can make us vulnerable to mental and other illnesses.

Some forms of stress are more common in women than in men: poverty, sexual abuse and assault, and domestic violence. Jobs traditionally filled by women, such as secretarial work, nursing, and teaching, that have a high level of responsibility and a low level of power raise a person's risk of depression. Women are also more likely to experience sexual harassment, which can increase their risk of anxiety and depression. Stressful experiences like illness, abandonment, and disasters cause bodily changes, sadness, irritability, relationship problems, and, sometimes, mental disorders. Mental disorders can also occur for no apparent reason.

Domestic violence is a factor in many kinds of mental illnesses. Women have often been blamed for their own victimization. One would hear questions like, "Why didn't she leave?" or "What did she do to deserve it?" As a society, we have begun to recognize the criminal nature of domestic violence and to develop legal and other support systems that recognize its impact. Doctors need to be aware of domestic violence and ask appropriate questions at every visit. Women are often ashamed of being victims, and it may take several visits before a woman feels comfortable enough to reveal her situation to her health care provider. These questions have to be asked in private because abusers often stick close to their victims during medical visits and punish them if they reveal the truth.

We have also learned a great deal about coping with stress, particularly through social support networks. Women who suffer from infertility, depression, or cancer are less likely to become depressed when they have strong support systems and/or they can join a group of others with similar experiences. A natural disaster is often easier to bear than a rape or assault because others are present and there is mutual support. Being active and helping others is the best way to overcome feelings of helplessness and powerlessness.

People with mental illnesses suffer more discrimination and have more difficulty obtaining health care than people with other kinds of illnesses. This is particularly true of schizophrenia, alcohol and substance abuse, and depression. There is a tendency to believe that these conditions can be overcome by determination or prayer. While both determination and prayer can be very useful in overcoming diseases, they are not treatments. A person with a disease should not be blamed for his or her own suffering. For example, some states in the United States have put pregnant women with alcohol and substance abuse problems in jail, ignoring the fact that many of them desire treatment. As a result, women with these treatable medical conditions are afraid to seek prenatal care for fear of punishment.

Diagnosing Mental Illness

An accurate diagnosis is the basis for successful treatment of any disorder. A health provider should ask, and a patient should be prepared to report:

1. What are your symptoms now?
2. What is the history of your symptoms?
   Under what circumstances did they start?
   How long have you had them?
   How have they changed?
   What has made them worse or better?
   What treatments have you had, and how did they work?

3. What is your personal history?
   Who is in your family?
   How was it for you growing up? Any problems?
   What and how did you do in school?
   What kinds of relationships have you had?
4. What is your sexual history?
   What were you taught?
   What do you know?
   What are your past and current sexual practices and concerns?
5. What is your family history, especially of similar symptoms?
   If others in your family had them, what, if anything, helped them?
6. What is your social history?
   Jobs?
   Personal habits like smoking, drinking, drugs?
   Marital/relationship status?
   Religion and spirituality?
7. What is your medical history?
   Reproductive history:
       When you started menstruating, any problems?
       Birth control?
       Conceptions?
       Abortions?
       Miscarriages?
       Pregnancies and deliveries?
       Sexually transmitted diseases?
   Illnesses?
   Surgeries?
   Hospitalizations?
   Past and current medications?

A complete mental health examination also includes a brief test of your mental functions: alertness, memory, concentration, abstraction, and level of general knowledge.

TREATMENT

Overall, mental health care is as effective as other kinds of medical care. All health care providers should spend time talking with patients, but in mental health, talking therapy—or psychotherapy—has developed into a specialized skill. For most mental illnesses, a combination of psychotherapy and medication works best. Several different types of clinicians—psychiatrists, social workers, psychologists, counselors—provide several kinds of psychotherapy: supportive, psychodynamic, interpersonal, and cognitive-behavioral.

Mental Health Conditions That Affect Women Differently from Men

Psychiatric disorders are diagnosed according to signs (what the doctor or someone else can see) and symptoms (what you feel) that are listed in the *Diagnostic and Statistical Manual of Mental Disorders*, now in its fourth edition (DSM-IV). It was created by the American Psychiatric Association, and we use the disorder definitions from DSM-IV in this chapter.

Gender differences in lifetime prevalence of psychiatric disorders

Disorder	Prevalence in percent		Female/male ratio
	Women	Men	
Bulimia	1.1	0.1	11.0
Anorexia nervosa	0.5	.05	10.0
Seasonal affective disorder	6.3	1.0	6.3
Panic disorder	5.0	2.0	2.5
Generalized anxiety disorder	6.6	3.6	1.8
Depression	21.3	12.7	1.7
Schizophrenia	1.7	1.2	1.4
Social phobia	15.5	11.1	1.4
Dysthmia	8.0	4.8	1.7
Bipolar disorder			
bipolar 1	0.9	0.7	1.3
bipolar 2	0.5	0.4	1.3
Drug abuse without dependence	3.5	5.4	0.7
Drug dependence	5.9	9.2	0.6
Alcohol abuse without dependence	6.4	12.5	0.5
Alcohol dependence	8.2	20.1	0.4
Antisocial personality	1.2	5.8	0.2

Adapted from Burt VK, Hendrick VC. *Concise Guide to Women's Mental Health*, 2nd Edition, Washington, DC, American Psychiatric Publishing, 2001.

MOOD DISORDERS

Mood disorders include major and minor depression, dysthymic disorder, bipolar (manic-depressive) disorders, and cyclothymia. The building blocks of mood disorders are mood episodes.

Major Depressive Episode

A person suffering from a major depressive episode suffers from five or more of the following symptoms for a two-week period. At least one symptom is either depressed mood or a loss of interest or pleasure in previously interesting or enjoyable activities:

♦ depressed mood most of the day, nearly every day
♦ decreased interest in or pleasure from most activities, most of the day, nearly every day
♦ significant weight loss when not dieting, weight gain, or change in appetite
♦ difficulty sleeping, or sleeping too much nearly every day
♦ agitation or retardation (being unable to sit still or slowed movements and speech)
♦ fatigue, loss of energy
♦ feeling worthless or guilty
♦ trouble concentrating or making decisions
♦ thoughts of death or suicide

The symptoms must cause considerable distress and/or interfere with home, school, or work responsibilities.

Grief
Grief after losing a loved one is not a disease. Some of the same symptoms occur during grief, but after about two months, the bereaved person should not be preoccupied with feelings of guilt or worthlessness and should be able to function at home and work. Significant depressive symptoms after two months are considered pathological grief.

Manic Episode
A manic episode is characterized by at least a week of an abnormally high or irritable mood or a shorter period if the symptoms are so severe that an individual has to be hospitalized, along with three or four of the following symptoms:

♦ inflated, unrealistic self-importance/sense of power
♦ decreased need for sleep
♦ talkativeness—chattering fast and constantly
♦ racing thoughts and ideas
♦ being easily distracted from a task
♦ increased activity
♦ excessive involvement in pleasant but potentially dangerous activities (shopping, sex)

These symptoms interfere with functioning, cause trouble in relationships, or require hospitalization. There are also mixed episodes of depression and mania.

Hypomanic Episode
These episodes are milder versions of mania. The person is functional, but her behavior differs from the usual.

Dysthymia
When a person's mood is depressed for most of the day, for most days, for at least two years, she has dysthymic disorder. While depressed, she must have at least two of the following symptoms:

- too much or too little appetite
- too much or too little sleep
- low energy, fatigue
- low self-esteem
- trouble concentrating or making decisions
- feelings of hopelessness

A person who has had dysthymia for many years may not notice and view it as part of her personality. Sometimes other people notice the symptoms rather than the person.

It is possible for a person with dysthymic disorder to have a major depressive episode; this is called double depression.

Atypical Depression
There is a form of depression, called atypical depression. It is more common in women, especially in their late teens and early 20s, and it causes increased appetite and too much sleep. Some women tend to become depressed at times of hormonal change: before menstruation, after childbirth, and at menopause. Hormonal-related depressions are discussed on page 245.

Seasonal Affective Disorder
The seasons influence some people's moods. Seasonal affective disorder (SAD) is classified by regularly occurring depressive symptoms during certain months of the year. Most often mood is depressed during the autumn and winter and lifts during the spring and summer. It seems to be the number of hours of sunlight, especially in the morning, that affects mood, evidenced by more cases in parts of the country where there is less light in the morning. It is three to six times more common in women than in men and can be treated with morning exposure to artificial light that mimics sunlight.

Risk Factors for Depressive Disorders
Risk factors for depression include being poor, abused, unemployed, uneducated, separated or divorced, and/or in poor health. However, it is

important to remember that depression, like other diseases, can strike anyone, no matter how fortunate. On the other hand, depression tends to be overlooked during difficult times, because people feel that the symptoms are linked to the circumstances. This is not true. When depression complicates an already difficult situation, it should be treated. In addition to relieving symptoms, treatment gives the individual a better chance of improving his or her circumstances.

After one episode of depression, there is a 50 percent chance of having another; after two episodes, the likelihood is closer to 70 percent; and after three episodes, it is 90 percent. Women tend to have more and longer-lasting episodes than men. A women is as at risk for chronic (lasting) depression if she becomes depressed early in life, has a family history of depression, had problems getting along as a child, and has poor quality of life overall.

Why Your Sex Matters in Depressive Disorders

Depression and dysthymia are two to three times more common in women than men, at least in Western cultures. The sex difference begins in adolescence and ends in later life. It was once believed that men and women had depression at the same rates, and the fact that women were diagnosed in greater numbers was because they were more likely to seek care. We now know that this is not the case, and the condition is actually more common in women. The incidence of depression peaks at age 44 for women, while for men it continues to rise throughout life. The lowest incidence rate for women is ages 45–65.

Depression tends to run in families. More often than not, depression and anxiety occur together; anxiety disorders are discussed in the next section.

Ten percent of childbearing-age women have depression. Major depressive disorder is classified as having one or more major depressive episodes, without any manic features. There are several variations of depression based on severity, repetition, and whether the depression occurs in a woman who has recently given birth to a baby (postpartum depression, discussed on page 247).

BIPOLAR DISORDER

Bipolar disorder is a condition in which episodes of depression and mania alternate; it used to be called manic depression. The incidence of bipolar disorder in men and women is about the same, but their clinical picture is different.

Why Your Sex Matters in Bipolar Disorder
Women with bipolar illness tend to cycle through ups and downs more rapidly than men and may be more vulnerable to the side effects of antidepressants, low thyroid function, and alcoholism. Women also tend to have more depressive than manic symptoms. Symptoms of bipolar disorder can worsen premenstrually, and women with bipolar disorder are especially vulnerable to episodes of depression or mania after childbirth.

When depression or mania becomes so severe that a person loses touch with reality, hears voices, or has bizarre thoughts, it is known as psychosis, discussed on page 240.

ANXIETY DISORDERS

Anxiety disorders include social anxiety, specific phobias, generalized anxiety disorder, post-traumatic stress disorder (PTSD), obsessive-compulsive disorder (OCD), and panic disorder, with or without agoraphobia. About 10 percent of the population suffers from anxiety disorders. Women are two to four times more likely than men to have an anxiety disorder in addition to obsessive-compulsive disorder. Genetics seems to play a role in the sex differences, but other factors are most likely involved as well.

A panic attack (like a major depressive episode, this is not a diagnosis in itself) is having intense fear or discomfort, reaching a peak within 10 minutes, with at least four of the following:

- palpitations (pounding or fast heart rate),
- sweating,
- trembling or shaking,
- feeling short of breath or smothering,
- feeling of choking,
- chest pain or discomfort,
- nausea or abdominal distress,
- feeling dizzy or lightheaded,
- feelings of unreality,
- fear of losing control or going crazy,
- fear of dying,
- numbness or tingling of the arms and legs, or
- chills or hot flushes.

Agoraphobia
Agoraphobia consists of anxiety about being in places or situations that are difficult or embarrassing to leave, or where help is not available in the event of a panic attack. Typical situations are being out of one's

home; on a bridge; or on a bus, train, or plane. The individual with ago-raphobia avoids situations that cause stress, gets extremely anxious if forced to be in the situation, or needs to have a companion to tolerate the situation.

Panic Disorder
Panic disorder consists of repeated panic attacks that result in the person worrying about having more attacks. People with panic disorder become concerned that the attacks will cause serious consequences such as a heart attack, or they change their behavior out of fear of attack (for example, not taking the bus). Panic disorder can occur with or without agoraphobia.

Specific Phobia
Specific phobia is a strong, lasting, unreasonable fear of one particular object or situation. Although the individual realizes that the fear is un-reasonable, she becomes extremely anxious or has a panic attack if ex-posed to the object or situation. As a result, she either experiences great anxiety or avoids the possibility of coming in contact with the object or situation. The phobia causes distress or interferes with her ability to maintain a social, work, academic, or domestic life.

Social Phobia
Social phobia is the fear of social or performance situations in which a person is observed by others or comes in contact with unfamiliar people. Although she realizes that her fear is unrealistic, having to be in these sit-uations makes her extremely anxious. She avoids these situations when-ever possible, so social phobia interferes with social relationships and normal routine. For example, the phobic cannot have a meal with friends for fear that her table manners will be embarrassing, or she is unable to stand up in church to make a routine announcement.

Generalized Anxiety Disorder
Generalized anxiety disorder (GAD) is characterized by an unrealistic amount of anxiety and worry about a number of things, occurring on most days. People with GAD are unable to control their anxiety, which interferes significantly with their lives. They have at least three of the following:

- restlessness or a feeling of being on edge
- tires easily
- trouble concentrating/mind going blank
- irritable

◆ muscle tension
◆ trouble falling or staying asleep

Obsessive-Compulsive Disorder

Obsessive-compulsive disorder (OCD) consists of either obsessions or compulsions. Obsessions are thoughts that intrude into an individual's mind often and against her will. The individual realizes that these thoughts are coming from her own mind, unlike hallucinations, which are perceived as coming from outside the mind. The individual tries to ignore or overcome them by deliberately having thoughts that counteract the obsessions. These thoughts are *not* simply exaggerated, everyday worries or other thoughts the person with OCD would normally have.

Compulsions are repeated behaviors that an individual feels she must carry out, either in response to an obsession (washing hands over and over again because of an obsession with germs, checking the front door lock over and over again because of an obsession with the possibility of a robbery) or according to strict rules (lining up all the fringe on the living room rug, tapping exactly seven times). If the individual tries to resist performing the behavior, she becomes overwhelmed with the fear that the obsession will occur—for example, someone will be hurt or they will catch a disease.

OCD is not a personality style (being anal); it is a disorder. Part of the time, the individual realizes that these obsessions or compulsions are not normal. The obsessions or compulsions cause the individual great distress, may take over an hour a day to carry out, and/or interfere with normal routine, social relationships, or work.

Men and women have approximately the same rate of OCD, but men tend to develop it earlier in life and to suffer from it longer and more severely.

Post-traumatic Stress Disorder

Post-traumatic stress disorder (PTSD) can occur following an experience or witnessing a life-threatening event. The experience causes the individual to feel terrified, horrified, or helpless. Common examples include natural disasters, terrorist incidents, serious accidents, and rape. After going through the experience, the individual has symptoms, lasting over a month, from the following three categories:

Re-experiencing (one or more of the following symptoms):

◆ upsetting memories of the event,
◆ upsetting dreams of the event,

- "flashbacks:" acting or feeling as if the event were happening all over again,
- becoming extremely upset at reminders of the event, or
- body signs of anxiety (sweating, fast heart rate, stomach upset) at reminders.

Avoidance and renumbing: PTSD may cause emotional numbness; people who experience this will not respond to events the way they did before the trauma. In addition, it causes three or more of the following symptoms:

- trying to avoid talking or thinking about the traumatic event,
- trying to avoid places, people, or activities that remind them of the event,
- being unable to remember some part of the traumatic event,
- losing interest in important activities,
- feeling detached from other people,
- being unable to feel love or other warm feelings, or
- a sense that one will not live out a normal life span/not making long-term plans.

Increased arousal; PTSD can cause increased arousal, with two or more of the following:

- trouble falling or staying asleep,
- irritability or fits of anger,
- trouble concentrating,
- being on the lookout for danger when there is none, or
- startling easily.

Acute Stress Disorder
Acute stress disorder is a version of PTSD that starts within four weeks of a traumatic event and lasts from two days to four weeks.

Preventing Anxiety
Both caffeine and nicotine can cause anxiety symptoms. Cutting back on caffeinated drinks and cigarette smoking is a good first step with mild anxiety. Anxiety can also be triggered by prescribed and over-the-counter medications, including decongestants, some herbal supplements, diet pills, and steroids. Medical conditions, including overactive thyroid, can mimic anxiety.

Why Your Sex Matters in Anxiety Disorders

Women are more likely than men to be diagnosed as anxious when a serious medical condition is actually causing their symptoms; a diagnosis of an anxiety disorder should not be made until there has been a complete medical evaluation. Women and men are equally likely to have panic or generalized anxiety disorder, but women are twice as likely to relapse after successful treatment. Alcoholism increases the risk of anxiety disorders, especially in women.

Why Your Sex Matters in PTSD

People tend to think of PTSD as a man's disease. It was first studied in male combat veterans, but, in fact, PTSD and acute stress disorder are twice as common in women as they are in men. At least part of the reason for the sex difference is that women and men tend to be exposed to different kinds of traumatic events. Women are raped 10 times more often than men, and studies show that close to 50 percent of women and men suffer from PTSD after being raped. Rape lowers the blood level of cortisol, a steroid hormone that helps regulate blood pressure and cardiovascular function, and decreases the body's use of protein, carbohydrates, and fat.

PTSD is associated with specific changes in the brain. Magnetic resonance imaging (MRI) of the brain reveals that, in PTSD, the hippocampus (part of the temporal lobe in the brain that plays a role in memory and emotion) becomes smaller. Men's traumas are more often physical assault, natural disasters, or combat. In addition to rape, women's are other kinds of assault and abuse and neglect in childhood. It seems that PTSD can develop as a result of a sequence of less severe traumas adding up over time.

Victims of domestic violence often develop PTSD. Their symptoms are often mistaken for other mental disorders, so the correct diagnosis is very important. For example, when a woman leaves an abusive relationship with the father of her children, he may demand custody on the grounds of the woman's psychiatric diagnosis. If the abuse caused or contributed to her symptoms, it becomes clear that her illness is due to his mistreatment, and the court is less likely to allow him custody of the children.

The risk of PTSD increases if a person has a pre-existing psychiatric disorder or a family history of PTSD. The symptoms and consequences of PTSD can increase the risk of depression, especially in women. Having a good support system provides some protection against PTSD.

Prevention and Treatment of PTSD

Now that the medical field recognizes and understands more about PTSD, work is being done to prevent symptoms after a person has been exposed to trauma. There is some evidence that cognitive behavior therapy, antidepressants, and benzodiazepines, also called minor tranquilizers, may be useful. In addition, urging individuals to talk in detail about the event immediately afterward, when she does not wish to, may make things worse.

SUBSTANCE ABUSE

Binging

Some people use drugs or alcohol in binges, in which large amounts of these substances are consumed within a few hours or days. Binges can cause serious complications, including death, but they do not make the body dependent on a drug or alcohol.

Substance (drug or alcohol) dependence is defined as three or more of the following:

♦ Tolerance: needing more and more of the substance to get the same effect, or getting less effect from the same amount.
♦ Withdrawal: symptoms that are experienced when drug use is discontinued or decreased. Symptoms can vary for each drug, and an individual may take another substance to avoid having withdrawal symptoms from the first one.
♦ Taking more of the substance, or for a longer time, than intended.
♦ Trouble stopping use of the substance, even when the individual wants to.
♦ Obtaining the substance takes a great deal of time and effort, often at the expense of relationships and financial security.
♦ Inability to complete other responsibilities and activities because of the substance.
♦ Using the substance even after realizing that it has caused another medical problem.

Why Your Sex Matters in Substance Abuse

Both men and women can develop complications with or addictions to alcohol or drugs, but there are sex and gender differences. Men are twice as likely as women to develop alcoholism. About 35 percent of men and 18 percent of women have some sort of substance abuse problem during their lifetimes. Roughly 20 percent of men and 8 percent of women suffer from alcohol dependence. Alcoholism and depression are often found together, but in women, the depression often develops first. Women who drink to ease their emotional turmoil often fail to realize that since alcohol is a depressant, it can make their problems worse. In addition, women are more likely to develop addictions to medications prescribed by a physician than are men, and more likely to abuse more than one drug.

After drinking the same amount of alcohol, the average woman has a greater percentage of alcohol in her bloodstream than a man. This is because women are usually smaller and have a greater proportion of body fat than men. Additionally, women's bodies produce less of an enzyme, called alcohol dehydrogenase, which helps breaks down alcohol in the body, so more alcohol circulates in women's bodies. Women are more likely than men to develop heart, brain, bone, and liver damage from drinking alcohol. Serious liver damage, from cirrhosis of the liver, can be fatal. Women who drink too much are also vulnerable to sexually transmitted diseases, unplanned pregnancy, and rape. A survey of college women revealed that one in 20 had been raped, and alcohol was involved in 75 percent of rape cases.

Women often get involved with alcohol or drugs through male partners and are more likely to have drug or alcohol problems when they live with substance-abusing partners. Once a woman is addicted, she may resort to prostitution to support her habit or to trading sex for drugs, both of which increase her risk of sexually transmitted diseases. On average, women begin drinking later and are more likely to drink alone at home. Male drinkers are more likely to get into fights when drunk than are women, who more often become quiet and sad. Fighting attracts attention, which may lead to treatment; being quiet and sad usually does not.

The use of drugs and alcohol during pregnancy is a particular problem. There is no consensus on the amount of alcohol a pregnant woman can safely consume without harming the fetus. Among the problems that alcohol can cause is fetal alcohol syndrome, which affects appearance, intelligence, and behavior. After birth, one of the major problems facing babies born to substance-abusing mothers relates to the child's unstable living situation.

Some women have been sent to prison for using drugs while pregnant. Punishment is not a good way to help pregnant women stop using drugs or alcohol. Most women in this situation want help, but if they are threatened with prison, they are less likely to go for prenatal care. Being in prison usually does not help the mother or the child in the long run.

Treatment for Substance Abuse

Although there are medications that are helpful in treating alcoholism, 12-step programs such as Alcoholics Anonymous often play a major role. The steps include accepting the fact that the person is an alcoholic, that the habit has caused harm to oneself and other people, and that a person can never drink safely. Most alcohol and drug treatment programs have been developed for men. Alcoholics Anonymous uses confrontation to force the individual to face up to the problem, while providing a group and network of people with similar experiences. Studies show that women are more comfortable and tend to do better in single-sex group therapy, and they respond better to treatment by nonjudgmental physicians. However, physicians are less likely to ask women patients about problem drinking than they are to question male patients.

EATING DISORDERS

Common eating disorders, which include anorexia nervosa, bulimia nervosa, overeating, and obesity, are 10 times more common in women than they are in men.

Anorexia is the inability to maintain a normal, healthy body weight, usually accompanied by an intense fear of becoming fat and a feeling that one is fat even when thin. Most patients with anorexia severely restrict what they eat, while others use excessive exercise or other bulimic behaviors to keep their weight abnormally low. Anorexia tends to begin earlier in life than bulimia, often at age 12 or younger. Anorexia is accompanied by loss of menstrual periods; other health consequences of anorexia include:

♦ abnormally slow heart rate and low blood pressure;
♦ osteoporosis;
♦ muscle loss and weakness;
♦ severe dehydration, which can result in kidney failure;
♦ fatigue and overall weakness;
♦ dry hair and skin; and
♦ growth of a downy layer of hair, called lanugo, all over the body, including the face, in an effort to keep the body warm.

Bulimia nervosa is characterized by a cycle of binging (eating much more food than normal within a limited period) and purging behaviors such as self-induced vomiting to undo the effects of binge eating. Bulimics feel unable to control these binges. Bulimia often starts with a diet and weight loss that gets out of hand. People with bulimia can be of normal or heavier-than-average weight, or they can maintain an unhealthy low weight.

Starving and purging cause a long list of serious medical complications, including high blood pressure, high cholesterol levels, heart disease, diabetes mellitus, and gallbladder disease. Repeated vomiting takes the enamel off the teeth, and loss of calcium causes osteoporosis. The longer the symptoms last, the less likely the woman is to recover. She often has other psychiatric disorders; depression is common. It takes a team of internists, psychiatrists, counselors, and dentists to treat these disorders; the first priority is to make the patient medically stable. If her body weight is 25 percent below normal, she should be hospitalized.

Both anorexics and bulimics are abnormally preoccupied with their body images. Many are humiliated by their diseases and go to great lengths to hide their condition from any health professional. Both anorexia and bulimia are serious and potentially life-threatening. About half of these patients recover fairly well. Thirty percent have some symptoms lasting into adulthood, 10 percent never get better, and 10 percent die of the disease.

New research using positron emission tomography (PET) scans is helping identify the brain changes that may help explain eating disorders.

Psychotic Disorders

Psychosis is loss of touch with reality, causing delusions or hallucinations, difficulty thinking and speaking logically, interference with normal emotions, and other symptoms. Delusions are false beliefs that persist despite evidence to the contrary. In paranoid psychosis, individuals are convinced that a particular group or person, or everyone, is out to hurt them. Hallucinating is hearing, seeing, smelling, or feeling something that is not there.

Schizophrenia
The most common psychotic disorder is schizophrenia, and the most common hallucination is hearing voices. People with hallucinations often hear voices criticizing or saying negative things about them. Sometimes people with schizophrenia hear more than one voice speaking to each other. "Command hallucinations" order the person to do something.

Why Your Sex Matters in Psychosis
The frequency of schizophrenia is about the same in men and women, but women tend to develop the illness at a slightly older age (20–29, even up to the mid-40s), have milder symptoms, and have a better chance of recovery. Before menopause, women often need and respond better to lower doses of antipsychotic medications than men do, which may be due to the protective effect of estrogen in the brain. There is some evidence that certain antipsychotic medications interfere with the menstrual cycle.

The most important sex-related issues in schizophrenia relate to sexual exploitation, pregnancy, and parenting. Women with untreated schizophrenia are at increased risk of sexual abuse, rape, and unplanned pregnancy. Some women with schizophrenia can be good mothers if they receive effective treatment and support.

SOMATOFORM DISORDERS

Somatoform disorders are conditions in which a person's emotional problems are expressed in the form of physical symptoms. These disorders are more common in women than in men. In the past, patients with these conditions, especially women, were often told that their symptoms were "all in their heads." We now know that the situation is much more complicated. The brain and other parts of the body interact all the time. We recognize that when we say we have butterflies in our stomach in a tense situation. It may be that the bodies of people with somatoform disorders are more sensitive and react more intensely to stresses than others, or that people with somatoform disorders are more acutely aware of body sensations. Somatoform disorders take different forms and seem to occur at different rates in different cultures.

Somatoform disorders are chronic. People with these types of disorders spend much more time getting medical care than the average person. Although no physical causes for their symptoms can be found, they are as disabled as people with severe medical and/or physical illnesses. Psychiatric disorders are physical, too—they are associated with brain changes. Generally, the disability can be reduced significantly, but the disorder cannot be completely cured.

Risk Factors
Risk factors for somatoform disorders include sexual and physical abuse, a family history of somatoform disorders, and a personal history of serious illness during childhood. Many people with somatoform disorders also have other psychiatric conditions, such as obsessive-compulsive disorder, mania, and schizophrenia. It is important to note that patients generally do not lie about or fake their symptoms. Pretending to be ill for personal gain, such as to avoid military service or get insurance payment, is called malingering.

There are four main types of somatoform disorders: somatization disorder, conversion disorder, hypochondria, and pain disorder.

Somatization Disorder
Somatization disorder begins before age 30 and lasts for many years. Patients have a wide array of symptoms that cause them to seek medical treatment or keep them from functioning well at work, school, or in social relationships. They must have all of the following symptoms, with

either no medical disease or a medical disease that is not serious enough
to explain them:

♦ four pain symptoms, such as lower back pain,
♦ two gastrointestinal symptoms,
♦ one sexual or menstrual symptom, and
♦ one neurological symptom (paralysis, convulsions, blindness, etc.).

Estimates vary, but anywhere between 0.2 and 2.0 percent of women
and less than 0.2 percent of men have somatization disorder. It seems to
run in families, with 10–20 percent of patients' mothers, sisters, and
daughters suffering from somatization as well.

Conversion Disorder
Onset of conversion disorder symptoms is usually very sudden and fol-
lows a stressful experience or life conflict. These symptoms often involve
the loss of one or more bodily functions (such as the sensation of a lump
in the throat, loss of sensation, blindness, deafness, or paralysis) in a man-
ner not compatible with medical or neurological disease. Diagnostic testing does not show a physical cause for the dysfunction. The disorder
typically begins before age 35, occurs in .01–0.5 percent of the population, and seems to be two to 10 times more common in women than in
men. Conversion disorder is more frequent in people who are not well ed-
ucated or who come from rural areas.

Hypochondria
The essential feature of hypochondria is a preoccupation, not with particular symptoms, but with the belief that one is ill and at risk of serious
consequences. Normal body sensations such as sweating, heart thump-
ing, or rumbling in the abdomen are misinterpreted as signs of disease.
Hypochondria occurs in 1–5 percent of the population and seems to be
equally common in men and women.

Pain Disorder
Pain disorder is another somatization in which the main symptom is unexplained pain that appears to be related to psychological conflict or distress. There are no known sex differences with this disorder.

Body Dysmorphic Disorder
Body dysmorphic disorder is also included among somatoform disorders. A person with body dysmorphic disorder is preoccupied with the

idea that there is something wrong with some visible part of her body, when either the body part is completely normal, or it is not nearly as unattractive as she believes it to be. It is equally common in men and women, and cultural influences play a role in what a person becomes preoccupied with. People with body dysmorphic disorder sometimes seek a series of plastic surgical procedures but are not fully satisfied with the results.

DISSOCIATIVE DISORDERS

Dissociation is a process in which an individual is not consciously aware of her own behavior for periods of time or feels as though she or her environment is not real. The most well-known dissociative disorder is called dissociative identity disorder, or "multiple personality." This diagnosis is somewhat controversial. It appears to be related to serious emotional trauma in childhood and is significantly more common in women than in men.

ATTENTION DEFICIT HYPERACTIVITY DISORDER

Attention deficit hyperactivity disorder (ADHD) usually begins in childhood, although there is increasing evidence that it can develop in adults as well. There is a strong genetic component, and it seems to be less common in girls than in boys, although there is some evidence that girls and women with ADHD have more severe symptoms and emotional impairments than do boys and men. Women may respond differently from men to some of the medications used to treat ADHD. It is important for health professionals to gather information from the patient's childhood, such as school records, rather than relying on her memory to make the diagnosis.

PERSONALITY DISORDERS

Personality disorders are distorted ways of feeling, thinking, and seeing the world that affect virtually every aspect of a person's life. Personality disorders are more severe than personality styles; the disorders often keep an individual from adapting successfully to her environment, from having satisfying relationships and stable jobs.

Unlike the other disorders mentioned in this chapter, personality disorders do not directly cause a patient distress. The person's way of thinking and feeling seems perfectly normal and reasonable to her, and she feels that any distress is caused by problem behavior of others. Ironically, expecting other people to behave in a particular way can often become a self-fulfilling prophecy. For example, when a person feels that those around her do not take care of her well enough and she is always demanding to be taken care of, people will start to pull away and avoid her, confirming what she was afraid of in the first place.

Why Your Sex Matters in Personality Disorders
There are several kinds of personality disorders; those diagnosed more commonly in women are dependent, histrionic, and, perhaps, borderline. Men are more often diagnosed with antisocial personality disorders.

- **Dependent personality disorder:** a person feels that she needs other people to carry out responsibilities that other adults do for themselves. She becomes distressed because others are not willing to take care of her.
- **Histrionic personality disorder:** a person is often described as a drama queen; dressing and behaving to attract attention, with an exaggerated reaction to the usual events of life.
- **Borderline personality:** a person has rapidly changing emotions, often with no obvious precipitant. She expects other people to be unfair and easily becomes angry. She often feels empty and desperate.

These types of personality disorders overlap one another and are often difficult to diagnose. They can be confused with cultural gender stereotypes and have become quite controversial.

Conditions Affecting Women Only

Menstruation, female-related fertility and infertility, pregnancy, birth, breastfeeding, and menopause are important markers in a woman's life. Some women seem to have mood symptoms at times of hormonal change: before menstruation, after childbirth, at menopause. There is also a cultural tendency to attribute a woman's moodiness to hormonal fluctuations, which often prevent women, their families and friends, and health care professionals from finding the true, underlying reason for distress.

Menstrual-Related Disorders

In the United States both women and men expect the menstrual cycle to cause psychological symptoms. In other countries, there are differences in the perception and expression of menstruation-related symptoms. Many women, if asked, report that they feel irritable, moody, and bloated for a few days before their period. This is called premenstrual syndrome, or PMS. It is not well defined, and more than 100 different symptoms have been attributed to PMS.

When health professionals ask women to record their PMS symptoms, more than half discover that their symptoms are not related to their monthly cycle. Menstruation tends to be implicated whenever a woman is angry, upset, or confused, but depression, anxiety disorders, personality disorders, and domestic violence can cause symptoms that many people attribute to PMS.

No treatment for PMS has been supported by careful scientific tests, but many treatments seem to help, including a healthy diet, reduced stress, adequate vitamins (particularly B vitamins), minerals (calcium), rest, and exercise.

Because PMS is so poorly defined, it is difficult to study scientifically. It is possible that 3–5 percent of menstruating women have such severe premenstrual symptoms that they interfere with their ability to work or with their relationships with friends and family. The American Psychiatric Association classifies this as premenstrual dysphoric disorder (PMDD). There may be a genetic component to this condition. The research definition of PMDD requires at least five symptoms occurring most of the time in the week before menstruation, during most cycles during the past year:

- ◆ depressed mood, hopelessness, feeling like a bad person,
- ◆ anxiety, tension,
- ◆ anger, irritability, conflict with others,
- ◆ sudden mood changes,
- ◆ decreased interest in one's usual activities,
- ◆ trouble concentrating,
- ◆ fatigue, lack of energy,
- ◆ changes in appetite/food cravings,
- ◆ changes in sleep,
- ◆ feeling overwhelmed or out of control, or
- ◆ physical symptoms: bloating, breast tenderness, headaches.

To meet the definition of PMDD, the symptoms must interfere with responsibilities or social activities and relationships and must be relieved within a day or two after menstrual bleeding begins, for at least two cycles. Women who have undergone hysterectomy but still have their ovaries can have PMDD; their menstrual cycles lack bleeding but can be tracked by means of blood hormone levels.

Some women seem to be vulnerable to depressive symptoms at times of hormonal change, including women with a history of depression. It is not the level of hormones, but the degree of hormonal change, that matters. Therefore, the diagnosis cannot be made on the basis of blood hormone levels.

EMOTIONAL REACTIONS TO INFERTILITY

Neither infertility nor pregnancy loss is caused by psychological conflict, but these conditions do cause stress and emotional pain and put pressure on relationships. In some cultures, a woman's value depends on her producing children.

PREGNANCY LOSS

The end of a pregnancy, whether spontaneous or induced, is a loss. But, with support, most women do as well psychologically after the loss as they did before. There is no specific psychiatric syndrome related to any form of pregnancy loss.

PREGNANCY

Pregnancy is not a risk factor for most psychiatric illnesses except schizophrenia and obsessive-compulsive disorder, which can be exacerbated when a woman is pregnant. About 10 percent of childbearing-age women have depression. There is a greater risk of depression in women who are teenagers, lack social support, have several children, have an unwanted pregnancy, or have had depression previously. Stopping antidepressant medication abruptly during pregnancy is also likely to precipitate a depressive episode. Depression can have a negative effect on the outcome of pregnancy, because depressed women are less likely to take good care of themselves during pregnancy. They are less likely to eat well, sleep well, rest, exercise, and follow medical advice. Depression during pregnancy often continues as postpartum depression (see the next section).

Treatment
Mild to moderate depression can be treated with psychotherapy. When medication is necessary, doctors must be cautious about prescribing it, since most medications do cross the placental barrier and can affect the growing fetus. No specific fetal defects have been linked to antidepressant medications such as SSRIs; the possible risks of medication have to be weighed against the risks of untreated depression. Abrupt discontinuation of medication can trigger withdrawal symptoms in the mother, and possibly the fetus, and it is very likely that the depression will recur. Some so-called mood stabilizers, including lithium used for the treat-

ment of bipolar disorders and anticonvulsants used as mood stabilizers, do increase the risk of fetal defects and complications.

After babies are born and are no longer receiving the medication through the placenta, there is some concern that they may experience withdrawal symptoms. In all cases one must consider the risk versus the benefit of medication use. The neonatal symptoms that have been reported with some medications are self-limited, and current data show no long-term effects. Discontinuing a medication before delivery could cause intrauterine withdrawal symptoms in the fetus, and it triples the risk of postpartum depression in the mother. Since this is an area of very active research, it is crucial to review the latest publications before making a decision about medication during pregnancy. Electroconvulsive treatment can be safely used when medication is not sufficient to treat severe depression during pregnancy.

POSTPARTUM PSYCHIATRIC DISORDERS

Postpartum depression and psychosis can be serious and life-threatening for both mother and baby. It is vital that they are diagnosed and treated immediately. There are three categories of postpartum psychiatric illness: "baby blues," postpartum depression, and postpartum psychosis.

"Baby Blues," which occurs in up to 90 percent of new mothers around the world, is a brief, self-limited period of moodiness that starts within a few days of delivery. It is most likely caused by rapid shifts in hormones in the immediate postpartum period. It resolves, without treatment, within a few days and has no lasting ill effects.

Postpartum depression occurs in about 10 percent of new mothers in the United States. It basically has the same signs and symptoms of a clinical depression during other times in life. The new mother who is depressed becomes preoccupied with thoughts that she is not a good mother and that something bad will happen to her baby. Her friends and family members are likely to be mystified, to tell her that this should be the happiest time of her life, and to remind her that she should be grateful she has a healthy new baby, thereby exacerbating her guilt and sadness. The risk of postpartum depression is higher when there have been obstetrical complications, or if the baby is born with medical problems. Untreated postpartum depression interferes with formation of the mother-baby relationship.

Treatment of Postpartum Depression
Issues in treatment for the breastfeeding mother are similar to those during pregnancy; psychotherapy should be tried in mild cases and medica-

tion added for more serious cases. Small amounts of psychotropic medications can get into breast milk but do not appear to cause significant harm. The psychological and physical advantages of breastfeeding must be weighed against the risks of medication.

Risk Factors for Postpartum Depression

Risk factors for postpartum depression are much the same as for depression during pregnancy. Postpartum depression can begin up to 12 months after the baby is born. Not only obstetricians, but family practitioners and pediatricians as well, should be on alert, and all new mothers should be screened. This is a highly treatable disease, and new mothers and their friends and family members have to be willing to report symptoms.

Postpartum psychosis is a medical emergency. It occurs in one to two of every 1,000 new mothers, and the risk is highest during the first three months after birth. Symptoms vary but may include agitation, disorientation, and difficulty sitting still. A woman with postpartum psychosis may have delusions or hallucinations focused on the baby. She may be convinced that the baby is Satan, or that she must send the baby to heaven. There is serious risk of infanticide. Many cases of postpartum psychosis are forms of mania, and the mothers are diagnosed with bipolar illness. When postpartum psychosis is suspected, the woman must be evaluated by a psychiatrist immediately. A woman diagnosed with postpartum psychosis must be hospitalized to protect her and the baby until her condition is stabilized. Close attention to her mental state allows the family and physician to make the diagnosis and begin treatment immediately. Unfortunately, the condition is likely to recur after future pregnancies.

Of course, it would be best if we could prevent postpartum psychiatric illness. There is active research in this area, but we have not reached any conclusions yet. Women with histories of depression, bipolar illness, or psychotic illness must be monitored carefully during and after pregnancy. If they are treated successfully with psychiatric medication, great caution should be exercised before discontinuing that medication.

MENOPAUSE

Menopause is not a disease; it is a phase in a woman's life cycle. As with PMS, there are many cultural implications in how this phase of life is viewed. Because many people consider menopause to be bad for women's mental health, it can be blamed for unrelated problems. These issues can stem from life circumstances that befall some women at about the same time as menopause: losing partners through death or divorce, age discrimination, abuse, the need to assume responsibility for ill or elderly relatives or grandchildren. In non-Western cultures, women often gain respect as they age; in Western cultures, women often lose respect. In some cultures, a woman's value depends on her sex appeal, and men may lose interest in aging women. As a result, women may see menopause as a dire sign of aging. The empty-nest phenomenon was thought to cause depression, but a woman's mental health tends to improve when her children grow up, and women who have never had children are not at increased risk of depression.

Research into the relationship between depression and menopause yields conflicting findings. Women with a history of previous depressions at times of hormonal change are vulnerable to depression at menopause. There is no correlation with blood hormone levels; however, small doses of hormones do seem to improve mood for these women. When menopause is related to surgical removal of ovaries, the abrupt change in ovarian hormone levels or the reason for the surgery (cancer, for example) can precipitate depression.

Treatment Issues

Some treatments for specific conditions have been covered in the sections describing those conditions. We also address some general issues in mental health care: varieties of mental health professionals, psychotherapies, medications, and other treatments.

MENTAL HEALTH PROFESSIONALS

Mental health professions include psychiatry, psychology, social work, and counseling. Most psychologists in clinical practice have either master's or doctoral degrees; licensing varies from state to state. Social workers may have either bachelor's or master's levels of training. "Counselor" includes a wide variety of professionals at various levels of training. Each of these kinds of mental health professionals can offer some kind of psychotherapy, or talk therapy, but they do not prescribe medications.

Psychiatrists are medical doctors who have completed college, four years of medical school, and at least four years of specialty training in mental health. Psychiatrists are trained to perform psychotherapy and to prescribe medications. They are also qualified to evaluate psychiatric aspects of medical illness, medical aspects of mental illnesses, and the effects of psychiatric and other medications. There are general psychiatrists as well as those who specialize in specific age groups (children or the elderly), specific conditions (depression, schizophrenia), or specific treatments (medication, psychotherapy). Psychologists with advanced degrees may specialize in certain age groups or conditions and are trained to do psychological testing and research as well as to administer psychotherapy. Many social workers and counselors focus on one clinical area: patients with medical illnesses, families, couples, or students in school.

PSYCHOTHERAPIES

Talking sessions between a patient and a trained psychotherapist can have powerful effects, including changing the brain; these changes can be demonstrated with new brain imaging techniques. Mental illnesses, as we have noted, can cause specific brain changes. Successful treatment, whether by psychotherapy or medication, returns the brain to normal. Psychotherapy can be provided individually (the most common), to couples, to families, or to groups of patients.

Most psychotherapy was originally classified as psychodynamic and focused on childhood experiences, unconscious feelings, and understanding the relationship between the therapist and patient. Another group of psychotherapies—cognitive-behavioral therapy and interpersonal therapy—focuses on the here and now, with a specified number of visits and a specific routine specified in a manual. Cognitive behavioral therapy helps the individual identify inaccurate and negative thoughts and behaviors and practice thoughts and behaviors that are more productive. Interpersonal therapy addresses problems in the individual's relationships. Psychotherapy can also be supportive, using a patient's emotional strengths to get her through a life crisis. Because manual-based therapies are short term and standardized, there is more evidence about their effectiveness than there is about the other kinds of psychotherapy. Recent evidence indicates that the other kinds have proven effectiveness as well.

Why Your Sex and Gender Matter in Choosing Treatment
Gender and sex issues play a role in a patient's choice of psychotherapy. Feminist therapists emphasize the effects of gender roles and sexism on women's psychological development and function. Some patients have a strong sex preference when choosing a therapist. Women who have been abused in any way by males often request female therapists. Preferences should be honored if possible, but patients should be careful about assuming that a particular type of therapist will behave as they expect. A patient may want to inquire about the gender views of a potential therapist and make sure the therapist does not have gender stereotypes or expectations that conflict with those of the patient. Sometimes it is necessary to interview two or more therapists before finding one who is a comfortable fit.

Potential patients may have to be very insistent with their health insurance companies to get adequate psychotherapy. Split treatment is when both psychotherapy and medication are indicated; a physician normally prescribes the medication, and a nonphysician provides counseling. Unfortunately, insurance plans seldom require that the two health professionals communicate closely with one another—or pay for them to do so. It is up to the patient to ensure that this vital communication occurs; the treatments often overlap, and changes in reactions to medication may appear to be psychotherapy issues and vice versa.

Why Your Sex Matters in Pharmacotherapy

Although women are 50 percent more likely to receive a prescription for an antidepressant during a general health care visit, sex issues and differences in medication treatment are not always taken into account. As with most prescription drugs, psychiatric medications were tested only in men until the mid-1980s, so there is not much information about long-term differences. We do know that women tend to weigh less and to have a higher proportion of body fat than men. Their stomachs empty more slowly, their hormones vary over their lifetimes and with their menstrual cycles, and their bodies handle medications differently. After age 65, depressed women seem to respond better to the newer SSRIs than to the older tricyclics. Women also may respond better than men to monoamine oxidase inhibitor antidepressants (MAOIs).

Sex makes a difference in medication side effects as well. Men and women both gain weight on certain antidepressants, but there are differences, and women, in particular, are less willing to tolerate this weight gain. If informed in advance, patients can pay extra attention to diet and exercise to maintain a desirable weight. SSRIs also cause sexual side effects (loss of desire, loss of orgasm). Antipsychotic medications can affect reproductive functions, interfere with the menstrual cycle, and cause the breasts to produce and secrete milk.

Electroconvulsive Therapy

Electroconvulsive therapy (ECT), the administration of electrical stimulation to the brain, has been called shock treatment. When first developed, it was used in large doses, without anesthesia, causing convulsions and loss of memory. Now patients are anesthetized, the electricity is applied to only one side of the brain, and smaller doses are used. ECT is a highly effective treatment for depression and is usually safer and produces results more quickly than most medications. Unfortunately, ECT is stigmatized from its use during earlier decades and its portrayal in movies like *One Flew Over the Cuckoo's Nest.*

New Experimental Treatments

Transcranial magnetic stimulation (TMS) consists of administering repeated, fast magnetic pulses to a specific area of the brain, from the outside of the head. Another new technique is stimulation of the vagus nerve, the longest cranial nerve in the body. Both of these treatments, which have shown promise in patients whose symptoms were not relieved by usual therapy, are under active study.

Alternative Therapies

Women are heavy users of herbal remedies, so-called nutraceuticals, and other alternatives to mainstream medicine. Traditionally, they are the caretakers for the family, often seeking what seem to be the safest and most natural ways for themselves and their family members to stay healthy. Unfortunately, these remedies are not always as safe as they appear to be, and many do not meet government standards. The kinds and proportions of active ingredients in herbal remedies vary from manufacturer to manufacturer and from batch to batch. As a result, there are conflicting results regarding the therapeutic effects of some herbal products, including Saint John's wort.

Another important consideration when using alternative therapies is medication interactions. Herbal preparations interact with each other and with standard medications, including hormonal contraceptives (oral, injected, implanted, or impregnated in an intrauterine device), and very little is known about their possible effects on pregnancy. Acupuncture, for example, can stimulate uterine contractions before term. As is the case with other combined treatments, all health professionals involved must be aware of any treatments the patient may be using.

Conclusion

Knowledge about sex issues in psychiatry has expanded significantly in the last decade. Critical questions have been raised about sex and gender differences in the occurrence and nature of mental illnesses and in responses to treatments. Discoveries in genetics, brain structure and function, pharmacology, and epidemiology have already answered some questions and have indicated paths for future research. We now have better tools for looking at the living brain and can actually see how men and women solve mental problems and react to emotional events. We can anticipate being able to make psychiatric diagnoses on the basis of these images.

Thanks to the efforts of the Society for Women's Health Research, scientists include women in clinical studies and are able to analyze their findings by sex. In the future, we will be able to match medications and dosages to sex and to women's hormonal phases. The field of medicine continues to work toward a better understanding of how social and biological forces interact in stress and in women's mental health. One hopes that research into how to overcome these forces will provide the best possible circumstances for girls and women to grow, thrive, and engage in healthy relationships and rewarding work in the future.

—CAROL NADELSON, MD, AND NADA STOTLAND, MD

CHAPTER 14

Oral Health

O ral health is an integral part of general health. New research is demonstrating the effect of female hormones on the oral cavity. Similarly, advances in dental science are showing links between oral diseases and systemic problems.

Female hormones affect the oral cavity throughout life; these changes occur during puberty, pregnancy, and menopause. This chapter discusses oral health during these critical times in girl's and women's lives, beginning with tooth decay and periodontal disease, two common oral diseases. The chapter also addresses oral problems associated with eating disorders, cleft lip/palate, temporomandibular disorders, and oral dryness and Sjögren's disease, problems encountered far more frequently in women than in men.

What Is Tooth Decay?

Tooth decay, or dental caries, is the most common disease of childhood. It is five times more common than asthma. While the prevalence of teeth decay has declined over the past 50 years, it still occurs in children and adults. The prevalence of tooth decay increases until the early 20s, decreases during middle adulthood (ages 35–55), and then increases slightly in older adulthood (over age 55).

Enamel, the outer layer of the teeth, is the hardest substance in the body, almost twice the hardness of bone. Tooth decay occurs when the *Strep mutans* bacteria attach to the teeth, metabolize the sugar that you eat, and produce acid. This acid breaks down the hard outer layer of enamel. When this process continues over time, the enamel becomes soft, and a cavity forms in the tooth.

This cavity requires a dental filling or restoration. The dentist removes the soft part of the tooth and replaces it with a filling material, such as composite resin, which is tooth colored, or silver dental amalgam. If the decay extends into the nerve of the tooth, a root canal may be required. This removes the nerve and blood supply in the center of the tooth. A restoration (filling) or a crown is necessary after a root canal, since there is often little natural tooth structure remaining.

PREVENTION

Tooth decay can be prevented by various measures. Fluoride in the water supply is the most cost-effective method of preventing tooth decay, and fluoride in toothpaste strengthens the teeth and makes them more resistant to acid breakdown. Sealants, a plastic coating applied to the chewing surfaces of the teeth, decreases tooth decay of the chewing surfaces of the teeth by protecting the surface from the bacteria that can hide in the pits and fissures of the tooth. Most children still do not have sealants on their teeth. Caucasian children are four times as likely to have sealants as African American children and twice as likely as Hispanic American children. As family income increases, the percentage of children with sealants increases. Parents should ask their dentists about sealants for their children's teeth. Changes in your diet can lower your risk for tooth decay by decreasing the amount of refined carbohydrates available for the bacteria to eat. Brushing and flossing can remove the number of bacteria in the mouth, as can antimicrobial mouthrinses.

What Are Periodontal Diseases?

Periodontal diseases are bacterial infections that destroy the gums and bone that surround the teeth. Gingivitis, a bacterial infection of the gums causing redness, puffiness, and/or bleeding, can usually be treated with daily oral hygiene and professional dental cleanings, called nonsurgical periodontal therapy. Periodontal disease is an infection of the bone supporting the teeth. Signs of periodontal disease include loosening teeth, bad breath, pus around teeth, or pain. Once it occurs, periodontal disease requires professional dental treatment to resolve it.

WHY YOUR SEX MATTERS

In addition to poor oral hygiene, increased bacterial levels, and smoking, pregnancy and various medical conditions more common in women—such as diabetes—can increase a woman's risk for periodontal disease. Research suggests that sex hormones may also increase a woman's risk for gingivitis.

Adolescence: Puberty and Menses
At puberty, estrogen and progesterone levels increase in girls. Studies have shown that increased levels of these sex hormones can result in an increased occurrence of gingivitis. This is because the sex hormones can make oral tissues more susceptible to the presence of these bacteria.

Good oral hygiene is essential during puberty and from the beginning of menses. Girls who may not brush regularly before puberty and not encounter any dental problems may notice redness or bleeding gums after they enter puberty if they do not brush and floss regularly. Daily, effective oral hygiene care with a toothbrush and floss can prevent gingivitis associated with puberty or menses. Regular professional cleaning at the dentist's office may also be necessary to treat persistent gingivitis.

Some young women can tell when they are getting their period by changes in their mouth. Women have reported mouth odor, presence of a herpes labialis (cold sore or fever blister on the lips), or mouth ulcers (also called an apthous ulcer and found on the inside of the mouth or on the tongue) before menstruation. If these conditions occur, tell your dental professional to see if she or he can provide treatment or relief. Numerous oral hygiene products are available to treat these conditions. Mouthrinses with antibacterial properties may assist with the mouth odor; topical anesthetics provide pain relief from mouth ulcers; and antiviral therapy is available for herpes lesions in the mouth.

Pregnancy
According to an old wives' tale, you lose one tooth for each child. Fortunately this is not true; teeth were designed to last a lifetime. The calcium in your teeth does not serve as a source of calcium for the developing fetus. The calcium in your bones is available for this purpose, which is why good bone health is important for women (see chapter 6). However, other oral problems can occur during pregnancy.

Gingivitis is the most prevalent oral problem associated with pregnancy; it can occur in 60–75 percent of all pregnant women. The hormonal changes that occur during pregnancy can exaggerate the inflammatory response to local plaque bacteria.

Pregnancy can also cause single, tumor-like growths on the gums between the teeth. This area of gum enlargement is referred to as a pregnancy tumor or pregnancy granuloma. It occurs most frequently on the front side of the top or bottom teeth and is benign. It may appear suddenly, is reddish or blue in color, and rarely grows larger than 2 cm (one inch) in diameter. Most pregnancy tumors are removed after delivery; however, if the lesion interferes with chewing or speaking, a dentist may need to remove it during pregnancy.

Periodontal Disease and Preterm Low Birth Weight Babies
In the United States, 10 percent of all births are low birth weight infants (less than 2500 grams or 5.5 pounds). The March of Dimes reported

that 25 percent of women who deliver a low birth weight baby have no known risk factors for preterm low birth weight (PLBW), such as age of mother, low socioeconomic status, alcohol and tobacco use, diabetes, hypertension, and genitourinary tract infections. New research is demonstrating a relationship between periodontal disease and PLBW. In one study, pregnant women with periodontal disease were seven times more likely to deliver a low birth weight infant.

A recent clinical trial of pregnant women with periodontal disease examined the effect of three different treatments on the women's giving birth to low birth weight babies. Results showed that the group receiving scaling and root planing decreased their risk of having a low birth weight baby by as much as 84 percent at 35 weeks. This new research suggests that periodontal disease may be a risk factor for PLBW infants. Although these results cannot be generalized to all pregnant women, this pilot research suggests that routine dental cleaning or scaling and root planing on pregnant women with periodontal disease may reduce the risk of a preterm birth.

Women considering becoming pregnant should see their dentist to ensure that their teeth and gums are healthy and infection-free. When they are pregnant, women should have their periodontal status assessed; if diagnosed with disease, they should undergo prophylaxis or scaling and root planing to decrease the infection and subsequent inflammation caused by gum disease.

Menopause
Menopause can cause changes in the oral cavity. Early studies reported women complaining of oral discomfort, burning sensations, altered taste perceptions, and dryness in the mouth. One study reported that while only 6 percent of premenopausal women complained of oral discomfort, 46 percent of postmenopausal women experienced oral discomfort. Another study found 80 percent of women complaining of a burning mouth and experiencing pain from three years before to 12 years after the onset of menopause. The causes of these oral problems are not well understood, and there are no clinical studies of the effect of hormone therapy on alleviating oral problems associated with menopause.

If you suffer from any of these problems during menopause, talk with your dentist. A thorough oral examination and diagnosis will help identify and eliminate potential causes. Many of the symptoms may have causes other than menopause. Treatment of burning mouth requires an understanding of the causes and managing them. Increased water intake, along with methods to stimulate salivary flow, may help.

Oral Health and Bulimia

Bulimia nervosa is estimated to affect 1–5 percent of the population, 90 percent of whom are women. Chronic regurgitation of gastric contents causes erosion or wearing away of the inside (tongue-side) of the teeth. The acidity of stomach contents essentially dissolves the inside surfaces of the teeth. Because of the characteristic wear patterns on teeth as a result of chronic vomiting, it is not uncommon for dental professionals to identify bulimia in a patient.

Bulimia can also increase the size of the parotid glands as a result of the stimulation from vomiting regularly. Since women who suffer from bulimia are usually thin, the increased swelling of these salivary glands can be quite noticeable. Oral hygiene habits, the extent of tooth erosion, and the frequency and amount of regurgitation appear to be related.

Cleft Lip/Palate

Cleft lip and palate are one of the most common birth defects, occurring in one of 600–700 live births. Folic acid intake can decrease the risk of this birth defect as well as the risk of neural tube defects. These defects occur early in the pregnancy, often before women know they are pregnant. As a result, current guidelines recommend that women who are considering becoming pregnant should take a folic acid supplement.

Temporomandibular Disorders

The temporomandibular joint is unique in that it is the only joint that rotates up and down and moves front to back and side to side, permitting your lower jaw to move for chewing, speaking, and swallowing. Problems with the temporomandibular joint result in disorders that fall into three categories:

- ◆ myofacial pain, or pain in the muscles that control jaw function, the neck, and/or shoulder muscles;
- ◆ internal derangement or problems of the joint, that is, a dislocated jaw, displaced disc, or injury to the condyle, a part of the lower jaw or mandible; and
- ◆ degenerative joint disease, such as osteoarthritis of the jaw joint.

WHY YOUR SEX MATTERS

It is not clear exactly how many women suffer from temporomandibular dysfunction (TMD); however, women are twice as likely to suffer from TMD as men. Women between ages 20 and 40 appear to be at greatest risk for TMD. Just as scientists are beginning to evaluate why women soccer players suffer more injuries from repeated stress on the knee ligament (anterior cruciate ligament injuries), perhaps repeated stress in the form of clenching and grinding the teeth may play a role in TMD.

TMD risk factors, symptoms, and treatments are discussed in chapter 15.

Dry Mouth/Sjögren's Syndrome

Consider saliva as a natural resource, one you do not appreciate until you do not have it. Saliva is necessary for chewing, speaking, swallowing, digesting. Its absence can make any or all of these oral functions much more difficult. Dry mouth, or xerostomia, occurs in approximately 10 percent of the population. In older adults, the prevalence may increase to 25 percent. The most common causes of oral dryness include multiple medications; medical treatments, such as radiation to the head and/or neck; or salivary gland disease, such as Sjögren's syndrome (see chapter 5).

In the absence of saliva, teeth are much more susceptible to tooth decay. Women with Sjögren's syndrome have a much higher rate of tooth decay because they lack the antibacterial properties in saliva. Because of this risk, women with Sjögren's syndrome should see their dentist more regularly. Dentists generally prescribe at-home fluoride mouthrinses to strengthen teeth and/or antibacterial mouthrinses. Chewing sugarless (xylitol) chewing gum stimulates salivary flow. Xylitol is a sugar alcohol that cannot be metabolized by the bacteria that cause tooth decay; it has been shown to decrease tooth decay rates in children.

—LINDA C. NIESSEN, DMD, MPH

CHAPTER 15

Painful Conditions

What Is Pain?

Everyone has felt pain at one time or another. The International Association for the Study of Pain defines pain as "an unpleasant and emotional experience associated with actual or potential tissue damage, or described in terms of such damage." It can be acute, meaning it comes on fast and does not last a long time. It can also be chronic, meaning it lasts a long time. You may have heard the "telephone switchboard" analogy of pain: touch a hot stove and a signal races from your finger along your spinal cord to your brain. Your brain perceives the danger and dispatches an urgent message to your hand. You yank your hand away.

Scientists now say pain is more complex than that, more like the Internet than an old-fashioned switchboard. A single stimulus may prompt multiple signals throughout the body. The pain you feel reflects an interaction among your basic cellular and genetic makeup, your current health, your emotional state, the situation in which the pain occurs, your past encounters with pain, and what you know and think about pain.

WHY YOUR SEX MATTERS

Your sex also influences how much pain you have, what type of pain it is, and how treatment affects you. Male and female brains process pain differently. Women experience pain differently from men, especially persistent and severe pain. In general, women report pain more often than men do and cope with it better than men. In one study that followed women and men after painful dental surgery, women described the surgery as significantly more painful than did the men, but 10 days afterward, women tolerated low levels of pain much better than did the men.

Estrogen influences women's pain response in many ways. Some women who live with chronic pain discover that the hormonal shift that comes with pregnancy and breastfeeding can act as a natural painkiller.

Pain treatment may work differently in men and women. The study of biological sex differences in the response to pain and treatment has just begun. Pain and analgesia involve activity in peripheral tissues beyond the central nervous system and at many levels of the nervous system. Differences in the biology at each of these sites could contribute to sex differences. In studies of postoperative dental pain, women were more sensitive than men to the analgesic effect of a certain class of pain-relieving medicine—kappa opioids.

In addition to the biological differences, social factors influence differences in pain in women and men. Menstrual cramps and childbirth themselves might help explain differences in how women and men perceive pain. Because women regularly experience pain that can be somewhat severe, they may be conditioned to recognize lower levels and tolerate higher levels of pain. Not only do women experience pain differently from men, they talk about it more. This does not, however, always result in more or better treatment. Society's attitudes toward men and women in pain may influence treatment. Some studies suggest that being female is a significant predictor of inadequate pain management. Women may experience undertreatment, as they are overrepresented in certain conditions associated with pain such as fibromyalgia and temporomandibular joint disorders. This may be due to perceptions that women complain more, they do not report their pain accurately, they are better able to tolerate their pain, or they have better skills in coping with pain. Some studies show that after surgery, men ask for and receive more morphine for their pain. It is thought that nurses and doctors assess a woman's pain at less than the level she reports it and may overestimate the pain of the "strong, silent" man. Women are more likely to seek treatment for their pain and less likely to receive it.

Many painful conditions, such as rheumatic and arthritis conditions, migraine, tension headaches, temporomandibular joint (TMJ) diseases and disorders, reflex sympathetic dystrophy syndrome (RSDS), and heartburn, are more common among women. This chapter discusses headaches, TMJ diseases and disorders, RSDS, and one painful condition that men do not experience: vulvodynia. (Other painful conditions experienced only by women, such as severe menstrual cramps [dysmenorrhea] and endometriosis, are discussed in chapter 18, and fibromyalgia is discussed in chapter 5).

What Are Headaches?

What hurts when you have a headache? Several areas of the head can contribute to pain, including a network of nerves that extends over the scalp and certain nerves in the face, mouth, and throat. Other contributors are delicate nerve fibers supplying muscles of the head and blood vessels found along the surface and at the base of the brain. Stress, muscular tension, dilated blood vessels, and other headache triggers can activate the ends of these nerves, called nociceptors, because they respond to intense stimulation. A number of chemicals help transmit nociceptive-related information to the brain. Some of these chemicals are natural painkilling proteins called endorphins, Greek for "the morphine within." One theory suggests that people who suffer from severe headache and other types of chronic pain have lower levels of endorphins than people who are generally pain free. An estimated 45 million Americans experience chronic headaches.

WHAT ARE MIGRAINE HEADACHES?

The most common type of vascular headache (those caused by abnormal function of the brain's blood vessels or vascular system) is migraine. Migraine headaches are usually characterized by severe pain on one or both sides of the head, often accompanied by nausea or an upset stomach, sensitivity to light and sound, and at times disturbed vision. Other symptoms of the type of migraine, previously called classic, include speech difficulty, weakness of an arm or leg, tingling of the face or hands, confusion, and the appearance of neurological symptoms 10–30 minutes before the pain starts. These symptoms, called an aura, can include flashing lights or zigzag lines or a temporary loss of vision. Aura symptoms last less than an hour and typically resolve before the head pain begins. The pain of a classic migraine headache may be described as intense, throbbing, or pounding and is felt in the forehead, temple, ear, jaw, or around the eye. Migraine starts on one side of the head but may eventually spread to the other side. An attack lasts up to three pain-wracked days. Migraine sufferers may experience a variety of headache presentations, including sinus pain, neck tension, and menstrual migraine or have an aura without headache.

Migraine with the greatest occurrence in the general population is not preceded by an aura. But some people do experience a variety of vague symptoms beforehand, including mental fuzziness, mood changes, fatigue, and unusual retention of fluids. During the headache phase of a migraine, a person may have diarrhea and increased urination as well as nausea and vomiting. With this type of migraine, pain can last three or four days.

Migraine can strike as often as several times a week or as rarely as once every few years, and it can occur at any time. Some people, however, experience migraines at predictable times—for example, near menstruation or every Saturday morning after a stressful week of work.

Research scientists are unclear about the precise cause of migraine headaches. There seems to be general agreement, however, that key elements are excitability of neurons and blood flow changes in the brain. People who get migraine headaches appear to have blood vessels that overreact to various triggers, including certain foods, strong or glaring light, intense odors, activity, emotions, or cigarette smoke. Triggers are not the same for everyone, and what causes a migraine in one person may relieve it in another. Triggers may be cumulative, and with exposure to multiple triggers, migraine may be more likely to occur.

Peak prevalence for migraine is ages 20–45 for both sexes. Migraine is often hereditary, and people who get migraines are thought to have an inherited abnormality in the regulation of blood vessels. They react abnormally to triggers such as stress and other normal emotions and to biological and environmental conditions.

In addition to the types discussed above, migraine headache can take several other forms, including:

- **Hemiplegic migraine**—migraine with temporary paralysis on one side of the body. Some people may experience vision problems and vertigo about 10–90 minutes before the onset of headache pain.
- **Ophthalmoplegic migraine**—pain is around the eye and is associated with a droopy eyelid, double vision, and other vision problems.
- **Basilar type migraine**—occurring primarily in adolescent and young adult women and often associated with the menstrual cycle, these migraines involve a disturbance of a major brain artery at the base of the brain. Preheadache symptoms include vertigo, double vision, loss of consciousness, and poor muscular coordination.
- **Benign exertional headache**—brought on by running, lifting, coughing, sneezing, or bending, this type rarely lasts more than several minutes.
- Headache-free migraine—characterized by such migraine symptoms as visual problems, nausea, vomiting, constipation, or diarrhea without head pain.

Why Your Sex Matters
Migraine headaches affect 28 million Americans, 75 percent of whom are women. The relationship between female hormones and migraine is still unclear. The National Headache Foundation estimates that 60 percent of women who get migraine headaches suffer from menstrual migraine headaches around the time of their menstrual period, which may disappear during pregnancy. Menstrual migraines are primarily caused

by estrogen. Other women develop migraine for the first time when they are pregnant, while some are first affected after menopause. Investigators are studying hormonal changes in women with migraine in the hope of identifying the specific ways these naturally occurring chemicals cause headaches.

Treatment

Drug therapy, biofeedback training, stress reduction, and elimination of certain foods from the diet are the most common methods of preventing and controlling migraine and other vascular headaches. Other strategies include proper sleep habits, exercise, acupuncture, massage, heat and cold applications, and avoidance of behaviors or situations that may trigger an attack. Drug therapy can be used to prevent the attacks or relieve symptoms after the headache occurs. In general, menstrual related migraines can be managed effectively with strategies similar to those used for non-menstrual related migraines.

WHAT ARE TENSION OR MUSCLE-CONTRACTION HEADACHES?

Tension headache is named not only for the role of stress in triggering the pain, but also for the contraction of neck, face, and scalp muscles brought on by stressful events. Ninety percent of all headaches are classified as tension/muscle contraction headaches, which can be divided into three categories, based on frequency of the attack. The pain is usually mild to moderate and feels like pressure is being applied to the head or neck. According to the National Headache Foundation, approximately 78 percent of adults experience a tension-type headache sometime in their lives, with a slightly higher prevalence among women.

Episodic tension-type headache occurs less than once a month and is usually triggered by temporary stress, anxiety, fatigue, or anger. This is what most of us consider to be "stress headache." It may disappear with the use of over-the-counter analgesics, withdrawal from the source of stress, or a relatively brief period of relaxation. Frequent tension-type headache occurs one to 15 days a month. Chronic tension-type headache occurs 15 or more days a month and evolves over time from episodic headache; it can last for weeks, months, and sometimes years. The pain of these headaches is often described as a tight band around the head or a feeling that the head and neck are in a cast. The pain is steady and is usually felt on both sides of the head. Chronic muscle-contraction headaches can cause sore scalps—even combing one's hair can be painful.

Occasionally, muscle-contraction headaches are accompanied by nausea, vomiting, and blurred vision, but there is no preheadache syndrome, link to hormones or foods, or a hereditary connection as there is with migraine. Research has shown that for many people, chronic muscle-contraction headaches are caused by depression and anxiety. Emotional factors are not the only triggers of muscle-contraction headaches. Certain physical postures that tense head and neck muscles can lead to head and neck pain. So can prolonged writing under poor light, or holding a phone between the shoulder and ear, or even chewing gum.

Risk Factors
Conditions associated with tension headaches include:

- depression,
- anxiety,
- teeth clenching or grinding,
- insomnia,
- sleep apnea, and
- arthritis in the neck.

Women are at greater risk of developing tension headaches than men.

Treatment
Treatment for muscle-contraction headache varies. The first consideration is to treat any specific disorder or disease that may be causing the headache. Acute tension headaches not associated with a disease are treated with analgesics. People with chronic muscle-contraction headaches may also be helped by taking monoamine oxidase (MAO) inhibitors or other antidepressants. Mixed muscle-contraction and migraine headaches are sometimes treated with barbiturate compounds. Nondrug therapy for chronic muscle-contraction headaches includes biofeedback, relaxation training, and counseling. People who suffer infrequent muscle-contraction headaches may benefit from a hot shower or moist heat applied to the back of the neck. Physical therapy, massage, and gentle exercise of the neck may also be helpful.

What Are TMJ Diseases and Disorders?

The temporomandibular joints or jaw joints are the small joints in front of each ear that attach the lower jaw (mandible) to the skull. They allow you to perform such functions as opening and closing your mouth, chewing, speaking, and swallowing. TMJ diseases and disorders, commonly called TMJ, refer to a complex and poorly understood set of conditions, manifested by pain in the area of the jaw and associated muscles. More than 10 million people in the United States suffer from

TMJ problems at any given time, 90 percent of them women are in their childbearing years.

TMJ patients experience one or more of the following:

- ♦ facial pain;
- ♦ pain in the jaw joint and surrounding tissues, including the ear;
- ♦ inability to open the mouth comfortably;
- ♦ clicking, popping, or grating sounds in the jaw joint;
- ♦ locking of the jaw when attempting to open the mouth;
- ♦ headaches;
- ♦ a bite that feels uncomfortable or feels "off;"
- ♦ neck, shoulder, and back pain; or
- ♦ swelling on the side of the face.

Medical research has not yet defined all the causes of TMJ diseases and disorders. Some possible causes are injuries to the jaw area, various forms of arthritis, dental procedures, genetics, hormones, stretching of the jaw that occurs with inserting a breathing tube before surgery, and clenching or grinding teeth. Most TMJ problems are temporary, lasting only weeks or months, and often resolve over time with or without treatment. Patients should avoid irreversible TMJ treatments that cause permanent, or irreversible, changes in the structure or position of the jaw or teeth, as they have not been proven to work and may make the problem worse. TMJ patients should be cautious in seeking a cure for their problems, but instead seek treatments that help manage their pain. Learning those pain management techniques that work best for you during flare-ups is a good way to approach dealing with your TMJ pain.

TMJ patients may also have co-morbidities associated with other body systems. Examples include:

- ♦ chronic fatigue syndrome;
- ♦ fibromyalgia;
- ♦ irritable bowel syndrome;
- ♦ multiple chemical sensitivity/allergies;
- ♦ tension and migraine headaches;
- ♦ a variety of cardiovascular symptoms, including mitral valve prolapse and arrhythmias; and
- ♦ sleep disturbances, possibly resulting in disruption of normal biological rhythms.

Neither the extent of the association nor the sequence of onset of the various symptoms is known, and little is known about the biological mechanisms that might link these disparate set of symptoms. Multidisciplinary research is essential to find a solution to these problems.

What Is Reflex Sympathetic Dystrophy Syndrome?

Also known as complex regional pain syndrome (CRPS, Type I), reflex sympathetic dystrophy syndrome (RSD) is a chronic pain condition that disproportionately affects women. An estimated 85 percent those affected with it are women. The key symptom of RSD is continuous, intense pain out of proportion to the severity of the stimulus or injury that gets worse rather than better over time. RSD most often affects one of the arms, legs, hands, or feet, and the pain often spreads to include the entire arm or leg. Typical features include:

+ dramatic changes in the color and temperature of the skin over the affected limb or body part;
+ intense burning pain;
+ skin sensitivity;
+ sweating; and
+ swelling, which is sometimes localized but often progressive.

The condition and symptoms can range from mild to severe. Some very mild cases may resolve with no treatment, while others can progress and become chronic and often debilitating.

Doctors are not sure what causes RSD. In some cases the sympathetic nervous system plays an important role in sustaining the pain. Another theory is that it is caused by a triggering of the immune response. This syndrome occurs after 1–2 percent of various fractures and after 2–5 percent of peripheral nerve injuries. Minor injuries, such as a sprain or fall, are frequent causes of RSD. In 10–26 percent of cases, no precipitating factor can be found.

Because there is no cure for RSD, treatment is aimed at relieving painful symptoms. Doctors may prescribe topical analgesics, antidepressants, corticosteroids, and opioids to relieve pain. Other treatments may include physical therapy, sympathetic nerve block, spinal cord stimulation, intrathecal drug pumps to deliver opioids and local anesthetic agents via the spinal cord, and psychological support.

From Living in Pain to Living for a Purpose

By Christin Veasley, director of research and professional programs, National Vulvodynia Association (NVA)

Over a decade ago, at the age of 15, I was struck by a car while riding my bicycle home from summer camp. I suffered massive internal trauma, and doctors weren't hopeful for my survival. I underwent several surgeries within the next 48 hours. One repaired my broken leg, another was done to find the cause of internal bleeding, and yet the most critical was performed to remove damaged areas of my liver. The physicians told my family that if it had not been for my age and athletic condition, I surely would have died.

After extensive rehabilitation and a few more minor surgeries throughout the next year, I was restored to the same physical shape that I was in before the accident. However, one very important thing in my life changed from that day forward—my attitude. I realized that life is an incredible gift from God, and I started not to take simple things for granted, as I had done before my accident. To do things as simple as breathe fresh air and put one foot in front of the other to step forward are marvelous gifts we don't think about twice unless forced, by accident or illness, to do so. Above all, I was thankful that I could now live a life free from physical pain. I had endured night after night of unimaginable pain that I thought would never go away. But it did, and I prayed that I would not suffer from any sort of physical pain ever again.

Three years later I was diagnosed with vulvodynia, a chronic pain syndrome that affects millions of women. Women with vulvodynia experience a variety of painful sensations in the vulva (the area of a woman's genitalia that surrounds the opening of the vagina) such as burning, stinging, and rawness. Women have described the pain they experience as a feeling of "acid being poured on my skin" or like "tiny pieces of glass are rubbing against my skin." Vulvodynia is idiopathic, which means that we don't know exactly what causes it. We do know that it is not an infectious disease, nor is it sexually transmitted. It is not a psychological manifestation. Many women are not able to engage in intercourse. Others are unable to sit for long periods of time or to wear normal clothing, such as jeans. Vulvodynia affects a woman's physical and social life to such an extent that some have taken their own lives because of it. There is no "cure" for vulvodynia, and since the causes of the condition are unknown, treatments can only be aimed at symptom relief and they vary in success.

The average woman with vulvodynia visits five health care providers in search of a diagnosis; a large percentage of these women remain undiagnosed, even after that many visits. I was fortunate that the first provider I visited was able to diagnosis me. But she did me a great disservice by telling me that there were not any treatments for the condition, which I later learned was not true. I left her office devastated and hopeless. I was 18 at the time and had no idea of the extent of the battle I was up against. I thought I would make an appointment, get a medication, and it would go away in a week's time like the common cold. It did not. Reality hit and I learned very quickly how relentless chronic pain is. It can take a long time to find a treatment or combination of treatments that provide relief. I felt a thousand different emotions and asked, "Why me?"

I've searched for the answer to this question for many years. I believe that some of us are given unpleasant and difficult things to deal with for the sake of a higher good. Many men and women take negative situations and turn them into positive initiatives, moving forward and fighting for better lives for themselves and others. Many are ordinary people, affected by a circumstance that prompted them to use their lives to fight racism, oppression, sexism, and disease. Why was my life any different? I was an ordinary person, affected by a circumstance and very capable of using my life to help others now and in the future.

I decided to learn all I could about vulvodynia—to try to fight the disorder with knowledge. This is when I came across an organization run by a group of women who had devoted their lives to helping others who were suffering and in need. I was given information about the National Vulvodynia Association (NVA) in 1995, shortly after it was created. I immediately joined and requested all of the information the organization had available. I was given the names of other women near me who were fighting the same battle. I went to the library and searched through medical journals and books to read and understand everything I could.

Shortly thereafter, I started volunteering my time to the NVA. I wanted to aid in its mission to educate affected women, the medical community, and the public about vulvodynia and to lessen the isolation and frustration apparent among those of us who were suffering needlessly. I became a support group leader and organized meetings for women to come together to learn more about the disorder and talk to each other for ongoing emotional support. Shortly after graduating college, I moved across the country to work at Johns Hopkins University with a researcher who was conducting studies on vulvodynia. A few years later, I began working for the NVA.

Through the years, I had tried almost all of the treatments available for vulvodynia—creams, antidepressants (not for depression but for *pain), biofeedback, physical therapy—all of which provided only minor relief. There was another option—surgery. But, after all the surgery I had undergone as a teenager, I didn't know if I could face any more. I decided to go through with it. Newly married to a wonderful man—who had first been my good friend from college, whom I could talk to about my pain without fear of losing his friendship—who later came to be my fiancé. He understood from the beginning that our relationship would face a unique set of difficulties. We would have to find ways to develop an intimate relationship with each other without having intercourse. Even though it has not been easy for either one of us or our relationship, he has supported me every step of the way and in every decision I have had to face.*

The surgery turned out to be a success. It took a few weeks to recover, and then I had to undergo additional therapy for a few more months. Although the pain was not completely gone right after the surgery, my husband and I were able to have intercourse for the first time. A year later, we welcomed our daughter, Grace, into the world. Today, almost five years after my surgery, I am doing well and the pain of vulvodynia is a distant memory.

Each step I've taken has given me hope that there will be a time when all those who suffer physical and emotional pain from vulvodynia will be able to speak freely about it. I know in my heart that I have traveled down this difficult road for a purpose and have decided to use my life to help others who needlessly suffer from the condition. Too many women have suffered for too long in silence, and we must speak out. Our voices hold more power than we realize, and when used together, have the capability to positively change the outcome of our circumstance and the circumstances of others who follow us.

(Reprinted with permission by Christin Veasley)

What Is Vulvodynia?

Vulvodynia literally means pain, or an unpleasant altered sensation, in the vulva (the area of a woman's genitalia that surrounds the opening of the vagina). Defined as chronic vulvar discomfort or pain and characterized by burning, stinging, irritation, or rawness of the female genitalia, in which there is no infection or skin disease causing these symptoms, vulvodynia affects as many as 14 million women at some point in their lives. Burning sensations are the most common, but the type and severity of symptoms are highly individualized. They can include stinging, stabbing, or knifelike pain. Pain may be constant or intermittent, localized or diffuse. It can be unprovoked or occur only on provocation (when the area is touched, such as with tampon insertion, gynecologic examination, intercourse, or riding a bicycle).

While a distinct area of redness may be visible, most often the vulva appears perfectly normal on physical exam. Vulvodynia is a diagnosis of exclusion; all conditions that could cause pain in the area, such as vaginal infection or dermatological disease, must be ruled out before vulvodynia can be diagnosed properly. Unfortunately, many doctors are unaware that this condition even exists and may mistakenly suggest to patients that their symptoms are psychological. It is common for women with vulvodynia to suffer for many years and to see many doctors before being correctly diagnosed.

Vulvodynia, like other chronic pain conditions, can profoundly affect a person's life. It typically affects her ability to engage in sexual activity and may interfere with daily functioning, for example, sitting at a desk, engaging in physical exercise, and participating in social activities. These limitations can negatively affect self-image and lead to depression.

Since vulvodynia is a pain condition that affects the vulva, many experts favor a multidisciplinary approach to its treatment. Treatment may involve visiting a gynecologist, dermatologist, neurologist, and/or pain management specialist. Treatment seeks to alleviate symptoms and may provide partial or complete relief. While some patients experience relief with a particular treatment regimen, others may not respond to it or may experience unacceptable side effects. No single treatment is appropriate for every patient, and it may take a considerable amount of time to find a treatment or combination of treatments that alleviates symptoms. Some current treatments include topical anesthetics (for example, lidocaine), oral antidepressant and/or anticonvulsant medications for their pain-blocking qualities (for example, amitriptyline), nerve blocks, physical therapy, and, in some cases, surgery.

—YVETTE COLÓN, MSW, ACSW, BCD;
TERRIE COWLEY; AND CHRISTIN VEASLEY

CHAPTER 16

Pulmonary Diseases

How We Breathe

The lungs and the other parts of the respiratory system help your body perform one of its most important tasks: breathing. They allow air and oxygen to enter the body and carbon dioxide, the major waste product, to leave it. This process is called gas exchange. The respiratory system also filters out potentially harmful substances before they can enter the body.

The upper airway portion of the respiratory system includes the nose, throat, and voice box (larynx) as well as the sinus tracts that drain into the nose. The lower airway includes the windpipe (trachea), bronchial tubes, and air sacs (alveoli).

The airways are equipped with gently beating hair-like cells (cilia) that sweep larger foreign particles out of the airways and trap them in mucus that can be coughed out of the body. The airways also protect against excessive cold, heat, and dryness.

Much like the branches of a tree, the airway divides as it enters the lungs into branches, called bronchial tubes, which allow air to flow into tiny air sacs. There are about 300 million air sacs in the five lobes of the lungs. Oxygen and carbon dioxide are transferred between the air and the blood system across a very thin membrane that separates the air sacs and tiny blood vessels, called capillaries.

The air we breathe is filled with harmful substances, from bacteria to pollution. To protect itself, the body has a very active immune system along the respiratory tract. It has cells that produce special antibodies that fight infectious agents that are inhaled into the airways as well as specialized immune cells, called macrophages, which help protect the body from toxic molecules or germs by ingesting and destroying them.

The lungs also serve as a chemical factory, producing hormones and other molecules essential to the smooth functioning of the body.

Muscles are also involved in the pulmonary system. The diaphragm, a long muscle that lies underneath your lungs, separates the chest cavity (heart and lungs) from the abdominal cavity (stomach, liver, spleen, intestines, gallbladder, pancreas, and sex organs). There are also small muscles attached to the outer edges of your lungs that help maintain optimum breathing ability.

Risks for Pulmonary Disease

More and more people are being diagnosed with diseases of the lungs, especially asthma. Tobacco use is a major factor. The best prevention is never to smoke, but it is equally important to protect yourself from passive smoke. If others are smoking around you, ask them to stop. If that is not possible, leave the area where people are smoking as quickly as you can.

Air pollution and poor ventilation systems in so-called modern buildings contribute to the increase in breathing problems, especially asthma. Many bacteria, viruses, and fungi (molds) also cause breathing problems.

Our emotions can also cause us to have breathing difficulties. Learning to manage stress is important for everyone, but it is especially important if you have any pulmonary disease. Use exercise, meditation, yoga, deep breathing, massage, or any other technique that works for you to reduce your stress level. While stress reduction may not prevent you from being diagnosed with a pulmonary disease, it may make living with the disease much easier.

What Are Pulmonary Disorders?

In this chapter we discuss four important conditions: shortness of breath, asthma, chronic obstructive pulmonary disease (COPD) and pulmonary hypertension. All of these conditions may be diagnosed earlier in women than in men, primarily because women usually seek medical advice before men do. Early diagnosis is generally beneficial, as corrective measures or treatment can begin earlier.

What Is Shortness of Breath?

Dyspnea (difficult breathing), the medical term for shortness of breath, is one of the most common complaints of people seeking help from a health care provider. It is not considered a disease, but rather a signal that something is wrong with the lungs or heart.

Like pain, dyspnea is subjective. For example, a runner who is used to running three miles a day in 25 minutes may have to complete the run in 30 or 35 minutes if dyspnea occurs. Another person may suddenly have difficulty breathing when climbing stairs or doing housework.

As we age, most people lose some forms of physical ability. An abrupt change in your ability to breathe, however, is never normal and needs to be checked out. Doctors may dismiss breathing changes in women, who are often told that their symptoms are a result of anxiety. If you have changes in your ability to breathe, make sure a doctor listens to you and checks out possible causes. It could be an early sign of something serious.

WHEN DYSPNEA SIGNALS DANGER

Dyspnea may be a sign that you have or are developing any of the following common, but serious, conditions:

- allergies,
- asthma,
- chronic bronchitis,
- COPD,
- emphysema,
- heart disease,
- lung cancer,
- pneumonia, or
- tuberculosis.

If you have shortness of breath, your doctor may first assess how well your lungs are functioning by using a simple test, called spirometry. You are asked to breath into a machine that calculates the strength of your lungs.

WHY YOUR SEX MATTERS

The most common parameter measured by spirometry is forced expiratory volume (FEV1). For reasons that are not yet understood, FEV1 declines more rapidly in women smokers than it does in men smokers. Because of this, smoking prevention and cessation is even more important in woman.

If your pulmonary function is lower than normal, your doctor should order more tests. These might include a computed tomography (CT) scan or a chest x-ray. The x-ray can determine if you have certain lung conditions, including asthma, bronchitis, tuberculosis, emphysema, or pneumonia. The CT scan can help determine if you have lung cancer and can clearly identify specific areas of emphysema.

TREATMENT FOR DYSPNEA

There is no specific treatment for dyspnea; it depends on the reason behind the shortness of breath. If your doctor cannot identify the underlying cause, there are other things that you can do to reduce the symptoms:

♦ exercise your pulmonary muscles by belly breathing;
♦ take part in daily exercise such as walking, cycling, swimming, yoga, aerobics, or other exercise; and
♦ participate in a weight reduction program, if you are over the ideal weight for your height.

What Is Asthma?

Asthma is caused by an inflammation of the lungs and upper and lower airways. Inflammation usually leads to spasm, an involuntary contraction of the bronchial tubes. The bronchial tubes can also become blocked by overproduction of thick mucus.

SYMPTOMS OF AN ASTHMA ATTACK

The range of symptoms for asthma varies greatly. Asthma can be very mild, with only minimal persistent symptoms and rare flare-ups, or it can be very debilitating, with constant symptoms and very frequent attacks that may be life threatening. Emotional factors seem to play a role and may contribute to the origin of asthma or may be the result of persistent trouble breathing or both.

Symptoms that should prompt a call to a physician include:

♦ progressive shortness of breath/wheezing,
♦ increased cough and mucus production,
♦ chest pain, or
♦ fever.

An immediate call for emergency help should be made if a person with asthma has:

♦ very rapid breathing rate;
♦ very rapid pulse rate;
♦ severe chest pain; or
♦ loss of consciousness.

Managing and Treating Asthma

Asthma is characterized by periods of stability with flare-ups of varying frequency and severity. The goals of management include avoiding or reducing the number of acute attacks and managing chronic or long-term symptoms. Asthmatics should have a yearly influenza immunization as well as immunization for pneumonia every five to 10 years.

Stress management is also very helpful. Many people find that daily meditation, yoga, and other regular exercise significantly improve their ability to live with asthma.

Some asthmatics have a problem with exercise and find that it can cause an attack. However, exercise is good for people with any lung disease, including asthma, because it exercises the muscles that help us breathe as well as the muscles that help us move. Using inhaled medications before exercise can usually minimize this problem.

Certain asthmatics are sensitive to aspirin, so this and similar drugs (NSAIDS such as ibuprofen) should be avoided. Always discuss your medications with a physician.

Maintaining adequate hydration is very important for avoiding attacks and managing flare-ups when they occur. Dehydation makes the mucus very thick and can trigger an asthma attack. By drinking six to eight glasses of water a day, asthmatics can help thin out the mucus in their lungs.

Steroids, potent anti-inflammatory agents, are the most important element in the treatment of asthma. Steroids can be very effective in the inhaled form and are usually much safer than those taken by mouth; however, they are very powerful drugs with many potentially serious side effects. Always follow the instructions on your prescription and tell your doctor if you have any questions.

Bronchodilators can also be helpful in managing asthma, but they can have side effects. Recently, long-acting inhaled medications (used twice daily) have proven to be very useful in maintenance therapy. They have replaced most of the older shorter-acting inhalers, which are now reserved for episodic treatment of wheezing and shortness of breath (rescue inhalers). Some people with asthma need to use their inhalers daily, others use them occasionally. If you have asthma that is triggered by an allergen such as seasonal pollen, you may only need to use your inhaler when you experience symptoms.

Antibiotics are used to manage a flare-up only if your doctor suspects you might have developed a bacterial infection. Side effects and the development of resistant bacteria can become a problem with frequent antibiotic use.

Much of the treatment of asthma is directed toward decreasing inflammation in the lungs. It is important to avoid things that may trigger inflammation. If you have asthma, try to learn what triggers your symptoms. Common triggers include:

♦ exposure to allergens such as pollen, dust, etc.;
♦ cigarette smoke;
♦ environmental pollutants; and
♦ viral or bacterial infections.

PREVENTING AN ATTACK

Prevention is always better than having an acute attack, and drugs are available to help manage asthma. It is especially important to avoid any known triggers, which might include such things as tobacco smoke, mold, or animal dander.

Asthma patients are often given a simple device, called a peak flow meter, that measures lung function. The results should be recorded daily. The goal is to abort an attack in its earliest stages. A significant decline in lung function often precedes an attack and should be reported to a physician immediately. The doctor might suggest increasing your dose of steroids to prevent or reduce the severity of the attack. The steroids are inhaled directly into the lungs, allowing them to work where they are needed. It is essential to learn to use your inhaler properly, or the medications will not work as expected.

WHY YOUR SEX MATTERS

In early childhood, more boys than girls are diagnosed with asthma. However, after puberty, the number of women diagnosed with asthma increases; by age 40, women outnumber men. The reasons for these differences are unclear, but boys tend to have smaller airways and, possibly, greater allergic susceptibility. In addition, female sex hormones may play a role after puberty. The obesity epidemic seems to be a significant factor in the recent increase of asthma in the general population. A study from New Zealand published in 2005 has shown a significant relationship between obesity and asthma in women, but not in boys or prepubescent girls. It is estimated that 28 percent of asthma in females, age nine to 26, may be attributed to obesity; therefore, weight control is especially important in women.

There is a strong association between prenatal exposure to maternal smoking and reduced lung function at birth in babies. Infants and children of women who smoke during and/or after pregnancy tend to wheeze more, have more respiratory infections and earaches, and are at greater risk of having asthma.

What Is Chronic Obstructive Pulmonary Disease?

Chronic bronchitis and emphysema are part of the disease complex called chronic obstructive pulmonary disease (COPD) and often occur together. Many people have a predominance of one type of COPD over the other, but most have elements of both.

Chronic bronchitis is caused by persistent inflammation of the bronchial tubes. The symptoms of chronic bronchitis, which include chronic cough and excess mucus production, often wax and wane, but with repeated attacks, there is a strong tendency for increasing shortness of breath.

Emphysema involves the actual destruction of lung tissue. The air sacs are destroyed, and large, nonfunctional balloon-like structures, called blebs, are formed. Symptoms of emphysema include progressive shortness of breath, coughing (with or without sputum), and wheezing. Progression can vary from very slow over many years to extremely rapid over a few months.

RISK FACTORS FOR COPD

Cigarette smoking is by far the most important cause of COPD, but genetic factors can play a role in some people. The most important genetic factor identified is alpha-1 anti-trypsin deficiency, which affects both sexes equally.

WHY YOUR SEX MATTERS

There is good evidence that women are more severely affected by cigarette smoking than are men. The American Lung Association finds that 80 percent of COPD deaths in women are directly attributable to smoking. If you smoke, it is important to find some way to quit. Even if you have tried to stop smoking many times before, discuss new approaches with your doctor.

It is important to understand that your lungs will not return to normal after quitting smoking. If you have started on the path to emphysema and have visible signs (blebs) on CT or x-ray, the affected portions of your lungs will not heal. By stopping smoking right away, you can prevent further damage to your lungs.

PREVENTING CHRONIC BRONCHITIS ATTACKS

Prevention strategies are the same as for asthma except that avoiding allergy triggers is less important.

TREATING COPD

Most people with COPD need to take medications daily. The same in-halants used to treat asthma are used in COPD, and antibiotics are used frequently. In addition, oxygen is often used to treat people with emphysema.

What Is Pulmonary Hypertension?

Pulmonary hypertension, a relatively rare syndrome, occurs when blood flow through the artery that connects the right ventricle of the heart to the lungs increases in pressure. This causes the right side of your heart to enlarge.

There are two forms of the syndrome: primary and secondary. If you are diagnosed with primary hypertension and do not have any of the conditions that might cause it, it is termed primary pulmonary hyperten-sion. Many people who took some of the diet drugs in the past 10 years or so developed primary pulmonary hypertension, and some forms of pulmonary hypertension are inherited. Primary pulmonary hypertension is diagnosed in women more frequently than it is in men. Secondary pul-monary hypertension happens in some people with emphysema, bronchi-tis, or some autoimmune diseases such as lupus and scleroderma.

Symptoms and signs of pulmonary hypertension include:

◆ shortness of breath,
◆ need to breathe harder and faster (hyperventilating),
◆ fatigue,
◆ weakness,
◆ lightheadedness or dizziness,
◆ coughing up blood,
◆ hands or feet having a bluish tint due to lack of good circulation,
◆ prominent veins in your neck,
◆ swelling in hands or feet due to fluid retention, and
◆ enlarged right side of your heart.

While there is no cure for pulmonary hypertension, some medications can lower pulmonary pressures and reduce symptoms, thereby increasing your ability to be active. Treatment may help to prolong your life span. Major treatments that help the vessels in the lungs expand include:

◆ **prostacyclin analogues** (common forms are prostacyclin, which is given as a continuous intravenous infusion, and treprostinil, which is given as a continuous infusion under the skin);

- **endothelin receptor antagonists,** provided in pill form, which counteract endothelin, a substance in blood vessels that causes the vessels to constrict;
- **high-dose calcium channel blockers,** which can help relax muscles in the blood vessels, are sometimes used in select patients;
- **sildenafil,** a drug used to treat male impotence, is being studied for use in patients with pulmonary hypertension; data will be reviewed by the Food and Drug Administration in the near future; and
- **low-dose blood thinners** (anticoagulants) such as warfarin are also effective in preventing small blood clots that may occur in many pulmonary hypertension patients.

Additional treatments can include diuretics to help remove excess fluid from body tissues, which may have been caused by high pressures in pulmonary blood vessels, and oxygen. In rare cases, a lung or heart-lung transplant may be an option.

WHY YOUR SEX MATTERS

Women may be at higher risk than men for the complication known as primary graft dysfunction. About 10 percent of lung transplant recipients have this condition, which can be fatal. A recent study found that women were nearly 60 percent more likely than men to experience this complication.

Preventing Lung Problems

Here are some other strategies that are important in maintaining good lung health:

- **Environmental**—The quality of the environment, both indoor and outdoor, is very important for lung health. We should all do what we can to support measures to clean our air, for our health and the health of our planet. Control of the indoor environment is essential as well. The home should be well ventilated and should be as free as possible from mildew, animal dander, dust, mites, and other allergens.
- **Smoking cessation**—It is crucial that everyone with breathing difficulties stop smoking. Nicotine addiction is very powerful, but it has been beaten by millions of people. Secondhand smoke should be avoided as well. Women can do a great deal to pre-

vent children from being exposed to passive smoke, and we can educate our children and friends about the dangers of smoking.

♦ **Hydration**—Drink adequate amounts of fluids every day. During a flare-up of lung difficulties, we breathe faster, which can rapidly lead to dehydration. Dehydration can cause retention of secretions and make management of attacks much more difficult.

In addition, chest physiotherapy and pulmonary rehabilitation/exercise training can help people with breathing problems. Several techniques and devices can be used with or without the supervision of a respiratory therapist. They help clear secretions and strengthen the breathing muscles. Be sure to ask your doctor or respiratory therapist for tips on these and other exercises.

Belly or yoga breathing helps to exercise the pulmonary muscles by allowing the entire capacity of the lungs to be filled with every breath and emptied with every exhalation. This also helps to clear toxic materials from the lungs.

To learn to belly breathe, lie on the floor with your hand on your belly (near or below your belly button). Slowly take a deep breath, letting the belly rise up as you inhale. Your shoulders should not move at all while you are doing this. When you exhale, squeeze all the muscles in your belly as tightly as possible to force all the air out of your lungs. Practice this type of breathing until you can do it in any position—lying down, sitting, or walking. In addition to strengthening your pulmonary muscles, you will strengthen your abdominal muscles.

Use of a handheld "threshold trainer"—an inexpensive, disposable device that exercises the respiratory muscles—has been shown to improve exercise capacity in people with chronic lung disease. These devices can be purchased at most medical supply houses.

Pulmonary rehabilitation programs, available at some hospital outpatient centers, often involve education about lung disease, evaluation of exercise capability, exercise training, nutrition counseling, and a psychosocial component. The group environment is an important part of the success of these programs, which have been shown to help people feel much better.

—MICHAEL E. KALAFER, MD, AND PEGGY McCARTHY, MBA

CHAPTER 17

Sexual Dissatisfactions

What Is Sexuality?

In the past, sexuality was thought to have one purpose, and that purpose was reproduction. Today, sexuality is seen as an important aspect of health and human behavior. Sexuality and sensuality enhance the quality of life, foster personal growth, and contribute to human fulfillment. When sexuality is viewed holistically, it refers to the totality of a being and includes all the qualities that make you who you are—biological, psychological, emotional, social, cultural, and spiritual—not just to the genitals and their functions. And people have the capacity to express their sexuality in any of these areas, without necessarily involving the genitals.

There are two commonly held views about sexual expression. The most common view is goal-oriented, which is analogous to climbing a flight of stairs. The first step is touching, the next step is kissing, followed by caressing, vagina-penis contact, intercourse, and then the last step of orgasm. The goal is orgasm, and if the sexual experience does not lead to orgasm, then one or both partners do not feel satisfied with the experience.

Another view of sexual expression is pleasure-oriented, which can be thought of as a circle, with each expression on the perimeter of the circle considered an end in itself. Whether the experience involves kissing, holding hands, cuddling, or oral sex, each, as an end in itself, is satisfying to the person or the couple. Stereotypically, most women are pleasure-oriented, and most men are goal-oriented, although the opposite can hold true. It is important for you and your partner to understand how you view sexual expressions.

Sexual Research and Women

Over the last three decades, interest in male sexuality has dominated the field of sexual research: there are more than double the number of studies published on men than there are on women. Since 1999, there has been a 30 percent increase in reported studies about women and their sexuality. One major reason for this was the U.S. Food and Drug Administration's (FDA's) approval of drugs for erectile dysfunction and the realization that money could be made from "sexual dysfunctions." However, it was soon obvious that women do not respond in the same way men do. Women are capable of experiencing sensual and sexual satisfaction from many forms of physical and psychological stimulation, not just from the linear pattern that most men do, and women have different biochemicals at the cellular level; therefore, drugs designed for men did not work in women.

Sexual Dissatisfaction

Not all sexual interactions are pleasurable and satisfying, and almost every woman experiences some sort of sexual dissatisfaction or problem related to sexuality sometime in her life. Sexual dissatisfactions can affect heterosexual and homosexual men and women at any age, regardless of whether they have physical or psychological problems. Most dissatisfactions have a biopsychosocial origin. A study conducted at the Yale School of Medicine and the Albert Einstein College of Medicine in 2005 found that 48 percent of women have "sexual dysfunction." Those with "sexual dysfunction" had decreased sensation in the clitoris compared to asymptomatic women. With any sexual dissatisfaction or problem, a multidisciplinary approach is always best. It is important to visit a physician to rule out physical disorders and an American Association of Sex Education Counselors & Therapists (AASECT)-certified sex therapist to determine if there are any psychosocial problems.

Female Sexual Disorders

Sexual desire disorders include:

♦ Hypoactive sexual desire disorder (HSDD), defined as the persistent or recurrent deficiency (or absence) of sexual fantasies, and/or desire for or receptivity to, sexual activity, which causes personal distress.
♦ Female sexual aversion disorder (FSAD), defined as the persistent or recurrent phobic aversion to and avoidance of sexual contact with a sexual partner, which causes personal distress.

A lack of sexual desire is quite common in women. Studies indicate a prevalence among 33 percent in women age 18–59, which may increase to 45 percent in women after menopause.

Sexual desire in men and women may depend on a hormone, testosterone, which is produced by the adrenal gland and ovaries in women. Currently, at least one pharmaceutical company is working on a testosterone patch for women who have had their ovaries removed for reasons including ovarian cancer and, therefore, experience low sexual desire. Doctors sometimes prescribe a medication that combines estrogen and testosterone that was approved to treat estrogen-resistant hot flashes. This oral medication, as with an oral testosterone, can negatively affect cholesterol levels. After physical causes for low desire have been ruled out, it often helps to talk with a sex therapist certified by AASECT .

SEXUAL AROUSAL DISORDER

Female sexual arousal disorder (FSAD) is the persistent or recurrent inability to attain or maintain sufficient sexual excitement, causing personal distress. It may be expressed as a lack of subjective excitement, a lack of genital lubrication/swelling, or other bodily response.

The medical community often equates this disorder to erectile dysfunction in men, so many drugs are being developed and tested for women. A woman who suffers from FSAD may find that she does not feel aroused or excited or does not have enough lubrication. Arousal disorders are reported by roughly one in five women, and the numbers may increase to roughly two in five as women approach and reach menopause.

Systemic or local hormone therapy may help. Estrogen alone can be used vaginally, and some vaginal products (ring and tablet) are not absorbed well by the body; those that are absorbed the least may be safer for women with cancer concerns. Kegel exercises (repeated voluntary contraction and relaxation of the pelvic floor muscles) are very helpful in bringing blood flow and lubrication to the genital area. Also, many over-the-counter, water-based lubricants are available and very helpful in providing additional vaginal lubrication.

ORGASMIC DISORDER

Orgasmic disorder is defined as the persistent or recurrent difficulty of, delay in, or absence of attaining orgasm following sufficient sexual stimulation and arousal, which causes personal distress. This disorder has been reported in an average of 24 percent of women before menopause and 39 percent of women after menopause. Recent research with twins indicates there may be a genetic basis to female orgasm.

Orgasm can be triggered by physical and/or mental stimuli. Every woman is different. Some women may be able to experience an orgasm with self-stimulation but not with partner stimulation. Others can experience orgasm through imagery alone, and some have even experienced orgasm after suffering from complete spinal cord injury.

Again, medical conditions and many prescription and over-the-counter medications may affect sexual response in all areas, and a biopsychosocial approach to this dissatisfaction is important. The strength of the pelvic floor muscles may be positively correlated with orgasmic response, so Kegel exercises may prove most helpful.

What Are Sexual Pain Disorders?

♦ Dyspareunia is defined as recurrent or persistent genital pain associated with sexual intercourse, which causes personal distress.
♦ Vaginismus is defined as recurrent or persistent involuntary spasm of the musculature of the outer third of the vagina that interferes with vaginal penetration, which causes personal distress.
♦ Noncoital sexual pain disorder is defined as recurrent or persistent genital pain induced by noncoital sexual stimulation, which causes personal distress.

Sexual stimulation of any kind should not cause pain. If you experience pain during sex play or before, during, or after vaginal intercourse, you need to get treatment. Again, a biopsychosocial multidisciplinary approach seems to work best for sexual pain disorders.

Why Your Sex Matters

Women can experience sexual arousal, orgasm, and satisfaction without desire, and they can experience desire, arousal, and satisfaction, without orgasm. If a woman is sexually satisfied without experiencing all of the liner phases of the sexual response cycle, should she be considered as having a sexual disorder?

Most health care providers who work with women and their sexual concerns will tell you that women's sexual experiences are more complex than having an orgasm or the presence or absence of vaginal lubrication. Women's sexual experiences encompass self-esteem, body image, relationship factors, pleasure, satisfaction, and many other variables. Again, women do not fit into a linear model that describes only one type of sexual response, and health care providers and patients need to recognize the variety of ways in which women experience sexual and sensual pleasure.

Classifying a Woman's Experience of Sexuality

This proposed classification system is based on a biopsychosocial understanding of women's sexual experience and does not "medicalize" a woman's sexuality. It includes:

- ♦ a capacity to experience pleasure and satisfaction independent of the occurrence of orgasm,
- ♦ desire for or receptivity to experience sexual pleasure and satisfaction,
- ♦ physical capability of responding to stimulation (vasocongestion) without pain or discomfort, and
- ♦ capability of experiencing orgasm under suitable circumstances.

If these descriptors, or ones similar to them, were viewed as characteristic of normal sexual function, then the persistent absence of or significant changes to any of them would most likely mean a person has a sexual dissatisfaction.

If you do experience any sexual dissatisfaction, please know that help is available to you. I wish each of you a healthy, pleasurable, and satisfying sensual and sexual life.

—BEVERLY WHIPPLE, PhD, RN, FAAN

CHAPTER 18

Sexual Health

This chapter reviews some of the more common female health issues, including vaginal infections, sexually transmitted diseases, uterine fibroids, menstrual disorders, and menopause. Disorders that can occur with pregnancy and infertility are also covered. Urinary tract infections are discussed in chapter 21.

Genital Health

Before we review the diseases that can affect the vagina, it is important to understand what a "healthy" vaginal environment is. The vagina is normally colonized by many different types of bacteria, the most predominant of which is lactobacillus, which produces hydrogen peroxide and helps to keep the vagina slightly acidic and healthy. When there is a shift in vaginal bacteria and one type overcrowds another, infection may result.

Vaginal discharge, a normal product of the cervix and vagina, comprises cervical and vaginal secretions, sloughed-off vaginal epithelial cells, and bacteria. The daily amount of discharge differs from person to person and may be in the 1–5 ml range within a 24-hour period. It ranges from clear to white in color and from thin to thick in consistency. The appearance of vaginal discharge is influenced by several factors, including menstrual cycle phase, ovulation, use and type of contraception, pregnancy, sexual activity, and medications.

Vaginal Infections

This chapter discusses the three most common causes of vaginitis, or inflammation of the vagina: bacterial vaginosis, candida, and trichomoniasis. Symptoms arising from these infections, including abnormal vaginal discharge or odor, itching, irritation, and/or pain with urination, account for a significant number of visits to the gynecologist each year.

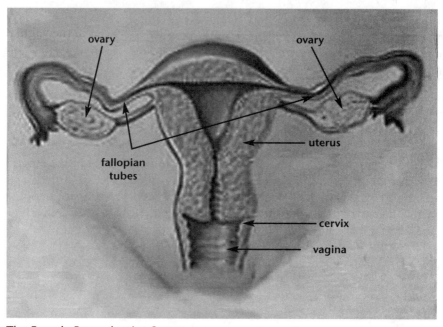

The Female Reproductive System
Source: MedlinePluse, a service of the U.S. National Library of Medicine and the
National Institutes of Health.

WHAT IS BACTERIAL VAGINOSIS?

The most common cause of vaginitis in women of childbearing age is bacterial vaginosis (BV). It occurs when the hydrogen peroxide-producing lactobacilli bacteria are overcrowded by other bacteria present. Symptoms include:

- ◆ "fish-like" vaginal odor, especially during menses or after unprotected vaginal intercourse;
- ◆ thin, gray-white vaginal discharge;
- ◆ pain during vaginal intercourse; and
- ◆ pain on urination (rare).

Diagnosis
The diagnosis of BV is usually made after a gynecological exam and lab tests of the vaginal fluid. BV is easy to recognize under a microscope, where the examiner sees "clue" cells on the slide. A clue cell is simply a vaginal epithelial cell studded with bacteria.

Treatment
BV is treated with antibiotics either taken orally or placed in the vagina. Metronidazole is the most effective antibiotic to treat bacterial vaginosis and is available for either oral or vaginal administration. The course of treatment is usually five to seven days, depending on the form of medication used. Both forms are equally effective.

An alternative to metronidazole is clindamycin. Often used as a first choice in patients allergic to metronidazole, it is not as effective. The vaginal preparation of clindamycin is more effective than the oral form. Approximately 30 percent of women on clindamycin have a recurrence of BV within three months of treatment. If left untreated, bacterial vaginosis can increase the risk of HIV transmission, pelvic inflammatory disease, and preterm delivery. For BV, it is not necessary to treat the sexual partner.

WHAT IS CANDIDIASIS?

Candida—yeast infection—is a fungus commonly found in the vagina. An infection usually occurs when there is an overgrowth of candida. The most common form in the vagina, *Candida albicans*, accounts for 85–90 percent of infections. Typical symptoms include:

♦ itching (most commonly noted on the vulva),
♦ redness of the vulva,
♦ thick, white, clumpy vaginal discharge,
♦ burning on urination,
♦ vaginal irritation, and
♦ pain during intercourse.

Risk Factors
Any woman is at risk for a yeast infection, but antibiotic use, immunosuppression, diabetes, and pregnancy all put a person at higher risk.

Diagnosis
A clinician who suspects a yeast infection based on the person's symptoms performs a pelvic exam to look for vaginal inflammation and white, thick discharge and examines the discharge under the microscope.

Treatment
Treatment administered to relieve symptoms consists of over-the-counter or prescribed regimens:

♦ oral fluconazole (one pill only),
♦ vaginal antifungals (three- to seven-day treatments), or

+ vaginal boric acid (for resistant cases of *Candida albicans* or for treatment of *Candida glabrata*).

If a woman self-treats with an over-the-counter medication and her symptoms do not resolve, she should see her health care provider. It is not necessary to treat the sexual partner.

WHAT IS TRICHOMONIASIS?

Trichomonas vaginalis is a sexually transmitted parasite, affecting two to three million American women annually. Infection in men is often self-limited and transient. Infection in women can be asymptomatic. When symptoms are present, they may include all or some of the following:

+ foul-smelling, thin pearly vaginal discharge,
+ frothy yellow-green vaginal discharge (seen in 10–30 percent affected women),
+ vulvar itching or burning,
+ pain on urination, and
+ redness of the vulva.

Diagnosis
A pelvic exam and swab of the area is normally performed by a physician who then looks at the vaginal discharge under a microscope. The presence of parasites, or trichomonads, seen moving on the slide indicates infection. On speculum exam, the cervix may occasionally have a "strawberry" appearance as a result of small point hemorrhages. When the clinical picture is consistent with trichomoniasis, but the microscopic exam does not find any parasites, a culture of the vagina can be examined. Asymptomatic infections, which can be diagnosed on a liquid-based Pap smear, should also be treated. Rapid DNA tests are also available for quick diagnosis in clinics where microscopes are not available. Women with *Trichomonas vaginalis* should also be tested for other sexually transmitted diseases.

Treatment
The treatment of choice is oral metronidazole in either a single two-gram dose or a seven-day course. It should be given to both the woman and her sexual partner. Sexual intercourse should not be resumed until the infection has cleared in both partners. Oral therapy is preferred over

vaginal therapy because it also treats the urethra and glands surrounding it. If left untreated, trichomoniasis infection can lead to infertility, increased transmission risk of HIV, and premature rupture of membranes in pregnancy.

Sexually Transmitted Diseases

Sexually transmitted diseases (STDs) are diseases transmitted through sexual contact. Today, STDs in women are one of the most troubling public health issues worldwide. STDs frequently affect men and women differently, and novel research in disease prevention and treatment specifically targeting women is currently underway. If left untreated, certain STDs can cause infertility, pregnancy complications, cervical cancer, and pelvic inflammatory disease.

When a sexually transmitted disease is diagnosed in either women or men, the following measures should be taken:

- testing for other STDs, including HIV;
- treatment of sexual partners (depending on the STD);
- use of barrier forms of contraception, such as condoms; and
- vaccination for hepatitis B, if not already done.

WHAT IS CHLAMYDIA TRACHOMATIS?

Chlamydia is one of the most commonly transmitted STDs in the United States, because the infection frequently does not cause any symptoms in women or men. Chlamydia can cause cervicitis, or inflammation of the cervix. In 50 percent of cases, symptoms may not be present. When women do experience them, they may include mucopurulent discharge from the cervix or lower abdominal pain.

Chlamydia can also lead to urethritis, inflammation of the lining of the urethra causing pain on urination, and Fitzhugh-Curtis syndrome, an inflammation of the liver capsule causing right-side upper abdominal pain. If left untreated, approximately 30 percent of Chlamydia infections progress to pelvic inflammatory disease (PID).

Prevention and Screening
The U.S. Preventive Services Task Force and the Centers for Disease Control and Prevention (CDC) recommend annual screening for sexually active women age 25 or younger and sexually active women over age 25 with risk factors.

Diagnosis

Traditionally, a diagnosis of *Chlamydia trachomatis* has required a pelvic exam with a speculum and a cervical swab. Newer, home tests for men and women can identify characteristic nucleic acids, substances present in all human cells, from either a male or female's urine specimen or from a self-administered vaginal swab.

Treatment

Treatment for Chlamydia is oral antibiotics. The most common regimens are azithromycin taken once orally or doxycycline taken orally for seven days. Erythromycin and the floroquinolone drugs are alternative therapy options. Sexual partners should also be treated.

WHAT IS NEISSERIA GONORRHOEAE?

Neisseria gonorrhoeae can affect any part of the genital tract, anorectal region, and throat and may spread to other parts of the body as well. Gonorrhea affects women and men differently. Often, women do not experience any symptoms, while men have them roughly 90 percent of the time.

The most common site of infection in women is the cervix. Symptoms associated with cervical infection, present 50 percent of time, include mucopurulent vaginal discharge and vaginal itching.

Gonorrhea can also affect the:

- urethra—infection of the urethra may cause pain with urination;
- anorectal region—only 3 percent of anorectal infections include such symptoms as anal itching, rectal discharge, rectal fullness, and pain on defecation; and
- throat—this infection rarely has any symptoms; those with symptoms have a sore throat and painful lymph nodes in the neck.

When left untreated, gonorrhea may lead to pelvic inflammatory disease (PID) or disseminated disease. PID occurs 10–40 percent of the time in untreated cervical disease, and disseminated gonorrhea occurs in 1–3 percent of patients. The latter is associated with arthralgia (severe pain in a joint) and infectious arthritis.

Diagnosis

Diagnosis of cervical gonorrhea is made by culture, which is considered to be the gold-standard test, and results are available within 48 hours. Other methods of diagnosis include:

♦ nucleic acid amplification test, with results available in hours, although it is more expensive, and
♦ DNA probe, which offers increased sample stability.

Treatment
Treatment of gonorrhea for men and women is the same. When a cervical, urethral, anorectal, or oral infection is confirmed, a single-dose regimen of antibiotics is administered. When treating gonorrhea, it is standard practice to also give antibiotics for the empiric treatment of Chlamydia. A study done between 1993 and 1995 found *Chlamydia trachomatis* co-infection in 42 percent of women with confirmed gonorrhea.

WHAT IS PELVIC INFLAMMATORY DISEASE?

One of the most serious complications of STDs in women is pelvic inflammatory disease (PID), an infection of the upper genital tract. It can affect the uterus, fallopian tubes, ovaries, or the capsule around the liver and is a common cause of hospitalization in reproductive age women. Recent research points out that recurrent PID increases a women's risk of developing chronic pelvic pain.

Symptoms
Symptoms may include one or more of the following:

♦ lower abdominal pain,
♦ pain with intercourse,
♦ abnormal vaginal discharge,
♦ fever, chills, and
♦ abnormal vaginal bleeding.

Risk Factors
Risk factors include:

♦ multiple sexual partners,
♦ nonbarrier contraception,
♦ being under 35 years old,
♦ history of STDs, and
♦ tobacco use.

Most cases of PID are caused by *Chlamydia trachomatis* or *Neisseria gonorrhoeae*. Other bacteria frequently involved in PID include anaerobes, mycoplasma, group B streptococcus, and *Gardnerella vaginalis*.

Diagnosis and Treatment
PID is not an easy diagnosis to make as the symptoms can mimic other ailments. In addition to a pelvic exam, the doctor may need to perform a sonogram, blood tests, or surgery to eliminate other possibilities. Once the diagnosis has been made, antibiotic therapy is initiated, usually done on an outpatient basis. Hospitalization may be required when the patient:

- is unable to keep down fluids and/or oral antibiotics;
- has a high fever;
- fails to comply with outpatient regimen;
- complies with the regimen, but it still fails;
- has an uncertain diagnosis; or
- has a pelvic abscess.

WHAT IS HUMAN PAPILLOMAVIRUS?

The human papillomavirus (HPV), also known as genital warts, has more than 100 strains, some of which are harmless; others are transmitted through sexual contact. Genital warts are most often caused by subtypes six or 11 of HPV. (Other high-risk HPV subtypes are associated with cervical cancer; see chapter 8). They typically present as multiple lesions on the external genitalia, including the vulva, penis, perineum, perianal skin, or scrotum. Occasionally, there may only be a solitary lesion present. They can also occur internally on the mucous membranes of the vagina, anus, urethra, cervix, or mouth. The appearance of genital warts ranges from flesh-colored, cauliflower-like lesions to red or brown dome-shaped, smooth lesions.

Symptoms
Most patients do not experience any symptoms. Occasionally, men or women with external genital warts may experience itching. When internal warts are present, they typically do not cause symptoms unless they are large. Symptoms of internal warts in women include vaginal pain, vaginal bleeding, and pain with intercourse.

Diagnosis
Diagnosis is usually made based on the appearance of the lesions. A biopsy may be performed if there is a question regarding the diagnosis, or if there is a poor response to therapy.

Treatment
Treatment of genital warts is based on the location, number, and size of the lesions. Treatment response rate for genital warts in men and women

ranges from 40 to 90 percent, depending on the type of therapy used. Treatment options for women include:

+ cryotherapy with liquid nitrogen,
+ imiquimod topical therapy,
+ interferon,
+ trichloroacetic acid,
+ podophyllin,
+ podofilox,
+ surgical removal, and
+ laser therapy.

If there is no response to medical therapy after three cycles, the diagnosis should be confirmed with biopsy and the treatment changed.

Prevention
Genital warts can be prevented by limiting the number of lifetime sexual partners, avoiding direct contact with sexual partners who are infected, and using condoms. Using condoms, however, does not always prevent transmission of the virus.

What Is Human Immunodeficiency Virus?

Human immunodeficiency virus (HIV) is a virus that progressively weakens the body's immune system. Acquired immunodeficiency syndrome (AIDS) is the most serious manifestation of HIV. Transmission of HIV infection occurs through sexual contact, infected blood or tissue exposure, from infected mother to infant during delivery and breastfeeding, blood transfusion, or organ transplantation.

Why Your Sex Matters
According to the CDC, the estimated number of AIDS cases in women increased by 15 percent between 1999 and 2003. In the United States, African American and Latino women are the most affected: HIV/AIDS is the fourth leading cause of death for women age 35–44 and the sixth leading cause of death for women age 25–34 in the United States.

Women are more susceptible to HIV; infected male-to-female transmission occurs more frequently than infected female-to-male transmission. Women with STDs other than HIV may be more likely to become infected. This occurs through lesions on the vulvovaginal/cervical mucosa or from the increased presence of white blood cells that occurs with certain sexually transmitted infections.

Diagnosis
Diagnosis of HIV is made by a blood test that identifies antibodies to the virus. If the initial screening test is positive, a confirmatory Western blot test is performed. These results typically take 24 hours. A rapid HIV test has been approved in the United States, results of which are available within 20 minutes.

Prevention and Treatment
Sexual abstinence is the most effective way to prevent HIV transmission. The second most effective preventive technique is consistent use of condoms. Diagnosis and treatment of STDs will aid in preventing HIV transmission. For the past 10 years, HIV/AIDS therapy has centered on antiviral drugs that attack HIV's ability to reproduce. These therapies are very effective for many patients, allowing them to live many years with the virus. While it was initially thought that these drugs could cure the disease, it has been discovered that the virus survives this therapy. Additionally, the drugs often have serious side effects and strict adherence requirements and can be very costly.

The Future
Unfortunately, the microbicide nonoxynol-9 has not proven effective in preventing HIV transmission in women and may potentially increase the risk of transmission. Nonoxynol-9 is considered a nonspecific microbicide and may actually break down vaginal and cervical epithelial cells, leading to erosions in the tissue and easier transmission of the virus. Researchers are looking for newer medications with fewer side effects and are developing drugs to reduce the adverse effects of current therapies. Additionally, research is progressing on new approaches to HIV/AIDS treatment. Currently, several microbicides are under investigation that could potentially target the HIV virus while not affecting the vaginal or cervical cells. Research is also underway on development of an HIV vaccine.

What Is Genital Herpes?

The herpes simplex viruses (HSVs) 1 and 2 are responsible for genital herpes, with the majority caused by type 2. The disease can be transmitted by viral shedding during the period when the virus is reproducing and can be easily passed to other people by skin-to-skin contact. This can occur even when there is no evidence of infection. Both men and women with genital herpes may transmit the virus during this time.

Symptoms

HSV can occur without symptoms. When they do occur, they can range from mild to severe. Classic symptoms of genital HSV include:

♦ painful genital ulcers;
♦ pain on urination;
♦ fever, headache, malaise; and
♦ tender, enlarged lymph nodes in the groin.

Many women may only experience genital abrasions, fissures, or itching without obvious ulcers. The first episode tends to more severe than recurrent episodes.

Diagnosis

Diagnosis is traditionally made by viral culture of the genital lesions. There are also type-specific blood tests that can distinguish between HSV type 1 and type 2.

Treatment

At this time, there is no cure for genital herpes. Therapy to suppress the virus is available and has proven to be quite effective in reducing the duration of symptoms and viral shedding. Oral antiviral therapy should be taken during the first episode. Topical antiviral medications are not effective, and their use is discouraged in genital herpes. Recurrent infection is more common in HSV type 2 than type 1. In a study published in 2004, daily suppressive therapy with valacyclovir was noted to prevent many genital HSV type 2 recurrences, reduce asymptomatic viral shedding, and decrease transmission to unaffected partners. Use of condoms decreases but does not completely eliminate the risk of genital HSV.

Informing a partner about genital herpes can be very difficult, but it should be done before initiating sexual activity.

Uterine Fibroids

Uterine fibroids (leiomyomas) are common tumors of the uterus made up of muscle and fibrous tissue. They are benign (noncancerous). Possibly as many as 80 percent of all women have uterine fibroids. While most of them have no symptoms, one in four ends up with symptoms severe enough to require treatment.

Symptoms

In some women, uterine fibroids may cause heavy vaginal bleeding, pelvic discomfort, and pain and put pressure on other organs. The heavy bleeding can cause anemia, and the pressure can result in constipation and hemorrhoids.

Risk Factors

There is no known cause for uterine fibroids and no known reasons why some women have severe symptoms from their fibroids while others do not. We do know that age, race, lifestyle, and genetics all likely play a part in the body's tendency to develop symptomatic uterine fibroids. The average age at which symptoms of fibroids develop is 35–50. African American women are two to three times more likely to present with symptomatic uterine fibroids and typically do so at a younger age than the rest of the population of women with uterine fibroids. Asian women have a lower incidence of symptomatic uterine fibroids. Obesity is associated with the presence of uterine fibroids.

Also, changes in a woman's hormone levels may affect fibroid growth: fibroids typically grow rapidly during pregnancy, when hormone levels are elevated, and shrink after menopause, when hormone levels are decreased.

Diagnosis

Abnormal vaginal bleeding and pelvic pain are symptoms of other conditions as well as uterine fibroids. Diagnosis can be made only after a thorough history and physical examination, which may include transvaginal ultrasound, magnetic resolution imaging (MRI), and endometrial biopsy. The exam may also include a hysteroscopy, which uses a slender rod to help the doctor see inside the uterus. During this exam the doctor can destroy endometrial lining by ablation—either cauterizing or lasering the tissue. Cryoablation involves freezing.

Treatment

The first step in treatment is often to alleviate the symptoms. Bleeding due to fibroids can be treated with hormones or surgery. Eating more whole grains, bran, and fruit and drinking lots of water may help alleviate the constipation. If treating the symptoms of uterine fibroids is ineffective, there are a variety of treatment options, including:

- ◆ Myomectomy—surgical removal of the fibroid; surgery can be performed through the navel and abdomen with the use of a laparoscope (a thin tube-like instrument with a light), through the vagina with a hysteroscope (a thin telescope-like instrument), or through an abdominal incision.

♦ Uterine artery embolization (UAE)—a minimally invasive, nonsurgical procedure performed by an interventional radiologist that involves placing a catheter into the artery and guiding it to the uterus. Small particles are then injected into the artery that block the blood supply feeding the fibroids, which then begin dying.

♦ Myolysis—appropriate for only a certain size of fibroids, this is performed by laparoscopic insertion of an instrument that sends a high-frequency electrical current to the fibroid, cutting off the blood flow. A similar procedure to myolysis is cryomyolysis, which uses liquid nitrogen at minus 180 degrees to freeze the fibroids.

♦ Magnetic resonance imaging (MRI) guided ultrasound therapy can be used to shrink the fibroid tumors.

Another option is hysterectomy. There are three types of hysterectomies:

♦ Subtotal hysterectomy involves only removal of the uterus.

♦ Total hysterectomy involves removing both the body of the uterus and the cervix (the lower part of the uterus). It can sometimes be done through the vagina (vaginal hysterectomy); at other times, a surgical incision in the abdomen is preferable. In a total hysterectomy and bilateral (both sides) salpingo-oophorectomy, the ovaries and fallopian tubes are removed along with the uterus and cervix.

♦ Radical hysterectomy is reserved for serious disease such as cancer. The entire uterus and usually both tubes and ovaries, as well as the pelvic lymph nodes, are removed through the abdomen.

Menstrual Disorders

WHAT IS PREMENSTRUAL SYNDROME/ PREMENSTRUAL DYSPHORIC DISORDER?

Premenstrual syndrome (PMS), a combination of physical and behavioral symptoms that interfere with daily functioning, usually occurs during the second half of the menstrual cycle. Symptoms typically resolve within four days from the onset of menses. The more commonly experienced symptoms are:

♦ abdominal bloating,
♦ fatigue,

- irritability/anxiety,
- acne,
- increased appetite,
- breast tenderness, and
- mood changes.

For a diagnosis to be made, these symptoms must occur during at least two consecutive cycles.

Treatment

Treatment of PMS includes both nonpharmacologic and pharmacologic therapies. For mild cases, behavioral changes, patient education and support, dietary changes, and exercise should be attempted. If there is no improvement, medications can be prescribed to address specific symptom(s).

PMDD

Premenstrual dysphoric disorder (PMDD), considered to be a severe form of PMS, is often a chronic medical condition that requires attention and treatment. Selective serotonin reuptake inhibitors (SSRIs) are generally the first-line therapy. There are strict diagnostic criteria for PMDD, and women must meet five of the 11 defined criteria during the second half of their menstrual cycle for at least two consecutive cycles. The symptoms must not be an exacerbation of a preexisting disorder, such as depression or psychosis. These criteria are:

- feeling of sadness or hopelessness, possible suicidal thoughts;
- feelings of tension or anxiety;
- mood swings marked by periods of teariness;
- persistent irritability or anger that affects other people;
- disinterest in daily activities and relationships;
- trouble concentrating;
- fatigue or low energy;
- food cravings or binge eating;
- sleep disturbances;
- feeling out of control; and
- physical symptoms, such as bloating, breast tenderness, headaches, and joint or muscle pain.

WHAT IS POLYCYSTIC OVARIAN SYNDROME?

Polycystic ovarian syndrome (PCOS) is a disorder in which the ovaries produce excessive amounts of male hormones (androgens) and develop multiple small cysts. The criteria necessary to make a diagnosis of PCOS have been a topic of heated debate for many years. In 2003, a group of European and American researchers and physicians revised the diagnostic criteria, which now state that women have two of the following:

♦ clinical or biochemical evidence of hyperandrogenism,
♦ menstrual irregularity due to oligo- or anovulatory cycles, and
♦ polycystic appearing ovaries on ultrasound.

Clinically, PCOS manifests as:

♦ fewer menstrual periods or none at all (oligo- or amenorrhea),
♦ hirsutism (excess body hair following a male pattern),
♦ male pattern balding,
♦ acne,
♦ infertility,
♦ insulin resistance, and
♦ obesity.

Diagnosis
Hirsutism, male pattern balding, and acne are clinical signs of hyperandrogenism; however, other causes must be ruled out before making a diagnosis of PCOS. The menstrual irregularities of PCOS usually begin following puberty. Women with PCOS should be screened for impaired glucose tolerance and type 2 diabetes because of the association with insulin resistance.

Treatment
Treatment of PCOS depends on the symptoms. Hirsutism is generally treated with laser hair removal, electrolysis, waxing, depilatories, or shaving. Oral contraceptives can be used to decrease acne and slow hair growth and can also prevent endometrial hyperplasia in those women without menstrual periods. Treatment for type 2 diabetes in PCOS patients is the same as treatment in patients without the condition.

WHAT IS DYSMENORRHEA?

Dysmenorrhea, or menstrual pain, affects approximately 50 percent of premenopausal women. There are two types of dysmenorrhea: primary (without pelvic disease) and secondary, when menstrual pain is accompanied with pelvic disease.

Primary dysmenorrhea is the most common gynecologic complaint among adolescent females. It is related to prostaglandin, a hormone-like substance released in the uterus and resulting in increased uterine tone and contractions. It usually begins one to two years after the onset of menstruation, when ovulatory cycles begin. The pain can have a significant impact on daily activities and is frequently the cause of many missed school days. Symptoms include recurrent crampy, lower abdominal pain. Primary dysmenorrhea may be associated with nausea, vomiting, diarrhea, and headache. It typically begins several hours before the onset of menstrual bleeding and may last up to three days. After ruling out any underlying pelvic disorders, diagnosis is made by a pelvic exam and by confirming the cyclic nature of the pain.

Treating Primary Dysmenorrhea

Nonsteroidal anti-inflammatory drugs (for example, ibuprofen or naproxen) are the most effective treatment in 80 percent of primary dysmenorrhea cases. They are typically taken at the onset of pain and continued every six to eight hours while the pain lasts. In those cases where NSAIDs do not provide relief or there is a contraindication to taking the medication, combined oral contraceptive pills may be used. These pills may be considered as first choice in those women who desire contraception in addition to relief of dysmenorrhea.

Treating Secondary Dysmenorrhea

Secondary dysmenorrhea may be caused by endometriosis, uterine fibroids, abnormalities of the uterus, or adenomyosis, among other conditions. Symptoms usually start years after the onset of menstruation. The pain may begin up to two weeks before menses, and diagnosis typically is made during a pelvic exam, ultrasound, or laparoscopy. Treatment depends on the type of disease.

WHAT IS ADENOMYOSIS?

Adenomyosis occurs when glands and the supporting connective tissue from the endometrial lining of the uterus grow into the muscle layer of the uterus (called the myometrium). It may cause pelvic pain one week before menses that can last throughout menstrual bleeding. Other symptoms associated with adenomyosis are heavy or prolonged menstrual blood flow and diffusely enlarged uterus. One-third of the women affected have no symptoms. Although adenomyosis may be present for years, symptoms tend to begin after age 40.

Diagnosis

Clinical diagnosis is often made when a woman has a diffusely enlarged uterus, pain during menses, and heavy menstrual bleeding in the absence of fibroids or endometriosis. However, a confirmatory diagnosis can be made only after a hysterectomy by examining the uterine tissue under the microscope. MRI is the most accurate imaging study for diagnosing adenomyosis.

Treatment
Treatment of adenomyosis depends on many factors, including age, future fertility, and desire for medical versus surgical therapy. The definitive treatment of adenomyosis is hysterectomy, surgical removal of the uterus. Other options include:

♦ endometrial ablation,
♦ hormonal therapy, and
♦ nonsteroidal anti-inflammatory drugs.

WHAT IS ENDOMETRIOSIS?

About five million American women and female adolescents have endometriosis, a sometimes painful and disabling condition in which tissue that lines the uterus is found outside the uterus, most commonly in the pelvis. As many as 30 percent of women who report infertility problems have endometriosis.

Risk Factors
The exact cause of endometriosis is unclear; however, there are several theories, including:

♦ reverse flow of menstrual blood and tissue through the fallopian tubes into the pelvis;
♦ inability of the body's immune system to destroy endometrial tissue outside the uterus;
♦ transport of endometrial tissue outside the uterus by blood and lymphatic vessels; and
♦ with stimulation, certain cells in the abdominal cavity develop into endometrial cells.

There is a genetic component to endometriosis with an occurrence rate of 7 percent in first-degree relatives.

Recent research indicates that women who have endometriosis are more likely than other women to have diseases such as chronic fatigue syndrome and fibromyalgia, as well as other painful conditions, such as irritable bowel disorder, interstitial cystitis, vulvodynia, temporomandibular disorder, and migraine headaches.

Symptoms

Endometriosis is not always symptomatic. When symptoms are present, they vary from patient to patient and do not necessarily correspond to the amount of endometriosis present. Clinical signs include:

♦ chronic pelvic pain,
♦ severe menstrual cramps (dysmenorrhea),
♦ pain during sexual intercourse (dyspareunia),
♦ infertility, and
♦ ovarian mass.

If the endometrial tissue affects the bladder or intestines, there can be painful urination or bowel movements and, sometimes, blood in the urine or stool.

Diagnosis

Diagnosis is made by direct visualization during surgery, preferably by laparoscopy. At the time of surgical evaluation, any endometriosis implants should be removed.

Treatment

Treatment depends on the ultimate goal of therapy: relief of pain, fertility, or removal of ovarian mass. Treatment options include:

♦ hormonal therapy,
♦ pain medication,
♦ laser ablation, and
♦ surgery.

What Is Menopause?

Menopause is defined as the permanent end of menses, when a woman has had no menstrual period for 12 months. The average age of menopause in the United States is 51. Before menopause, women may experience irregular menstrual cycles for up to five years; this period is known as perimenopause and is defined by both ovulatory and anovulatory (ovulation fails to occur) cycles. If menopause occurs before age 40, it is called premature ovarian failure.

Throughout the perimenopausal phase, the follicle stimulating hormone (FSH) becomes slightly elevated while the luteinizing hormone (LH) generally stays within the normal range. Following menopause, there is a significant increase in both FSH and LH due to the rapid depletion of ovarian follicles. Although testosterone production continues in the ovaries after menopause, the serum level is less than the pre-menopausal level.

SYMPTOMS

Symptoms of perimenopause include:

◆ hot flashes,
◆ night sweats,
◆ mood disturbances,
◆ vaginal dryness, and
◆ reduced skin elasticity.

TREATMENT

The Women's Health Initiative (WHI) study was an important landmark, causing many clinicians to reevaluate hormone therapy (HT). This comprehensive study of oral estrogen-progesterone hormone therapy showed a small increased risk of breast cancer, blood clotting disease, stroke, and coronary artery disease. A second arm, following women on oral conjugated equine estrogens alone, found increased risk of blood clotting and stroke, but no increased risk of breast cancer or coronary artery disease. Women receiving estrogen-progesterone and those receiving only estrogen had an elevated risk of urinary incontinence. Most significant, the data confirmed that hormone therapy should not be used long term to prevent cardiovascular disease.

On the plus side, the studies showed that hormone therapy can lower a woman's risk for osteoporosis and colon cancer. The studies were not designed to measure the quality-of-life benefits from taking hormones during the transition to menopause, such as fewer hot flashes, night sweats, and mood swings and less vaginal dryness.

Since the initial halt of WHI, academicians and health care professionals have taken a closer look at the data to determine how they relate to women undergoing the menopausal transition. WHI did not study women going through menopause; rather it looked at women who were postmenopausal by at least a decade on average.

Many have come to believe that beginning hormone therapy around the time of menopause seems to be far different in terms of cardiovascular risk than beginning many years later. New studies are underway to determine the risks and benefits of hormone therapy in the population of current users. The first of these, issued in June 2005, stated that peri- and postmenopausal women who have moderate to severe vasomotor symptoms associated with estrogen deficiency may benefit from HT.

The decision to take HT requires a thorough discussion between a woman and her health care provider. Both the risks and benefits of therapy should be reviewed as well as the woman's personal and family medical history. If HT is initiated, it should be started at the lowest dose and used for the shortest amount of time necessary to treat the vasomotor and other symptoms of menopause. But the lowest dose and the time a woman spends on hormone therapy are not the same for every woman. Treatment should be customized to individual needs.

The following are alternatives to systemic HT for treatment of:

Vasomotor symptoms of menopause, including hot flashes and night sweats:
  ♦ clonidine (usually used to treat high blood pressure),
  ♦ selective serotonin reuptake inhibitors (SSRIs),
  ♦ phytoestrogens, and
  ♦ acupuncture

Vaginal atrophy:
  ♦ vaginal lubricants and moisturizers, and
  ♦ vaginal estrogen,

Prevention of osteoporosis:
  ♦ calcium and vitamin D,
  ♦ weight-bearing exercises,
  ♦ selective estrogen receptor modulators, and
  ♦ bisphosphonates.

Disorders of Pregnancy

What Is Miscarriage?

Miscarriage, or spontaneous abortion, is defined as a loss of a pregnancy before 20 weeks' gestation. Approximately 15–20 percent of known pregnancies end in miscarriage. The majority of cases are isolated and do not recur; the recurrence rate is 20 percent in subsequent pregnancies. The most common cause of miscarriage is fetal chromosomal abnormalities, which account for 50 percent of all miscarriages.

There are six types of miscarriages:

  ♦ threatened—vaginal bleeding with or without pain, cervix is closed, loss of pregnancy does not always occur;

- inevitable—vaginal bleeding, abdominal pain, cervix is dilated, loss of pregnancy is imminent;
- incomplete—partial expulsion of pregnancy tissue: vaginal bleeding, abdominal pain, cervix is dilated;
- complete—expulsion of all fetal and placental tissue;
- septic—vaginal bleeding, abdominal pain, fever, chills, dilated cervix, pus-like vaginal discharge; and
- missed—in utero demise of the fetus without expulsion.

Recurrent pregnancy loss is defined as three or more spontaneous abortions before 20 weeks of pregnancy.

Symptoms
Symptoms of miscarriage include vaginal bleeding and lower abdominal pain.

Treatment
Treatment for spontaneous abortions depends on the clinical scenario as well as patient preference. Traditionally, inevitable, missed, and incomplete abortions have been treated with a dilation and curettage (D&C). Waiting for these types of abortions to pass on their own is also common if the patient is healthy and clinically stable. However, if surgery and expectant management are not desired, and the patient is stable from a clinical standpoint, medical therapy can be administered. This is usually done by placing misoprostol—a prostaglandin drug that causes cramping and the expulsion of the pregnancy—in the vagina. Some women do require D&C following medical therapy.

WHAT IS COMPLETE MOLAR PREGNANCY?

Complete molar pregnancy, which occurs in one in 1,000 pregnancies in the United States, arises from an abnormality of fertilization. There is no fetus in a complete molar pregnancy.

Symptoms
Clinical signs of complete molar pregnancy include:

- vaginal bleeding,
- multiple ovarian cysts (theca lutein cysts),
- hyperthyroidism,
- uterine size greater than gestational age,
- pre-eclampsia before 20 weeks,

- hyperemesis gravidarum (extreme nausea and vomiting of pregnancy),
- passage of tissue from the vagina that has a grape-cluster or vesicle-like appearance, and
- abnormally elevated levels of a hormone normally produced during pregnancy (human chorionic gonadotropin [HCG]).

Risk Factors
Risk factors include maternal age under 20 or greater than 35, a history of molar pregnancy, and never having given birth (nulliparity).

Diagnosis and Treatment
Evaluation includes an ultrasound exam that shows no fetal or embryonic tissue, no amniotic fluid, and a uterine mass that has a "snowstorm" pattern appearance. Since molar pregnancies are associated with a high level of HCG, the doctor also performs a blood test.

When the doctor diagnoses molar pregnancy, she or he performs a suction D&C. If a woman is finished with childbearing and desires permanent sterilization, the doctor can perform a hysterectomy instead. The rationale behind hysterectomy is that approximately 20 percent of women with complete moles can develop persistent gestational trophoblastic disease, requiring chemotherapy. Gestational trophoblastic tumor is a rare cancer in women in which malignant cells grow in the tissues that are formed following conception. This disease, which is not always easy to find, can be detected during an internal (pelvic) examination, an ultrasound, or a blood test looking for high levels of a hormone, called beta HCG (beta human chorionic gonadotropin), that is present during normal pregnancy. If a woman is not pregnant and HCG is in the blood, it can be a sign of gestational trophoblastic tumor. Following treatment, serum beta-HCG is closely monitored to ensure that it returns to the prepregnancy level.

What Is Ectopic Pregnancy?

An ectopic pregnancy occurs when an embryo or fertilized egg implants in a site other than the uterine cavity. Implantation occurs within the fallopian tubes in 98 percent of ectopic pregnancies; other locations include the cervix, abdominal cavity, and ovary. In general, these pregnancies do not survive, but they can pose significant risk to the woman. Ectopic pregnancies can cause rupture of the organ in which they are implanted, which can lead to internal bleeding, shock, and—potentially—death if not treated quickly. With early detection of an ectopic pregnancy, treatment can be carried out before these complications occur, However, 50 percent of women have no symptoms other than those typically present in an early pregnancy.

Symptoms
When symptoms are present, they include abdominal pain and vaginal bleeding. Symptoms of rupture of the fallopian tube include severe abdominal pain, dizziness, and loss of consciousness.

Risk Factors
Risk factors for ectopic pregnancy include:

♦ prior ectopic pregnancy,
♦ prior pelvic inflammatory disease (PID),
♦ cigarette smoking,
♦ prior surgery of the fallopian tubes,
♦ diethylstilbestrol (DES) exposure, and
♦ increasing maternal age.

Diagnosis and Treatment
Diagnosis begins with a transvaginal ultrasound and measure of HCG. Treatment can be either medical or surgical. Medical treatment is an injection of methotrexate, a folic acid analogue, if:

♦ no intrauterine gestational sac or fluid collection is seen on the transvaginal ultrasound,
♦ the unruptured mass is less than or equal to 3.5 cm, and
♦ there are no contraindications to taking methotrexate.

Women are advised to discontinue folic acid supplements for one week after methotrexate treatment and to avoid foods rich in folate for two weeks after methotrexate administration. Additionally, alcohol can interact with methotrexate and cause liver damage, so it should be avoided during treatment. As with other conditions in which excessive bleeding is a concern, aspirin should be avoided as well.

WHAT IS GESTATIONAL DIABETES?

Gestational diabetes, commonly referred to as diabetes of pregnancy, is defined as an intolerance to carbohydrates that begins or is first detected during pregnancy. Approximately 2.5 percent of pregnancies are complicated by gestational diabetes. When left untreated, gestational diabetes can lead to:

- heavier than normal infant,
- Cesarean section,
- excessive amniotic fluid,
- neonatal hypoglycemia,
- perinatal death, and
- pre-eclampsia.

Diagnosis
Gestational diabetes is diagnosed by a screening test between the 24th and 28th weeks of pregnancy. During the test, pregnant women drink a 50 gram dose of glucose and have their blood drawn one hour later. A serum glucose result of 140 mg/dL or higher on the screening test is considered abnormal. Women who display an abnormal value have their fasting glucose drawn and then drink a 100 gram dose of glucose. Their blood is then drawn each hour for the next three hours. If there are two or more abnormal values, women are diagnosed with gestational diabetes. Screening can be performed earlier in the pregnancy if women will be age 35 or older at the time of delivery or if they have risk factors for diabetes, such as prepregnancy overweight, parent or sibling with diabetes, previous large baby, or previous perinatal loss. Treatment of gestational diabetes can be achieved with either diet or insulin.

WHAT IS PRE-ECLAMPSIA?

Pre-eclampsia, often called toxemia, is defined as the onset of high blood pressure and increased protein in the urine after the 20th week of pregnancy in women who previously had normal blood pressures. It occurs in approximately 5 percent of pregnancies. Pre-eclampsia ranges from mild to severe. If left untreated, eclampsia—defined as a new onset seizure in a woman with pre-eclampsia—occurs in less than 1 percent of cases.

Symptoms
Symptoms of pre-eclampsia include

- headache,
- visual changes,
- body swelling, and
- upper abdominal pain.

Risk Factors
Risk factors of pre-eclampsia are:

- pre-eclampsia in a previous pregnancy;
- maternal age younger than 20 or older than 35;
- family history of pre-eclampsia;
- multiple gestation; and
- history of high blood pressure, kidney disease, or diabetes.

Diagnosis and Treatment
Pre-eclampsia is diagnosed by systolic blood pressures greater than or equal to 140mmHg or diastolic blood pressures greater than or equal to 90mmHg, along with 0.3 grams of protein in a 24-hour urine collection specimen. The definitive treatment for pre-eclampsia is delivery. Expectant management with observation can be carried out only when the patient is remote from delivery and medically stable.

What Is Infertility?

Infertility is defined as inability to conceive after one year of unprotected intercourse. It affects 15 percent of couples trying to conceive. More than six million couples in the United States are affected by infertility, yet fewer than half seek infertility evaluation and treatment, despite the fact that modern treatments can help the majority of them.

RISK FACTORS

Every couple is at risk for infertility. In general, women who suffer from infertility are very healthy in every other way. One common risk factor for infertility is age; as women age, their incidence of infertility increases. A woman's fertility peaks in her late teens and early 20s and declines yearly between 30 and 43. Two-thirds of women over age 40 have trouble conceiving on their own. In addition to difficulty conceiving, the miscarriage rate goes up significantly when a woman is older than 35.

Other risk factors include:

- irregular menstrual cycles,
- history of pelvic inflammatory disease (PID) or Chlamydia,
- history of cancer treatment in either partner,

◆ smoking by either partner,
◆ pelvic surgery, and
◆ endometriosis.

CAUSES OF INFERTILITY

A couple's infertility can be caused by many things or be unexplained. Known causes include:

◆ anovulation (a menstrual cycle in which ovulation fails to occur);
◆ tubal obstruction;
◆ decreased sperm counts;
◆ ovarian failure;
◆ endometriosis;
◆ hormonal imbalance, such as hyperprolactinemia or thyroid dysfunction; and
◆ genetic factors, such as chromosomal rearrangements or deletions in the Y chromosome.

OPTIMIZING FERTILITY

Knowing their most fertile time can be a challenge for some women. Those with regular cycles ovulate approximately 14 days before their next expected menstrual period. Over-the-counter urine test strips are available to detect the lutenizing hormone surge that occurs one day before ovulation. It is best to try a couple of days before and the day of ovulation. Intercourse every other day is as effective as daily intercourse for most couples.
   Other things couples can do to improve fertility are:

◆ avoiding or quitting smoking;
◆ maintaining a healthy body weight;
◆ avoiding the use of vaginal lubricants;
◆ avoiding the use of medications that could impair fertility, such as nonsteroidal anti-inflammatory agents (ibuprofen or naproxen) in women and calcium channel blockers in men; and
◆ having regular intercourse around the time of ovulation.

WHEN TO SEE A FERTILITY SPECIALIST

Ideally, all women should speak with their physician before becoming pregnant. Preconception counseling is most important for women with medical conditions that might be affected by pregnancy. Infertility evaluation should be considered after a year of unprotected intercourse, or after six months if the woman is older than 35. Couples with the known risk factors mentioned above may need evaluation even before six months.

—LEAH S. MILLHEISER, MD; RUTH B. LATHI, MD;
LINDA C. GIUDICE, MD, PhD

CHAPTER 19

Sleep Disorders

S leep is a basic human need, as important for good health as diet and exercise. Sleep lays the groundwork for a productive day ahead. Although most adults need seven to nine hours of sleep each night to function well the next day, on average, women get 6.9 hours a night during the week, and only 30 percent get eight hours or more, according to the 2005 National Sleep Foundation (NSF) *Sleep in America* poll. Women also report that they are more likely than men to have difficulty falling and staying asleep and to experience daytime sleepiness at least a few nights or days a week. Daytime sleepiness that interferes with daily activities is not normal and may be a major sign of sleep deprivation, a sleep disorder, or an underlying medical condition.

Both quantity and quality of sleep are essential to optimum functioning. Although continuous sleep is ideal, it is not uncommon to experience disruptions from a variety of underlying causes. For example, more women than men suffer from nighttime pain. In one study, one in four women reported that pain or physical discomfort interrupted her sleep three nights a week or more. Women are twice as likely to experience depression as men, and they are more prone to arthritis and headaches, all conditions that can result in fragmented sleep. Research has shown that too little and poor-quality sleep results in not only daytime sleepiness, but also more accidents, problems concentrating, poor performance on the job, difficulty getting along with others, and, possibly, more illness and weight gain.

Why Your Sex Matters

Biological conditions unique to women can affect how well they sleep; the changing levels of hormones women experience throughout the month and over their lifetimes have an impact on sleep. Based on a study of nearly 40,000 people in Taiwan, better-educated women are more likely to report having a good night's sleep with fewer disruptions.

Your Monthly Cycle and Sleep

On average, women report disrupted sleep for two to three days each menstrual cycle. These changes can be linked to the rise and fall of hormone levels in the body. The hormone, progesterone, which rises after ovulation, may cause some women to feel sleepy or fatigued. However, poor-quality sleep is more likely at the beginning of the menstrual cycle when bleeding starts. During the last part of the monthly cycle, premenstrual syndrome (PMS) symptoms, including bloating, headaches, moodiness, irritability, disruptions, and abdominal cramps, may contribute to difficulty sleeping well. The most common sleep-related problems reported by women with PMS are insomnia, hypersomnia (sleeping too much), and daytime sleepiness. The most common problem, insomnia, consists of difficulty falling asleep or staying asleep, waking up too early, or having unrefreshed sleep. Women are more likely than men to experience symptoms of insomnia and poor-quality sleep at least a few nights a week.

Pregnancy and Sleep

Physical symptoms that occur during pregnancy (body aches, nausea, leg cramps, fetus movements, weight gain, and heartburn), as well as emotional changes (depression, anxiety, worry), can interfere with sleep. Overall, women have lower quality of sleep during their last trimester than early in pregnancy. Progesterone levels rise during pregnancy, causing increased feelings of sleepiness. Heartburn, leg cramps, and sinus congestion are common reasons for disturbed sleep, as is an increased need to urinate (the fetus puts pressure on the bladder). As might be expected, mothers of newborn babies experience a lot of postpartum sleeplessness and daytime sleepiness, which may contribute to the postpartum blues many mothers experience.

Pregnant women who have never snored before may begin doing so during pregnancy. About 15–30 percent of pregnant women snore because of pregnancy-related weight gain and increased swelling in their nasal passages, which may partially block the airways. Snoring may also lead to high blood pressure, which can put both the mother and fetus at risk. If the blockage is severe, sleep apnea may result, characterized by loud snoring and periods of stopped breathing during sleep. This can result in a lack of oxygen, which disrupts sleep and may affect the unborn fetus. If loud snoring and severe daytime sleepiness (another symptom of sleep apnea and other sleep disorders) occur, consult your physician. During pregnancy, as many as 25 percent of women develop symptoms of restless legs syndrome, which may be due to lower levels of folic acid, anemia, or other unknown factors.

Menopause and Sleep

Menopause is a time of major hormonal, physical, and psychological change for women. From perimenopause—the transition phase—to postmenopause, women report a marked increase in sleeping problems. Most notable among them are hot flashes, insomnia, and sleep-disordered breathing. Hot flashes may interrupt sleep, and frequent awakenings cause next-day fatigue.

In general, postmenopausal women are less satisfied with their sleep than premenopausal women; as many as 61 percent of postmenopausal women report insomnia symptoms. Snoring has also been found to be more common after menopause. Snoring, along with pauses or gasps in breathing, are signs of a more serious sleep disorder, obstructive sleep apnea. Both age and weight gain, assessed as body mass index (BMI) (see chapter 1) are strong predictors of sleep apnea. However, after age 50, obesity becomes a less important risk factor for sleep apnea than it is in younger women.

The Most Common Sleep Disorders in Women

INSOMNIA

Insomnia is the most common sleep complaint; at least one-third of American adults say they have it occasionally and 10–15 percent on a chronic basis. Women consistently report that they are more likely than men to experience difficulty falling asleep, frequent awakenings, waking too early and being unable to fall back to sleep, and unrefreshed sleep. And although they generally sleep longer, according to NSF polls, more women than men rate the quality of their sleep as fair or poor. Insomnia can be short term when it is in response to a current situation, such as the loss of a job or loved one, a dramatic event, or another situation that may cause stress or anxiety. Women often experience a great deal of stress—and sometimes depression—along with the discomfort associated with the biological changes that occur before and during menstruation, pregnancy, and menopause.

Although these bouts of short-term insomnia may occur, women have to be careful that they do not develop poor sleep habits or attitudes and insomnia becomes long term. Chronic insomnia is a sleeping disorder that is characterized by occurrence three or more nights per week for a month or longer and results in serious daytime impairment. Effective medications are available; a combination of behavioral change and medications works best for the long-term.

SLEEP APNEA

Sleep apnea is a serious, potentially life-threatening breathing disorder that affects 18 million adults in America. Women are more likely to experience symptoms of sleep apnea as they age. In general, sleep apnea is associated with increased blood pressure, a risk for cardiovascular disease and stroke.

Why Your Sex Matters in Sleep Apnea

Physicians may overlook sleep apnea in women because women with this condition may have different symptoms from men. Women with sleep apnea are more likely to have depression and insomnia, less likely to have been told that they stop breathing during sleep, and more likely to have thyroid disease than are men.

Sufferers often experience sleep apnea as partial or full obstruction of airflow through the airway as often as 10 times an hour and throughout the night, leading to pauses in breathing and frequent arousals. Sleep apnea is characterized by the following signs and symptoms:

◆ loud and regular snoring;
◆ pauses or interruptions of airflow during sleep and loss of oxygen;
◆ repetitive arousals, often unnoticed or appearing as snorts or gasps, during sleep;
◆ falling asleep at inappropriate times during the day, such as while driving, working, or talking;
◆ early-morning headaches;
◆ depression, irritability, and sexual dysfunction; and
◆ learning and memory difficulties.

Recent studies have found that women are less likely to be diagnosed with sleep apnea; yet they do better with treatment. The most effective treatment for sleep apnea is the use of a continuous positive airway pressure (CPAP) machine that forces air through a mask attached to the nose so the patient can breathe well and prevent arousals and disrupted sleep.

RESTLESS LEGS SYNDROME

Restless legs syndrome (RLS) is a neurological movement disorder that affects as many as 12 million Americans. It is characterized by uncomfortable and unpleasant leg sensations associated with an urge to move that occur while your body is at rest and are worse at night. Because the unpleasant feelings occur at rest and are relieved by movement, RLS sufferers have difficulty sleeping. Because of these difficulties sleeping, RLS can lead to daytime sleepiness, mood swings, anxiety, and depression.

RLS most recently has been associated with iron-deficiency anemia as well as pregnancy or diabetes. Up to 15 percent of pregnant women develop RLS during their third trimester. RLS may include the following signs and symptoms:

◆ the urge to move the legs, which is often accompanied by uncomfortable sensations in the foot, calf, or upper leg (these sensations are usually described as a creeping or crawling feeling and may be experienced as a tingling, cramping, or burning sensation);
◆ the need to move the legs to relieve the discomfort by stretching, bending, or rubbing the legs, tossing or turning in bed, or getting up and pacing the floor;
◆ a tendency to experience the most discomfort late in the day and at night;
◆ continuous nighttime sleep disruption; and
◆ daytime fatigue.

Medications are available to treat RLS, and women with this disorder should avoid alcohol, nicotine, and caffeine. A healthy diet and moderate exercise can also be helpful.

About 80 percent of RLS sufferers may also experience periodic limb movements: jerking or kicking the legs and sometimes the arms. Although this can be very disturbing to the bed partner, limb movements are very common in all sleep disorders. They also occur with many medications and with disrupted sleep in general. Limb movements alone should not require treatment.

NARCOLEPSY

Narcolepsy is a chronic neurological disorder that affects the region of the central nervous system that regulates sleep and wakefulness and affects approximately one in 2,000 people. Persons with narcolepsy experience excessive daytime sleepiness and have involuntary sleep attacks at inappropriate times (for example, while having dinner, talking, driving, or working).

Narcolepsy symptoms, which frequently appear in teen years, may include the following:

♦ sudden episodes of loss of muscle tone in response to an intense emotion such as laugher or anger, called cataplexy. The loss may range from slight weakness (such as limpness at the neck or knees, sagging facial muscles, or inability to speak clearly) to complete body collapse;
♦ inability to talk or move when falling asleep or waking up;
♦ vivid, often unpleasant, dream-like experiences that occur while dozing or falling asleep;
♦ disrupted nighttime sleep with frequent awakenings;
♦ performance of routine tasks with little awareness or memory of the action; and
♦ learning and memory difficulties.

Recent scientific breakthroughs have led to new understanding of the cause of this condition, and new treatments have given doctors more ways to help manage its symptoms.

NOCTURNAL SLEEP-RELATED EATING DISORDER

Nocturnal sleep-related eating disorder (NS-RED), an uncommon condition, is one of a class of sleep disorders called parasomnias. People with NS-RED eat food during the night while they appear to be asleep. Since parts of the brain that control memory are asleep, people with NS-RED cannot remember nighttime eating. One study indicates that more than 66 percent of sufferers are women. NS-RED can be caused by medications, psychological issues, or sleep disorders.

When to See a Doctor

Many sleep problems can be improved by following the tips below and changing your sleep habits, reducing stress, improving your diet, or exercising. If sleep problems persist, you should seek professional help. Your doctor will determine the cause of your sleep problem and may refer you to a sleep disorders center. Most centers are staffed with sleep specialists who will ask you questions about your sleep problems and may monitor your sleep overnight. They will then provide you with a diagnosis and treatment program so you can get better sleep and have a productive, safe, and healthy quality of life.

NSF's Top 10 Healthy Tips for Better Sleep

♦ Maintain a regular bed and wake time schedule, including weekends.
♦ Establish a regular, relaxing bedtime routine, such as soaking in a hot bath or hot tub and then reading a book or listening to soothing music.
♦ Create a sleep-conducive environment that is dark, quiet, comfortable, and cool.
♦ Sleep on a comfortable mattress and pillows.
♦ Use your bedroom only for sleep and sex. It is best to remove work materials, computers, and televisions from the sleeping environment.
♦ Finish eating at least two to three hours before your regular bedtime.
♦ Exercise regularly; it is best to complete your workout at least a few hours before bedtime.
♦ Avoid nicotine (cigarettes, tobacco products); used close to bedtime, it can lead to poor sleep.
♦ Avoid caffeine (coffee, tea, soft drinks, chocolate) close to bedtime; it also can keep you awake.
♦ Avoid alcohol close to bedtime, which can lead to disrupted sleep later in the night.

—Patricia A. Britz, MEd, MPM, and
Barbara A. Phillips, MD, MSPH

CHAPTER 20

Stroke

What Is a Stroke?

A stroke is a form of cardiovascular disease that affects the arteries traveling toward and inside the brain. A stroke results when one of these vessels becomes blocked and the brain is deprived of blood and oxygen. Stroke is the third leading cause of death in the United States, the most common cause of disability, and costs more than $40 billion in 2004. The impact of stroke will increase as our population ages, making prevention and treatment of stroke one of the most important public health issues for women.

WHY YOUR SEX MATTERS

Each year about 700,000 Americans have a stroke, and nearly 40,000 more women than men die of a stroke. Sixty-two percent of all deaths from stroke in the United States occur in women.

Heart disease and stroke take more women's lives than the next five leading causes of death combined (cancer, chronic lower respiratory diseases, diabetes, Alzheimer's disease, and unintentional injuries). Women are less likely to have a stroke than men in early and mid-adulthood. However, women's strokes occur later in life, perhaps explaining the alarming statistic that women account for more than 60 percent of total stroke deaths. Although mortality from heart disease appears to be declining in men, this advance has not been evident in women (470,000 deaths per year in 1970, compared with 500,000 per year in 2001). Both stroke incidence and mortality appear to have increased in women over the past three decades, perhaps because of women's overall increased life span.

Most international studies demonstrate that women enjoy lower stroke incidence than men until late in life. However, women may have worse early outcomes from injury when stroke does occur. In 2002, 38.5 percent of people who died from stroke were men, and 61.5 percent were women. Six months after the stroke, women are more likely to be dead or dependent on institutional care. The reasons for these differences have not been investigated; but as women have strokes later in life than men do, other co-morbid medical conditions likely contribute to poorer outcome. In addition, elderly women may have less family support, as many have outlived their spouses.

Women may experience stroke symptoms different from those common in men, and there is some evidence that women are less likely to receive some of the standard diagnostic tests that can help determine the most appropriate treatment.

A recent analysis of more than 19,000 patients in the International Stroke Trial revealed that women patients were older and sustained worse strokes than men, had a higher incidence of the abnormal heart rhythm known as atrial fibrillation, and had higher systolic blood pressures. Additionally, women who have strokes are less likely to receive some standard tests to help diagnose the type of stroke and determine treatment. Similar findings have been well documented in women experiencing heart attacks.

Symptoms of Ischemic Stroke

Ischemic strokes are caused by the sudden blockage of an artery that supplies the brain, causing an unexpected and catastrophic loss of blood and oxygen to the brain. These are the most common type of stroke. Symptoms occur quickly because the brain is utterly dependent on a constant supply of oxygen. Because each part of the brain controls different functions, the symptoms a person experiences depend largely on the particular region of the brain that is injured. For example, if a blockage occurs in the left middle cerebral artery (a common location), the person may be unable to speak or to understand language. If the blockage occurs in deeper arteries of the brain (known as lacunar stroke), the result is more subtle, such as slurring of speech.

Other symptoms are possible, such as severe headache, dizziness, visual changes, or weakness in the arms or legs. Therefore, any new and severe symptom that affects balance, vision, or speech must be recognized as "brain attack." Similar to a heart attack, a brain attack is a true emergency and requires immediate treatment.

Treatment of Acute Ischemic Stroke
The only proven treatment currently available for acute ischemic stroke is the clot-buster drug, tissue plasminogen activator (TPA). TPA breaks up or melts the clot within the blocked vessel and restores blood flow to the brain. This is nothing more than a plumbing issue, but with very dire consequences. If there is a blockage in the pipe, the blood cannot get through, and without the blood, the brain will die. TPA melts the clot, thereby relieving the blockage and restoring blood flow.

TPA is currently only approved for treatment within three hours of the onset of symptoms. This critical fact limits the usefulness of the drug, because many patients do not arrive in the emergency department within the three-hour window of treatment. Equally problematic is the woman who wakes up with stroke symptoms and is unsure how much time has elapsed.

New data suggest that women may actually *benefit more* from TPA than men do. Women treated with TPA have improved recanalization rates (the clot is more likely to be melted) and have improved functional outcomes at 90 days, compared to treated males. This emphasizes the importance of early identification of stroke symptoms so appropriate treatment can be given.

It is vital that women recognize signs of acute stroke and seek treatment quickly. Never delay calling 911 thinking that symptoms will improve. Calling a primary care physician can delay treatment, as does traveling to the hospital in a personal vehicle rather than by ambulance.

For patients seeking treatment outside of the three-hour window of treatment, other options for opening a blocked blood vessel may be available. For example, blood clot retrieval devices are available at certified hospital stroke centers. Women and their families need to know where these specialty services are available and how to access them quickly. Irreversible brain damage can only be minimized after stroke with rapid treatment and restoring blood flow.

WHAT ARE OTHER TYPES OF STROKES?

Not all strokes are ischemic. A second major type results from bleeding from a blood vessel in the brain, known as a hemorrhagic stroke. This type is often related to high blood pressure. Determining whether a stroke is ischemic or hemorrhagic is vital to receiving the appropriate care. Hemorrhagic strokes can not be treated with TPA, because the drug can enhance bleeding and worsen the damage. To distinguish this type of stroke, a brain scan, known as computerized tomography (CT), is done as soon as the patient arrives in the emergency department.

Other strokes are cardioembolic in origin. In approximately 20 percent of cases, a clot forms in the heart as a consequence of a blood-clotting disorder or an irregular heart rhythm, known as atrial fibrillation. The clot then dislodges from the heart and blocks a brain blood vessel. Treatment for this type of stroke consists of anticoagulation medication (blood thinners).

Last, stroke or brain attack is not necessarily a one-time event in a woman's life. Recurrent stroke in women requires controlling the risk factors, including adequate blood pressure, glucose and cholesterol control, and smoking cessation. Treatment with aspirin or other antiplatelet agents can prevent recurrent stroke.

RISK FACTORS

Traditional risk factors for heart disease and stroke, similar in men and women, include:

♦ hypertension,
♦ high cholesterol,
♦ smoking,
♦ diabetes,
♦ previous transient ischemic attack (TIA), or "mini-stroke," and
♦ physical inactivity/obesity.

Women in the perimenopausal period who have diabetes may require special attention. Diabetic women age 55–64 are at higher stroke risk than are age-matched males.

Risk Reduction

First, talk with your physician to determine your personal risk for stroke. Women are considered low, moderate, or high risk for stroke depending on their individual risk factors, and treatment recommendations differ based on this assessment. For example, high-risk women should be treated with daily aspirin, low-risk women should not. The American Heart Association has developed guidelines for stroke risk-reduction in women.
All women should:

♦ stop smoking,
♦ increase physical activity,
♦ treat high cholesterol aggressively,
♦ control blood sugar,
♦ control blood pressure (below 135/85),
♦ maintain a healthy weight, and
♦ eat a heart-healthy diet.

High-risk women should discuss appropriate treatments with their physicians. These may include blood thinners for atrial fibrillation or treatments for carotid artery narrowing and blockage, high blood pressure, or high blood sugar.
In the spring of 2005 research from a 10-year study of nearly 40,000

women found that aspirin cuts the risk of stroke for women, but not for men. While the benefits of aspirin may not outweigh the risks for healthy women in their 40s and 50s, the balance shifts enough to make it worthwhile for many women once they hit their 60s. The major risk from taking aspirin is bleeding, which can cause serious problems, including rare but deadly bleeding strokes. Women with high blood pressure and problems with stomach bleeding may be at particular risk and should discuss aspirin use with their physicians.

Hormone Therapy

How estrogen and progesterone hormone therapy (HT) affect stroke risk and outcome is much debated. Research suggests that women are relatively protected from stroke before menopause, implying that female hormones are protective. Consistent with this idea, laboratory evidence has overwhelmingly shown that estrogen treatment reduces brain injury in animal and cell models of stroke. However, the benefit of using these hormones in women after menopause has not been demonstrated consistently. Several recent trials have cast significant doubt on the effectiveness of postmenopausal HT to prevent stroke. The highly publicized Women's Health Initiative found a small but significant increase in stroke risk in healthy older women receiving combined progesterone-estrogen or estrogen-only therapy. Current guidelines recommend against HT for prevention of stroke in either healthy women or women with previous stroke.

Additional Special Factors for Women

As mentioned above, over their lifetime, women are more likely than men to be functionally dependent on others and institutionalized as a result of stroke. It is not clear if this is due to differences in biological response to treatment or to differences in sociological-cultural factors. In some European studies, women appear to be undertreated after a stroke compared to age-matched men. Men over 85 years of age were more likely than women of the same age to be treated with antiplatelet therapy. A large study of primary care in Ireland demonstrated that women were less likely to receive prescriptions for blood pressure medications shown to reduce stroke risk, or to be advised to take aspirin, to prevent stroke. This was true even for women with known cardiovascular disease. In contrast, women were more likely than men to receive antianxiety medication.

There are also differences in surgical interventions for stroke in women. Women are less likely to be operated on for carotid artery disease. Large studies have shown that carotid endarterectomy (CEA) may not be as successful in women as in men. CEA reduced stroke and death at five years by only 17 percent in women, compared to a 66 percent reduction in men. In part, this result reflects a greater incidence of complications after surgery in women (3.6 percent) than in men (1.7 percent). Women receiving CEA also sustained a higher incidence of intraoperative stroke and enjoyed only half the long-term benefit that men did, especially when they had disease without symptoms.

Recent work has also evaluated women with symptoms of carotid artery disease (mild stroke or transient ischemic attack with resolving symptoms). For these women, CEA was beneficial only if initiated rapidly, within two weeks after their symptoms began. These studies illustrate potentially important sex-based differences in efficacy of stroke treatment. Clinical trials are needed to determine best treatment practices for women.

Tests done in scientific labs have shown differences between how men and women react to the loss of blood to the brain. Recent research on human stroke in animal and cell models emphasizes that the response to injury can be different in women. In part, this may be related to differences in how male and female brains react to injury and when their brain cells begin to die. Data from genetically engineered mice support this concept and suggest the potential for sex-specific treatments in brain injury.

What Do I Do If I Have
Symptoms of a Stroke?

♦ *Call 911!*
♦ Expect treatment with TPA if eligible (within time window, no bleeding, or moderate stroke that is not spontaneously improving).
♦ Consider referral to a specialized stroke center for large and sudden strokes.

—LOUISE D. MCCULLOUGH, MD, PHD, AND
PATRICIA D. HURN, PHD

CHAPTER 21

Urinary and Bladder Health

How the Urinary Tract Works

The urinary tract is responsible for the production, storage, and expulsion of urine, one of your body's waste products. The two kidneys, located just underneath the lowermost ribs to the left and right of the spine, filter the blood and remove waste products. They also help balance a number of essential minerals for the body, including sodium, chloride, and calcium. The bladder functions as the storage unit for urine, after it has been transported by the ureters to the bladder. The ureters are two, hollow, one-way tubes connecting each kidney to the bladder. When the appropriate conditions are found (namely, a bathroom) the urine is then emptied by urinating through the urethra, another hollow tube that connects the bladder to the outside world. The urethra normally ends near the tip of the penis in men and on the inside at the top of the vagina in women. Refer back to figure 1 in chapter 8.

What Are Urinary Tract Infections?

Normal urine is sterile and contains no bacteria. However, bacteria from the rectal area and vaginal area (known as the perineum) may multiply and migrate up the urethra into the urine and cause an infection in the urinary tract (including the kidneys, bladder, or urethra, or prostate in men). A bladder infection is known as cystitis (or lower urinary tract infection) and is the most common form of urinary tract infection (UTI). UTIs are often categorized as simple (uncomplicated) or complicated. Simple UTIs are infections that occur in a normal bladder. Complicated UTIs occur in abnormal bladders or when migration of bacteria and subsequent infection occur in the kidney (an upper urinary tract infection) or the prostate gland. An infection with bacteria resistant to multiple antibiotics, or one in which the patient has multiple other medical conditions, is also considered a complicated UTI.

UTIs are responsible for more than seven million visits to physicians' offices each year and about 5 percent of all visits to primary care physicians. The majority of those who suffer from UTIs are women. Approximately 40 percent of women and 12 percent of men experience at least one symptomatic UTI during their lifetime. UTIs result in loss of time from work and increased medical expenses, in addition to the pain and suffering they cause.

UTIs are rarely caused by viruses and are due almost exclusively to certain types of bacteria. Yeast rarely infects the urinary tract; a UTI caused by yeast would be considered a complicated infection.

RISK FACTORS

Just as some people are more prone to get colds, some people are more prone to get UTIs. You are more likely to get a UTI if your urinary tract has an abnormality or if you have recently had a catheter in place. If you are unable to urinate normally because of some type of obstruction, you also have a higher chance of developing a UTI. Disorders such as diabetes also put people at higher risk for UTIs because of both disease-specific changes in the bladder and of elevation of sugar (glucose) in the bladder, which bacteria use as a food source. Anatomical abnormalities in the urinary tract due to minor and major congenital (birth) defects or previous surgery may also lead to UTIs.

WHY YOUR SEX MATTERS

Women are more prone to UTIs for a variety of reasons. Their urethras are shorter than men's, which means that bacteria have less distance to travel to reach the bladder. The location of the urethra within the perineum provides bacteria a warm, moist environment in which they can flourish before gaining access to the urethra. Some women have urinary tracts that allow bacteria to adhere to the lining of the urethra and bladder more readily and thus are genetically predisposed to UTIs. Sexual intercourse also increases the frequency of UTIs in women. It is interesting to note that the woman's own bacteria are responsible for the infection. The use of condoms with spermicidal foam and diaphragms for birth control are also associated with an increase in UTIs in women. Spermicidals disturb the normal "good" bacteria in the vagina that protect the urinary tract from infection, and diaphrams also change the anatomic relationship of the bladder and urethra thereby increasing the likelihood of infection. The risks of these birth control methods have to be weighed against the positive benefits they provide—protection from sexually transmitted diseases and unwanted pregnancies. Women who have gone through menopause undergo a change in the lining of their vagina and urethra and lose estrogen's protective effect against harmful bacteria.

SYMPTOMS

When you have a UTI, bacteria irritate the lining of the bladder and urethra, which may become red, irritated, and actually bleed. The irritation can cause pain in your abdomen, pelvic region, and lower back and a sensation of burning in the urethra while urinating. You may feel like emptying your bladder more often and have the sensation of incomplete bladder emptying. You may even try to urinate but only produce a few drops. Although urine can be cloudy naturally, you may also find that your urine is regularly cloudy or smells unpleasant.

An upper urinary tract infection or kidney infection can produce high fevers, chills, back pain, and nausea and vomiting. Such infections require immediate medical attention. They usually follow lower UTIs (cystitis) and are generally preventable if the cystitis is treated.

DIAGNOSIS

If you have symptoms of a UTI, your doctor may do a simple chemical analysis (dip stick) of the urine or examine it under a microscope to look for the presence of bacteria or infection-fighting white blood cells. If you are having fevers along with UTI symptoms or persistent symptoms despite therapy, then you may need further tests, such as an ultrasound or computed tomography (CT) scan to assess the urinary tract. Visualization of the bladder using a special scope may also be recommended (cystoscopy).

TREATMENT

A simple UTI can be treated with a short course of antibiotics; few infections may need to be treated for several weeks. Even though a few doses of medication may relieve your symptoms, you should complete the full course prescribed for you to rid the urinary tract of the offending bacteria. UTIs may recur if the antibiotics are not taken as prescribed. You should also drink plenty of liquids (to wash out offending bacteria) and avoid foods that irritate the bladder such as acidic fruits, sodas, or coffee. Complicated UTIs may require stronger and longer antibiotic courses. Sometimes intravenous treatment in the hospital is necessary.

PREGNANCY AND UTIs

Urine infections are common during pregnancy. The bladder may not empty as well during pregnancy, allowing bacteria to remain inside and multiply. Also, pregnant women are less likely to experience the telltale burning and pelvic pain that heralds the onset of a UTI. Because of the position of the uterus, and especially the pressure it places on the ureter from the right kidney, the right kidney becomes blocked and cannot empty as well during pregnancy, also increasing the risk. Several of the antibiotics that treat UTIs have been used extensively in pregnant women and do not cause any problems in the fetus. Some antibiotics are safe to use during certain stages of pregnancy but not others, so it is important to check with your doctor before self-medicating. If UTIs occur repeatedly in pregnancy, you may need to have an ultrasound scan of your kidneys to determine there are no kidney stones or other anatomic abnormalities that could be the culprit.

PREVENTION

There are some simple steps you can take to help avoid UTIs. You should drink plenty of fluids at regular intervals throughout the day. Urinate when you need to and try not to hold it in for extended periods (void every three to four hours). Take time to empty the bladder completely when you do urinate. After urinating, wipe from front to back to prevent bacteria around the anus from gaining access to the vagina or urethra. Avoid constipation as it changes the ability of the bladder to empty correctly. Drinking a large glass of water before sexual intercourse and urinating afterward may decrease the risk of a UTI, because the process can flush out any bacteria that were introduced during intercourse. Sometimes a small dose of antibiotic before intercourse can help prevent a UTI from occurring.

Women who have gone through menopause and have lost their normal estrogen output have a change in the lining of the vagina that allows hostile bacteria to survive. If this is the cause of increased UTIs, you should discuss hormone therapy with your doctor.

SUI Is Treatable

By Bonnie Blair, winner of Olympic gold medals for speed skating at the 1988, 1992, and 1994 Winter Olympics and member of the U.S. Speedskating Board of Directors

Bonnie Blair—who was known as the fastest woman on ice—was not used to being slowed down. After winning gold medals for speed skating at the 1988, 1992, and 1994 Winter Olympics, she hung up her skates and became a motivational speaker and a member of the U.S. Speedskating Board of Directors.

She married fellow Olympian David Cruikshank and became a mother of two. After the birth of her first child and her initial attempt at running, she realized she had a physical problem. "After giving birth to my son, I was so excited to have the chance to run again—until I got about a block away and my shorts were soaked. Why had this happened to me?"

Her experience, which may resonate with the estimated 11 million women in the United States who live with stress urinary incontinence (SUI), upset and embarrassed her. She was too embarrassed to talk with her doctor or husband and tried to cope by wearing dark shorts, using feminine pads, and limiting her intake of fluids.

A year later, she finally talked to her doctor about the problem. Her doctor diagnosed her with stress urinary incontinence, a condition that occurs when the pelvic muscles that support the bladder and urethra become damaged or weakened. Weakened pelvic muscles cannot hold the urethra in its correct position. As a result, the urethra can lose its seal and allow urine to escape with any movement from the diaphragm that puts stress on the bladder, such as coughing, sneezing, laughing, or exercising.

Bonnie discussed her options with her physician and tried different treatments, including Kegel exercises, weights, and electrical stimulation to strengthen her pelvic muscles. When none of these options worked, Bonnie and her doctor agreed on a simple, minimally invasive surgery that involves insertion of a strip of mesh-like tape under the urethra to create a supportive sling. This procedure provides support and allows the urethra to remain closed when appropriate, preventing urine loss during sudden movements and exercise.

For Bonnie, who has a long list of accomplishments to her credit, her triumph over SUI is one she wants to share with others. "My experience is similar to many women who have given birth, which is why I want to encourage women to talk to their doctors so they can treat and beat SUI like I did.

"Now I can jump on the trampoline with my kids without fear I might have an accident. Even my family has noticed a difference in my attitude," she says.

Bonnie's advice to other women with SUI is to talk with their doctors about treatment options. "It's not something you have to learn to cope with. SUI is treatable."

(Reprinted with permission by Bonnie Blair)

What Is Urinary Incontinence?

Urinary incontinence, the involuntary loss of bladder control, affects as many as 13 million people in the United States, occurring twice as often in women as in men. It occurs most often because of problems with the muscles or ligaments associated with the bladder and urethra, typically if your bladder muscles suddenly contract (or squeeze) or if the muscles or ligaments around the urethra suddenly relax. Bladder control means more than just telling yourself to wait to urinate until you get to the bathroom. It takes teamwork from organs, muscles, and nerves in your body. Your bladder is a muscle; when it stores urine, it relaxes, and when you urinate, it tightens to squeeze urine out of the bladder.

Additional muscles help with bladder control as well. Two sphincter muscles surround the urethra, which carries urine from your bladder down to an opening in the front of the vagina. The sphincter muscles keep the urethra closed by squeezing like rubber bands. Pelvic floor muscles support the uterus, or womb, and the rectum and bladder. They also help keep the urethra closed.

When your bladder is full, nerves in the bladder signal the brain, and you get the urge to urinate. Once you reach the toilet, your brain sends a message down to the sphincter muscles and the pelvic floor muscles telling them to relax. The brain also tells the bladder muscles to tighten up to squeeze urine out of the bladder.

The different types of urinary incontinence include:

- **Stress incontinence**—Leaking small amounts of urine caused by an increase in abdominal pressure during physical activities such as coughing, laughing, sneezing, lifting, straining, getting out of a chair, or bending over. A common form of incontinence in women, stress incontinence is treatable.
- **Urge incontinence**—Also referred to as overactive bladder, this type of incontinence usually is accompanied by a sudden, strong urge to urinate and an inability to get to the toilet fast enough. It can occur during the night or on awakening or when you touch water or hear it running (as when washing dishes).
- **Functional incontinence**—Not being able to reach a toilet in time because of physical disability, obstacles, or problems in thinking or communicating that prevent a person from reaching a toilet.
- **Overflow incontinence**—Leaking small amounts of urine because the bladder does not empty properly; this condition is rare in women but common in men with enlarged prostates.

- **Mixed incontinence**—A combination of types of incontinence, most often when stress and urge incontinence occur together.
- **Transient incontinence**—Leaking urine temporarily due to a medical condition or infection that goes away once the condition or infection is treated. It can be triggered by medications, UTIs, mental impairment, restricted mobility, and severe constipation.

RISK FACTORS

Trouble with bladder control can stem from nerve injury, birth defects, strokes, or multiple sclerosis, but it can be as simple as physical changes associated with the aging process. Older women generally have more bladder control problems than younger women do, but bladder issues happen in younger women as well. The loss of bladder control, however, is not something that has to happen as you age. It can be treated and often cured, whatever your age. Certain types of medications can cause or exacerbate incontinence, including diuretics, sedatives, narcotics, antidepressants, antihistamines, calcium channel blockers, and alpha blockers. The WHI study indicated that estrogen-progesterone and estrogen-only hormone therapy raises the risk of urinary incontinence.

WHY YOUR SEX MATTERS

Some women experience incontinence during pregnancy. The added weight and pressure of the fetus can weaken pelvic floor muscles and ligaments, affecting your ability to control your bladder. Sometimes the position of your bladder and urethra can change because of the position of the fetus, which can also cause problems. After delivery, urinary incontinence often goes away by itself. However, vaginal delivery can weaken bladder control muscles and ligaments, and pregnancy and childbirth can damage bladder control nerves. Bladder control problems do not always show up right after childbirth.

Menopause can cause bladder control problems for some women. During menopause, the amount of estrogen in your body starts decreasing, which can cause the bladder control muscles to weaken.

DIAGNOSIS

To diagnose the problem, your doctor should ask about your symptoms and for a complete medical history, including medications you are taking, surgeries you have had, pregnancy history, and illnesses. You will also be asked how often you empty your bladder, how and when you leak urine, and when you have accidents. You should then have a physical exam to look for signs of any medical conditions that can cause incontinence. A test may be done to determine how much your bladder can hold and how well your bladder muscles function. For this test, you are asked to drink plenty of fluids and urinate into a measuring pan, after which any urine that remains in the bladder is measured. There may be blood and urine tests as well as. Possible tests include:

♦ Stress test—you relax, then cough hard.
♦ Ultrasound—sound waves are used to take a picture of the kidneys, bladder, and urethra.
♦ Cystoscopy—a thin tube with a tiny camera is placed inside the urethra to view the inside of the urethra and bladder.
♦ Urodynamics—pressure in the bladder and the flow of urine are measured using special techniques.

You may be asked to keep a diary for a day or a week to record the times you urinate and the amounts of urine you produce.

TREATMENT

There are a number of ways to treat incontinence, including:

♦ **Pelvic muscle (Kegel) exercises.**
♦ **Electrical stimulation**—brief doses of electrical stimulation can strengthen muscles in the lower pelvis in a way similar to exercising the muscles. This treatment can reduce both stress incontinence and urge incontinence.
♦ **Biofeedback**—biofeedback uses measuring devices to help you become aware of your body's functioning. It can be used with pelvic muscle exercises and electrical stimulation to relieve stress incontinence and urge incontinence.
♦ **Timed voiding or bladder training**—two techniques that help you train your bladder to hold urine better.
♦ **Medications**—Medications can reduce many types of leakage and help tighten or strengthen pelvic floor muscles and muscles around the urethra. Some can also calm overactive bladder muscles.
♦ **Implants**—substances such as collagen (a natural fibrous tissue from cows) or other bulking agents are injected through a needle into tissues around the urethra to add bulk and help the urethra stay closed. This treatment reduces stress incontinence. Before

getting a collagen urethral injection, you need to have a skin test to make sure you are not allergic to this substance.

◆ **Catheterization**—a catheter is a small tube that you can learn to insert yourself through the urethra into the bladder to drain urine.

◆ **Pessary**—a stiff ring inserted by a health care provider into the vagina, a pessary presses against the wall of the vagina and the nearby urethra. The pressure helps to hold up the bladder and reduce stress leakage. This can raise your risk of vaginal and urinary tract infections, however. A newer generation of catheters and pessaries is made from naturally derived material rather than material derived synthetically.

◆ **Urethral inserts**—a urethral insert is a small device that you place inside the urethra, remove when you urinate, and then put back in until you need to urinate again.

◆ **Urine seals**—urine seals are small foam pads that you place over the urethra opening. The pad seals itself against your body, keeping you from leaking. You remove and discard it after urinating and place a new seal over the urethra.

◆ **Bladder pacemaker**—a new technology is using a pacemaker to control bladder function. This technology consists of a small electrode inserted in the patient's back close to the nerve that controls bladder function. The electrode is connected to a pulse generator, and the electrical impulses control bladder function. There is a greater than 60–75 percent improvement or cure rate with this technology.

◆ **Other surgery.** Different types of surgery can be done, depending on the kind of incontinence problem you have. Some surgeries keep the urethra from dropping or rotating, which prevents urine leakage. Other surgeries use implants to help the bladder function better.

◆ **Newer, minimally invasive procedures,** known as sling procedures, can be helpful for some people. In this procedure, the surgeon removes a strip of tissue from the abdomen, or may use a small amount of stable woven material, and fashions a sling that is placed under the urethra and bladder neck to compress the urethra during stress maneuvers.

In addition to treatment options, if you are overweight, you should lose weight, since extra weight can cause bladder control problems. Certain foods and drinks, such as caffeine, can cause incontinence. Alcohol, carbonated beverages, decaffeinated coffee or tea, chocolate, citrus fruits, tomatoes, and acidic fruit juices may also irritate your bladder. You can often reduce incontinence by restricting these foods and liquids in your diet.

What Is Interstitial Cystitis?

Interstitial cystitis (IC) is a chronic inflammatory condition of the bladder whose cause is unknown. Unlike a UTI, known as "common" cystitis, which is caused by bacteria and can be treated with antibiotics, IC is not caused by bacteria and does not respond to conventional antibiotic therapy.

POSSIBLE CAUSES

There are no known specific causes of IC. Theories include a defect in the lining of the bladder (epithelium), a toxic component in the urine, neurogenic inflammation, or some type of immune response. Some studies have indicated a hereditary or familial risk factor.

Several biomarkers for IC are currently under investigation. Antiproliferative factor (APF) is a very promising biomarker that is found exclusively in the urine of people with IC. APF, a low molecular weight protein that appears to inhibit growth of the bladder lining, has been isolated and sequenced. This discovery could lead to a definitive test and, possibly, to new targeted treatments.

WHY YOUR SEX MATTERS

IC can affect people of any age, race, or sex; however, 90 percent of cases occur in adult women. Studies estimate that there may be more than 700,000 cases of IC in the United States, but this may be an underestimation because IC is often undiagnosed or misdiagnosed. Although it is considerably less well known, the incidence of IC is similar to that of Parkinson's disease or type I diabetes.

SYMPTOMS

Some or all of these symptoms may be present:

- ♦ Frequency—in early or very mild cases, urinary frequency is sometimes the only symptom. In severe cases the frequency can reach up to 60 times in a 24-hour period.

◆ Urgency—the sensation of having to urinate immediately may be accompanied by pain, pressure, or spasms.
◆ Pain in the lower abdominal, urethral, or vaginal area—pain also is frequently associated with sexual intercourse. Men with IC may experience testicular, scrotal, and/or perineal pain, and painful ejaculation.

Some patients also report muscle and joint pain, migraines, allergic reactions, and gastrointestinal problems. It appears that IC has an unexplained association with certain other chronic diseases and pain syndromes, such as vulvar vestibulitis, fibromyalgia, and irritable bowel syndrome.

Diagnosis

Most IC patients have difficulty obtaining a diagnosis. In fact, studies have shown that it can take approximately five to seven years to receive a correct diagnosis of IC. It is important to note that IC is not a psychosomatic disorder, nor is it caused by stress. A series of steps is necessary to make a proper diagnosis: a urologist must have your urine tested to determine if a bacterial infection is present, rule out other diseases or conditions with similar symptoms, and perform a cystoscopy with hydrodistention under general anesthesia if no infection is present and no other disorder is discovered. Cystoscopy with hydrodistention can show the pinpoint hemorrhages on the bladder wall that are the hallmark of IC. During this procedure, a biopsy of the bladder wall may be performed to rule out other conditions such as carcinoma in situ. If hydrodistention under anesthesia is not performed, the diagnosis of IC may be missed, and an in-office cystoscopy can be painful for those who have IC.

Treatment

Many IC patients are helped by one or more of the following treatments:

◆ A diet low in acidic/irritating foods, and avoiding beverages such as coffee, tea, carbonated, and/or alcoholic drinks, may be helpful in reducing IC symptoms.
◆ Oral medications can be helpful; the U.S. Food and Drug Administration has approved one oral medication (pentosan polysulfate sodium) to treat IC. It is thought to work by repairing a thin or damaged bladder lining. Other oral medications such as anti-inflammatory agents, antispasmodics, bladder analgesics, antihistamines, and muscle relaxants may be helpful. Low-dose

tricyclic antidepressants have been shown to help with both the pain and frequency of IC.

♦ Bladder distention, in which the bladder is stretched by filling it with water under general anesthesia, is used as a diagnostic tool and can also be therapeutic in some cases.

♦ Medications instilled directly into the bladder (bladder instillations), such as dimethyl sulfoxide (DMSO) or heparin, may be helpful. These medications are believed to work as anti-inflammatory agents. DMSO and/or heparin is often combined with steroids, local anesthetics, and/or other ingredients to form a bladder "cocktail."

♦ Surgery helps a small minority of patients whose symptoms are severe and who do not respond to other IC treatments. In some cases, however, IC symptoms persist. Several types of surgery have been used to treat IC, including cystectomy and urinary diversion. Laser surgery should be reserved solely for the Hunner's ulcer form of IC.

♦ Anticonvulsants such as gabapentin and clonazepam are being used to treat chronic pain, as are some muscle relaxants. Short-acting opioid analgesics may be used to treat moderate, intermittent IC pain; long-acting analgesics are useful in treating chronic, severe IC pain.

Some other measures that can improve the quality of life and reduce the incidence and severity of flare-ups include stress reduction techniques such as visualization or biofeedback, bladder retraining, physical therapy, and exercise.

A number of experimental medications and devices are being tested to treat IC, including neuromodulation devices, which are implanted in the region of the spine, and various asthma and allergy preparations (leukotriene inhibitors, for example).

SOME OTHER FACTORS FOR WOMEN

There is a definite, although poorly understood, link between IC and other diseases, many of which are also more common in women. Allergies, irritable bowel syndrome (IBS), sensitive skin, vulvodynia, and fibromyalgia are the most common conditions associated with IC.

Several studies have found that a subset of IC patients has an increased number of bladder mast cells, and many of these patients also have systemic allergies. Mast cells are thought to trigger the pain and inflammation of IC and are also associated with allergies. These patients may be helped with histamine-blocking agents.

Research also has found that IC and IBS share some of the same characteristics, which could help to explain why these two diseases are found to co-exist with such frequency (see chapter 9). Since the intestines and the bladder have similar mucosal linings, perhaps a similar defect occurs in the linings of both of these organs.

One study indicates that 68 percent of women with refractory (not responding to standard treatments) vulvodynia have IC (see chapter 15). One theory is that vulvodynia, fibromyalgia, and IC share a common connection through increased or up-regulated pain perception in the central nervous system.

Currently, some urologists are developing multimodal approaches to treating IC and related diseases. These physicians work in conjunction with other specialists in related fields of medicine to provide wide-ranging treatment strategies for patients' varying symptoms. As more and more research points to relationships between various diseases processes, it will be easier to find comprehensive help for the array of symptoms IC patients experience, in the bladder and beyond.

—LINDSEY KERR, MD; ATTILA BARABAS, MD; AND
VICKI RATNER, MD

PART 3

WHERE TO GO FOR HELP

CHAPTER **22**

Medical Research— How You Can Participate and How You Can Learn More

My Body on the Line
Take Me, for Example

By Meredith F. Small, professor of anthropology, Cornell
University

*I am lying on an exam table at Strong Memorial Hospital in Rochester,
N.Y. I stare at the ceiling and try to keep my legs apart while nurse practitioner Kay Rust threads a catheter through my urethra and instills a
cool liquid into my bladder. This is not part of any usual exam, and I
would rather be just about anyplace else on earth. But I lie here quietly
because I volunteered for a National Institutes of Health (NIH) double-
blind clinical trial, and even with that catheter sliding up my urethra, I
am convinced this is the right place to be.*

*I have a condition called interstitial cystitis (IC), an inflammation of
the bladder lining that results in a frequent and urgent need to urinate;
sometimes it also results in pain. There is no known cure for this condition and no sure way to ease the symptoms. But researchers are conducting a variety of studies on treatments that show promise. My particular
clinical trial is testing the efficacy of instilling a weakened cow tuberculosis bacteria, bacillus calmette guérin (BCG), directly into the bladder;
BCG has been used successfully for 30 years to treat bladder cancer. In
a pilot study, some IC patients experienced marked improvement.*

*So here I am, a biological anthropologist, helping researchers figure
out whether this treatment might really work.*

*Across the country, volunteers like me are participating in more than
24,000 clinical trials funded by the NIH; thousands more trials are conducted and paid for by medical research facilities, drug companies, and*

makers of medical devices. Those of us who have offered our bodies up to science understand that testing on human subjects is the only way that medicine can move forward. Lab work and animal tests can go only so far in trying to predict what works in homo sapiens; sooner or later humans have to take their own medicine and see if it works.

Clinical trials aren't just science, they are a social experiment. Who is willing to step up and be a subject so the rest of us can get effective and safe treatments? If not I, who should lie on that table? What about you?

Facing the Placebo Question

The process of a clinical trial is, by design, rigorous. First, researchers must find subjects. I was recruited during my first appointment with Robert Mayer, a urologist and specialist in IC at Strong Memorial. After we had discussed the various options available—I had already tried most of them—Mayer brought up the BCG trial. As a scientist, I knew that a clinical trial aims to produce trustworthy results by removing as much human bias as possible. But was my faith in science strong enough to put my own body on the line?

I took home all the information about the trial, read what was involved and spent some time on the Internet looking up BCG. Then I sought the opinion of a physician friend. (He voted yes.) In the end, I decided to go for it. The risks were small, and—who knows?—it might just work.

I had also made a promise to myself and my family that I would try anything to make this condition better, and this trial was an "anything."

As in most trials, once subjects are recruited, they are randomly divided into two groups, treatment and placebo. In other words, I had a 50–50 chance of going through all this treatment only to discover that I had received the placebo. In this trial, that possibility was not such an issue because, after the results of the placebo-controlled study were in, every subject in this trial was to be given the real thing. The researchers figured that the results of the pilot study were good enough, and BCG involved no real risk, so it was worth giving it to all of us at the end.

But that's not always standard procedure. Some studies have built-in stopping points where preliminary results are reviewed: if the treatment is clearly advantageous, the trial is halted and everyone is given the medication. In other trials—for example, a cancer or HIV trial—it can be harder for subjects to accept the chance of receiving a placebo as a way to move science forward. In such cases, participation requires having your eyes wide open.

Volunteers also need to be committed. For my trial, I gave up 14 afternoons to drive two hours each way to Rochester and back, and I spent many more hours monitoring and recording my reaction to the treatment.

I also had to keep logs of my medications, down to each aspirin or vitamin C tablet. At various times I even had to chart the number of times

I went to the toilet and measure how much I peed. This might sound obsessive, but that diary is a baseline record of my toilet needs; I now know when things get better or worse.

Focusing on the log also gave some purpose to all those visits to the bathroom—I wasn't just urinating, I was contributing to science.

A Call for Patience

Participation in a clinical trial also takes patience. Findings may not be apparent for months or years, which in the case of terminal illnesses, is often deathly slow. IC won't kill me, but I would certainly like some relief. Travel is torture: Waiting out an airline delay strapped in my seat is simply not possible; long car trips become even longer with hourly stops. The pain, when it comes, affects my relationship with my husband and daughter. Some days at work I just put my head down and cry.

I would love medical research to happen faster. But participating in a trial decreased my frustration with the pace because I saw firsthand just what it takes—all the visits, all the exams, all the treatment and the mountains of data to be analyzed. By doing it, not just reading about it, I gained respect for the process.

Even so, lying on that table I still often asked myself: Is this the only way to make progress in dealing with IC?

Until 50 years ago, there was no gold standard for judging new treatments or medications. Physicians relied instead on their powers of observation and memory: If it was common to give this or that treatment, they used it and then watched to see if it worked. The standard of care was based on history, not testing.

But in 1946 researchers in England tested the effect of the new antibiotic streptomycin on tuberculosis. All the patients in the study received the standard of care for that time—bed rest—but half were also given the antibiotic. Equally important, no one working on the study knew which patients were on the drugs; the staff and the patients were doubly "blind" to the treatment and therefore could not project an outcome in either direction.

The results were striking. Fifty-one percent of those on streptomycin improved, compared with only 8 percent of those on bed rest alone.

The double-blind clinical trial rapidly became the gold standard for medical science and a standard for government approval for medications.

Beyond the science, I quickly became a fan of clinical trials. The process, I learned firsthand, is not as dispassionate as the rules imply.

Royal Treatment

I really didn't mind the afternoons in Rochester. In fact, I looked forward to them. For once, people wanted me to talk endlessly about my condi-

tion. Instead of hiding it or being embarrassed, I could complain as much as I wanted.

For a year and a half, a team of physicians, nurses and administrators monitored my health in person, by telephone and by e-mail. I didn't take a pill or feel an ache without this team's knowing what was going on with my body. For the only time in my life, I received the health care of presidents and kings.

For example, when I tried a medication for the acute pain that comes with this condition, it gave me occasional heart palpitations. I was quickly sent for an EKG and consultation with my primary care physician. And on the next visit to Rochester, my team was all over me. Suddenly I had Dr. Mayer, Nurse Rust and the program administrator waiting in turn to take my pulse. They could have left this up to my regular doctor, but they didn't.

I also learned that I was not just a subject in one isolated clinical trial, but contributing to a wider understanding of IC. All the notes and urine samples would also serve to fill in gaps about the natural history of IC, which in turn will point researchers toward the next step.

"Any type of medical research is a learning experience," explained my urologist, Robert Mayer. "During clinical trials, we gather all sorts of information that is fundamental to understanding the condition, as well as the treatment."

Still I worried that the study might end up being useless to the IC community if the results weren't positive or if the treatment worked only for a few people. I answered my concerns this way.

As health consumers, we are left with three options. You could let your doctor sort through the studies and decide what is best for you. Or you could bone up on your condition, read about the possible treatments and then weigh the evidence yourself.

Or you could just jump in there and be involved.

In my case, I am not waiting for any body of evidence, but trying to produce it. This kind of participation takes not just dedication, but a certain kind of enthusiasm, even in the fact of negative results.

Moving On

A recent letter just informed me that I had been given the placebo in Phase One of the study. In any case, whatever went in there hadn't reduced my symptoms a bit. Even after I received the real substance in Phase Two, there was no improvement in my bladder. This month, the study results were published in the Journal of Urology. There, I learned the treatment appeared to help 21 percent of the subjects, compared to 12 percent in the placebo group who saw improvement. So BCG may offer relief to some patients with interstitial cystitis, if not to me. Researchers, though, continue their search for a more effective treatment.

Meanwhile, I am in contact with the research group in Rochester. I miss them. Maybe all that enthusiastic participation did nothing for my particular bladder, but it did a lot for me. I was treated well, listened to, and I felt like part of the process. It gave me hope.

For that reason alone, I'd offer up my body to science any day . . .

(Reprinted with permission by Meredith F. Small)

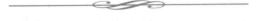

What Is Medical Research?

As you have seen from the preceding chapters, medical research helps us learn more about how our bodies work, why we get sick, and what we can do to get and stay well. The main goal of medical research is to improve our health. This is the reason that the Society for Women's Health Research promotes more research in areas that pertain to women.

There are four basic types of medical research:

♦ Observational studies examine the health of the same group of people over time.
♦ Epidemiological studies try to find patterns of diseases in large groups of people.
♦ Intervention studies explore ways to change behaviors that can affect health.
♦ Prevention studies seek ways to keep people from getting sick.

Studies that involve drugs, vaccines, and medical devices are called clinical trials; they can be classified as either intervention or prevention studies. In the United States, clinical trials are regulated by the U.S. Food and Drug Administration (FDA), which requires that manufacturers prove that their products are both safe and effective for their intended uses before they can be sold. Clinical trials begin only after laboratory research and/or studies in animals show that the new product is safe for more testing and likely to be effective in people. The FDA requires three phases of clinical trials:

♦ Phase I clinical trials include a very small number of people (usually 20–100) and last up to one year. Researchers look primarily at the best dose to be used in further testing.
♦ Phase II clinical trials begin answering the question whether the treatment actually works as scientists believe it will. These studies are also designed to confirm the best dose and start looking at safety questions, including unintended results. They usually include up to several hundred people and last one to two years.

♦ Phase III clinical trials measure how well the investigational treatment works; it may be compared to a treatment that is known not to be effective (placebo) or to treatments that are currently used. Dosage and safety questions continue to be explored. These studies last two to four years and include several hundred to several thousand volunteers.

Because clinical trials involve only a relatively small number of people, sometimes the FDA requires that manufacturers continue clinical trials after it approves the new treatment. This type of postmarketing study is referred to as Phase IV clinical trials. Sometimes manufacturers choose to conduct postmarketing studies even if the FDA does not require them; they may want to see if the treatment works for other diseases or conditions or to test different ways to package the medicine (for example, time-release capsules).

Why Your Sex Matters

Throughout this book, you have seen some of the sex differences in disease and how a person's sex can affect disease prevention and treatment. For example, flexible sigmoidoscopy is not as effective for women as it is for men as a screening test for colon cancer; women seem to develop lung cancer at younger ages than men; and women suffer from depression and anxiety disorders two to three times more often than men.

These differences have been detected because people just like you participated in clinical trials or other studies. As you have seen, there is still much we do not know, and the health of women and men alike will improve when we learn more. For example, one study indicates that women may tend to retain or recover language abilities much more readily after a stroke because of how their brains are wired. Learning whether this is true and why may lead to better therapies for all stroke victims and new therapies for boys and girls with such learning disabilities as dyslexia. Another example is that researchers and manufacturers are developing promising new diagnostic techniques, such as sex-specific EKGs, that may ultimately improve outcomes in women.

What You Can Do

You can participate in medical research. Nearly every woman can qualify for a medical research study at some time in her life. If you are healthy, you may be needed for an observational study or an early clinical trial. If you are healthy but at risk for a disease, you can volunteer for a prevention study. And if you are sick, you may be eligible for a clinical trial to study how a behavioral change or investigational treatment may help you. If you are not eligible for any studies, you may know someone who is and can encourage her to participate.

You may not benefit directly from your participation, but you are helping to discover whether a behavior, vaccine, or treatment is effective. If it is, you will receive that benefit. Even so, participation in medical research is not the same as getting medical care, and you should not substitute it for care from the appropriate health care provider. Many people who participate in medical research do so for the indirect benefits, knowing that they are helping researchers learn more about health and disease.

How You Can Learn More about Participating

If you are interested in participating, you probably have many other questions about matters such as privacy, qualifications, risks, the study itself, costs, and reimbursement. The Society for Women's Health Research sponsors an educational program, "Some Things Only a Woman Can Do," that provides the answers to these and many other questions. You can order the free educational package at www.womancando.org or by either mailing or faxing the Society: 1025 Connecticut Ave., #701, Washington D.C. 20036; fax: 202–833–3472.

How You Can Learn More about Women's Health Research

The new field of sex-based biology is developing rapidly, with new research about sex differences in health and disease emerging every month. The Society encourages you to continue to learn what may be new in women's health. The Society's web site, www.womenshealthresearch.org, contains the latest research news on women's health. It also provides links to the many voluntary health agencies that offer support and fund research on many diseases and conditions. You can sign up for a free subscription to the Society's electronic newsletter at the Society's site.

National Institutes of Health

In the United States, the first source for up-to-date information about the latest medical research, including many of the studies on matters that concern women, is the National Library of Medicine (NLM), part of the National Institutes of Health (NIH). Located at 8600 Rockville Pike, Bethesda, Maryland, the NLM is the world's largest medical library. You can look at materials in the library's reading room or request them on interlibrary loan. The main reading room hours are:

♦ Winter—Mon., Tues., Wed., Fri: 8:30 a.m.–5:00 p.m.; Thurs.: 8:30 a.m.–9:00 p.m. (reference assistance available until 8:00 p.m.); Sat.: 8:30 a.m.–12.30 p.m.
♦ Summer—Mon. through Fri.: 8:30 a.m.–5:00 p.m.; Sat.: 8:30 a.m.–12.30 p.m.

Begun as a one-room Laboratory of Hygiene in 1887, NIH today is one of the world's foremost medical research centers and our nation's focal point for health research. It consists of the Office of the Director and 27 institutes and centers, each of which conducts research at NIH and funds research elsewhere. These institutes and centers look at different populations, diseases, scientific disciplines, research methods, and professions. Each one maintains a Web site that provides the latest news about the research it conducts or funds. Use the list below as a starting point; because many conditions are studied by multiple disciplines, you may find it necessary to look at more than one institute or center's site.

POPULATIONS

Women's Health: The Office of Research on Women's Health (ORWH), in the Office of the Director, strengthens and enhances research related to diseases, disorders, and conditions that affect women. It ensures that women are represented appropriately in biomedical and biobehavioral research studies supported by NIH and develops opportunities for and supports recruitment, retention, reentry, and advancement of women in biomedical careers. Information about the ORWH can be found at http://www4.od.nih.gov/orwh/.

The National Heart, Lung, and Blood Institute (NHLBI) has administrative responsibility for the NIH Woman's Health Initiative (WHI), a 15-year project consisting of a randomized controlled clinical trial and an observation study as well as a study of community approaches to developing healthful behaviors. The clinical trial and the observational study, consisting of more than 167,000 women, age 50–79, has sought to answer questions on benefits and risks of hormone therapy and the role of diet changes and calcium/vitamin D supplements in disease prevention. Information about the WHI can be found at http://www.nhlbi.nih.gov/whi/

Minorities: The National Center on Minority Health and Health Disparities (NCMHD) is at http://www.ncmhd.nih.gov.

Aging: The National Institute on Aging (NIA) is at http://www.nia.nih.gov.

CONDITIONS/DISEASES

Addiction: National Institute on Drug Abuse (NIDA), at http://nida.nih.gov

AIDS: National Institute of Allergy and Infectious Diseases (NIAID), at http://niaid.nih.gov

Alcoholism: National Institute on Alcohol Abuse and Alcoholism (NIAAA), at http://www.niaaa.nih.gov

Allergy: NIAID, at http://niaid.nih.gov

Alzheimer's disease: NIA, at http://www.nia.nih.gov

Arthritis: National Institute of Arthritis and Musculoskeletal and Skin Diseases (NIAMS), at http:/www.niams.nih.gov

Asthma: NIAID, at http://niaid.nih.gov

Autoimmune diseases: NIAID, at http://niaid.nih.gov

Balance: National Institute on Deafness and Other Communication Disorders (NIDCD), at nidcd.nih.gov

Brain and degenerative diseases: National Institute of Mental Health (NIMH), at http://www.nimh.nih.gov

Cancer: National Cancer Institute (NCI), at http://www.nci.nih.gov

Deafness: NIDCD, at http://www.nidcd.nih.gov

Digestive disorders: National Institute of Diabetes and Digestive and Kidney Diseases (NIDDK), at http:/www.niddkd.nih.gov

Drug abuse: NIDA, at http://www.nida.nih.gov

Endometriosis: National Institute of Child Health and Human Development (NICHD), at http://www.nichd.nih.gov

Eye health: National Eye Institute (NEI), at http://www.nei.nih.gov

Heart disease: National Heart, Lung, and Blood Institute (NHLBI), at http://nhlbi.nih.gov

Infectious diseases: NIAID, at http://www.niaid.nih.gov

Infertility: NICHD, at http://www.nichd.nih.gov

Kidney, bladder, and urinary tract health: National Institute of Diabetes and Digestive and Kidney Diseases (NIDDK), at http://www.niddk.nih.gov

Mental health: NIMH, at http://www.nimh.nih.gov

Oral and dental health: National Institute of Dental and Craniofacial Research (NIDCR), at http://www.nidcr.nih.gov

Osteoporosis: NIAMS, at http:/www.niams.nih.gov

Pain: National Institute of Neurological Disorders and Stroke (NINDS), at http://www.ninds.nih.gov

Parkinson's disease: NINDS, at http://www.ninds.nih.gov

Pulmonary diseases: NHLBI, at http://nhlbi.nih.gov

Pregnancy: NICHD, at http://www.nichd.nih.gov

Sexual health: NICHD, at http://www.nichd.nih.gov

Sexually transmitted infections: NIAID, at http://niaid.nih.gov

Skin diseases: NIAMS, at http:/www.niams.nih.gov
Sleep disorders: National Center on Sleep Disorders Research, housed in NHLBI, at http://www.nhlbi.nih.gov
Stroke: NINDS, at http://www.ninds.nih.gov
TMJ: NIDCR, at http://nidcr.nih.gov

TREATMENT

Alternative therapies: National Center for Complementary and Alternative Medicine (NCCAM), at http://www.nccam.nih.gov
Nursing care: National Institute of Nursing Research (NINR), at http://www.ninr.nih.gov
Nutrition: NIDDK, at http://www.niddk.nih.gov
Vaccines: NIAID, at http://www.niaid.nih.gov

In addition to the Web sites of the various National Institutes of Health, one of the most authoritative sites is the one maintained by NLM, which publishes the Index Medicus®, a monthly guide to articles in 4,000 journals, at http://medlineplus.gov/ or http://medlineplus.gov/esp (Spanish). MedlinePlus contains:

♦ Health Topics, which link to health information from NIH and other sources and include current news items about the topic;
♦ Medical Encyclopedia, with 4,000 articles about diseases, tests, symptoms, injuries, and surgeries and an extensive library of medical images;
♦ Current Health News; and
♦ Medical Dictionary.

BEYOND NIH

Clearly, the Internet has emerged as an important source of health information for consumers. Overall, the Pew Internet and American Life Project found that 80 percent of adult Internet users in the United States (93 million) use the Internet to obtain health-related information. But the amount of information available is overwhelming.

Today, more than 70,000 Web sites contain health information, a figure that continues to grow exponentially. Not only are we turning to Internet Web sites for primary health information, but we also have access to online communities, such as chat rooms, bulletin boards, listservs (virtual conversations that come directly into your e-mail), and the newest entrant, blogs.

On the one hand, this is great. The more access you have to information, the more control you feel you have over your health. However, the sheer plethora of information out there means that online health searching can be bewildering, confusing, and in many instances, downright wrong. That is why it is so important to carefully evaluate the source of any medical information you receive online. NIH suggests you ask the following questions about health-related Web sites:

- **Who runs this site?** The information should be clearly available (check the "about us" link) and should be marked on every page. Be wary of individual's Web sites; the person running the site may not have the medical background necessary to provide accurate information. Instead, look for government Web sites (they end in .gov), university Web sites (they end in .edu), and nonprofit Web sites (they end in .org).
- **What is the purpose of the site?** This should be clearly stated on the home page (or by a link from the home page).
- **Where does the information come from, and what is the basis of the information?** The original source should be clearly labeled if it is not original information. Look for references.
- **How is the information selected?** Is there an editorial board? Do the individuals running the site have professional and scientific qualifications? Is the information reviewed by a qualified individual?
- **How old is the information?** Things change quickly in medicine; high-quality health care sites should be reviewed at least once a year.
- **How does the Web site choose links to other sites?** Reliable Web sites usually have a policy regarding links.
- **What information is the Web site collecting about you?** If you have to register to use the Web site, beware; the owner is collecting information about you, and you should ask why. Some sell this information to other marketers, some use it to market directly to you.
- **How does the Web site manage interactions with users?** Make sure there is a way for you to contact the Web site owners with questions or concerns.

You should also look for the gold standard when it comes to health information on the Web: the HONcode from the nongovernment, nonprofit Health on the Net Foundation. Web sites approach the foundation and ask to be certified. To be able to display the blue-and-red seal, sites must adhere to the foundation's eight principles, which address the authority of the information provided, data confidentiality and privacy, proper attribution of sources, transparency of financial sponsorship, and the importance of clearly separating advertising from editorial content. Today, some 3,000 sites are HONcode subscribers, including the Society for Women's Health Research.

—SUZANNE STONE AND DEBRA GORDON

CHAPTER 23

The Society for Women's Health Research and the Future of Women's Health

The Society for Women's Health Research (SWHR) is changing the way research is conducted in the United States and the way researchers examine sex-based differences in health and disease. We champion increased funding for research on women's health, encourage interdisciplinary scientific inquiry through Society-sponsored research networks and professional conferences, and urge that sex-based analyses be included as an integral part of clinical studies and their published results.

Advocacy

Without a substantial, ongoing commitment of both private and federal funds for promising medical research, lifesaving treatments for disease will not be developed. The Society is recognized as a spirited and tireless advocate for increased funding for research into women's health and for sex-based research.

Society spokespersons testify before the committees in the U.S. Senate and U.S. House of Representatives responsible for funding the National Institutes of Health (NIH) and meet regularly with members of Congress. SWHR also holds regular Capitol Hill briefings to educate members and staff, to ensure that vital women's health issues are on the national agenda and in the public spotlight and that our government responds effectively to the urgent needs of American women.

To keep women's health issues among our lawmakers' top priorities, the Society established the national Women's Health Research Coalition, which now comprises more than 600 advocates from a broad range of academic, medical, and scientific institutions as well as health-related associations and organizations. Coalition members receive a monthly Hotline newsletter and legislative action alerts, and they advocate for the Society's legislative priorities during an annual Capitol Hill Day and throughout the year. The Coalition's major initiatives include:

- increasing funds for women's health research equal to the rate of increases for all biomedical research;
- ensuring adequate funding for the government offices that support women's health research, including NIH and its Office on Women's Health Research, the Centers for Disease Control and Prevention (CDC), and the U.S. Food and Drug Administration (FDA);
- encouraging permanent authorization for women's health offices within these and other agencies, including the Department of Health and Human Services; and
- advocating expansion of an NIH program that supports the career development of junior research faculty members.

The Society also advocates with scientists at the NIH and elsewhere in the federal government for

- continued inclusion of women in clinical trials for both basic and clinical research,
- inclusion of women in the early phases of research studies,
- a database to coordinate the inclusion of women in clinical trials at the FDA, and
- improved collaboration across research disciplines at NIH to realize the benefits of sex-based biology.

Due to its science-based, nonpartisan approach, the Society has become a credible, balanced source of information for health care providers, academicians, and legislators.

Interdisciplinary Scientific Inquiry

CONFERENCES

The Society's annual conference on Sex and Gene Expression (SAGE) focuses on basic research into the molecular and cellular biology of sex differences. SAGE conferences explore the frontiers of how biological sex influences the expression of genetic information throughout life. The conferences provide an opportunity for dialogue between leading, established scientists and outstanding new researchers to exchange information about cutting-edge research.

Isis Fund for Sex-Based Biology Research

The Society established the Isis Fund for Sex-Based Biology Research to foster interdisciplinary basic and clinical research on sex and gender differences. Named for the powerful Egyptian goddess, the Isis Fund Networks address interdisciplinary questions in the biology of sex differences by bringing together experts in various scientific fields who have research interests in, or relevant to, sex-based biology and have in an interest and capacity for developing collaborative research relationships with other leading researchers.

Sex, Gender, Drugs, and the Brain
The neuroscience network, the Isis Fund Network on Sex, Gender, Drugs, and the Brain, began in 2002, with initial funding from Ortho-McNeil Pharmaceutical. Network participants are addressing the broad question: How do sex differences in the brain influence responses to neuropharmaceuticals, and how should such differences be taken into account in the development of new neuropharmaceuticals? Other collaborative studies are focusing on postpartum depression and genetic determinants of drug responses. Participants present symposia at major scientific meetings and publish on the topic of sex, gender, drugs, and the brain.

Sex Differences in Metabolism
Participants in the Isis Fund Network on Sex Differences in Metabolism, established in 2003, have agreed "to promote research on the developmental influences on metabolic disorders, in order to understand their sex-dependent etiology and subsequent pathophysiology." They are identifying common research interests, which include the following:

- What are the steroidal effects on food intake and body weight homeostasis?
- Are there sexually dimorphic aspects in the etiology of metabolic syndrome?
- How does sexual dimorphism develop?
- Is sexual dimorphism of hormones and enzymes involved in anabolism or catabolism of endogenous and exogenous substrates?

Initial funding for this network was provided by Aventis Pharmaceuticals.

Breast Cancer
To be funded by a grant from the Komen Foundation, the third Isis Network will begin in 2006 and will address the question, "What causes breast cancer?" The network will apply a unique interdisciplinary approach to this question.

Improving Women's Health

At the heart of all of the Society's efforts is improving women's health. To this end, it educates women, the medical community, and policymakers about major health issues and supports relevant legislation. Its education efforts include a Web site, quarterly newsletter, and biweekly e-newsletter. Additionally, the Society annually conducts consumer education campaigns on a variety of topics, has a press service distributing news on women's health to more than 10,000 media outlets, conducts periodic media briefings and roundtables, and holds workshops for clinicians.

Much Remains to Be Done

Women are different from men, and those differences are often beyond the obvious, especially when it comes to our health. Because of the efforts of the Society for Women's Health Research, we now know definitively that men and women are different when it comes to health; that prevalence, course, prevention, and treatment of various conditions may differ; and that understanding these differences is important. But this is still a relatively new science, and there is still much we do not know.

Since 1990, when the Society was founded, we have worked to ensure that women are not forgotten in medical research. As a result of the Society's work, women's health is becoming a priority on the national agenda. For the most part, sex differences are now widely recognized and included as critical factors in medical research studies.

Yes, the Society has made great strides . . . but there is much more to do. Because understanding these differences will ultimately lead to better health for all—men as well as women, for ourselves and our loved ones. It has taken too long to get to this point, but we cannot rest on our laurels. We must continue to challenge the scientific medical community and keep the importance of these issues front and center.

The Society is dedicated to making that message benefit all of us. We welcome your support.

—PHYLLIS GREENBERGER, MSW, CEO AND PRESIDENT,
SOCIETY FOR WOMEN'S HEALTH RESEARCH

ABOUT THE EDITORS

Phyllis Greenberger, MSW, is the first president and CEO of the Society for Women's Health Research. *The Medical Herald* selected Greenberger as one of the twenty most influential women in medicine today. She has been quoted in numerous publications including *The New York Times, The Washington Post, The Washington Times, The Wall Street Journal,* and *US News and World Report* and frequently testifies before Congress advocating for additional research and funding for women's health.

Jennifer Wider, MD, received her medical degree from the Mount Sinai School of Medicine in 1999. During medical school, she interned at a CBS local news affiliate and "20/20," and after graduation was a senior editor at "Medscape/CBS Health Watch." She has been a guest on CBS News, National Public Radio and various cable channels. She currently reports on health and medical issues for the Society for Women's Health Research.

INDEX